DATE DUE

DEMCO 38-296

Public Health
and Aging

Public Health and Aging

Edited by

Tom Hickey

Marjorie A. Speers

Thomas R. Prohaska

The Johns Hopkins University Press

Baltimore and London

© 1997 The Johns Hopkins University Press

blished 1997

iversity Press
es Street
21218-4319
Ltd., London

ble from the British Library.

-in-Publication Data

Public health and aging / edited by Tom Hickey, Marjorie A. Speers, and Thomas R. Prohaska.
   p.   cm.
   Includes index.
   ISBN 0-8018-5558-6 (alk. paper). — ISBN 0-8018-5559-4 (pbk. : alk. paper)
   1. Community health services for the aged—United States.
2. Preventive health services for the aged—United States.   3. Aged-Medical care—United States.   I. Hickey, Tom, 1939–
II. Speers, Marjorie A.   III. Prohaska, Thomas R.
   [DNLM: 1. Public Health—United States.   2. Chronic Disease—in old age.   3. Health Policy—United States.   4. Health Services for the Aged—United States.   WA 300 P976 1997]
RA564.8.P83   1997
362.1'9897—dc20
DNLM/DLC
for Library of Congress   96-29282
                                        CIP

Printed in the United States of America on acid-free recycled paper
06   05   04   03   02   01   00   99   98   97   5 4 3 2 1

Contents

Foreword, by Fernando Torres-Gil, ix

Preface, xiii

List of Contributors, xix

I

The Role of Public Health in an Aging Society, 1

1   The Public Health Paradigm, 3
     Robert L. Kane

2   Understanding the Aging and Public Health Networks, 17
     Alan L. Balsam and Carolyn L. Bottum

3   Behavioral, Social, and Socioenvironmental Factors Adding Years to
     Life and Life to Years, 37
     George A. Kaplan

4   Issues of Resource Allocation in an Aging Society, 53
     Robert H. Binstock

II

Aging and Chronic Illness, 73

5   Variability in Disease Manifestations in Older Adults: Implications for
     Public and Community Health Programs, 75
     Robert B. Wallace

6   Disability Outcomes of Chronic Disease and Their Implications for
     Public Health, 87
     Marcel E. Salive and Jack M. Guralnik

7   Evidence of Modifiable Risk Factors in Older Adults as a Basis for
     Health Promotion and Disease Prevention Programs, 107
     Gilbert S. Omenn, Shirley A. A. Beresford, David M. Buchner, Andrea LaCroix,
     Mona Martin, Donald L. Patrick, Jeffrey I. Wallace, and Edward H. Wagner

III

Program Planning and Development for Older Populations, 129

8   Integrating Research into Program Planning and Development, 131
     Terrie Wetle

9   Surveillance, Needs Assessment, and Evaluation, 144
     Susan L. Hughes

10   Conceptual, Measurement, and Analytical Issues in Assessing Health
     Status in Older Populations, 163
     Anita L. Stewart and Ron D. Hays

11   Heterogeneity and Multiple Risk Factors in Aging Populations:
     Implications for Research, 190
     Pearl S. German and Sam Shapiro

12   On the Economic Analysis of Interventions for Aged Populations, 207
     Ronald J. Ozminkowski and Laurence G. Branch

IV

Challenges for Intervention and Services, 235

13 Postponing Disability: Identifying Points of Decline and Potential Intervention, 237
S. Jay Olshansky and Mark A. Rudberg

14 Aging, Bioethics, and Public Health: Issues at the Intersection of Three Multidisciplinary Fields, 252
Rosalie A. Kane

15 Implications of an Aging Society for the Preparation of Public Health Professionals, 275
Thomas R. Prohaska and Steven P. Wallace

16 Implications of an Aging Society for the Organization and Evaluation of Public Health Services, 293
Elizabeth A. Kutza

V

Conclusion, 309

17 Toward a Synthesis of a Public Health Agenda for an Aging Society, 311
Ronald Andersen and Nadereh Pourat

Index, 325

Foreword

The United States needs a national public health agenda for aging. The trends are clear: The number of people age 65 and older has increased tenfold in this century, and will easily double in the first part of the next century; most Americans can expect to live to the age of 75, if not longer; and the fastest-growing segment in our population are those over the age of 85—the ones most likely to require services from the public health and aging networks. The compelling evidence of growing numbers of at-risk and chronically impaired older adults stands on its own. However, there are major gaps in what we know about the epidemiology of major chronic illnesses such as cancer and Alzheimer's disease in the older population. Based on their respective strengths, professionals in the fields of aging and public health need to develop a shared agenda for cross-cutting efforts to address the growing health challenges of an aging society. There is a great need to translate what we know at this point into effective strategies for intervention.

There will also be greater diversity among aging Americans. More people will be active and productive well past the traditional retirement age. Many more will have greater buying power and contribute significantly to the national economy. At the same time, the number of people who will be frail and vulnerable will also increase, with obvious implications for specialized public health and aging services. Thus, one of the most important challenges for public health and aging professionals will be to improve the access to services for an increasingly diverse older population. Growing numbers of older persons from the African American, Hispanic, Native American, Asian, and Pacific Islander communities will mean more minority older persons. There will also be greater geographic dispersion in the older population across urban, suburban, and rural settings.

A second challenge will be to promote and sustain collaborative initiatives and efforts. Public health and aging initiatives must go beyond the restrictive organizational structures and jurisdictions that have built up over many decades. We no longer have the luxury of maintaining separate infrastructures and organizational networks.

A third challenge is to recognize the complementary strengths of the aging and public health networks at national and local levels. The aging network is a well-established infrastructure of state- and community-based services representing over 670 area Agencies on Aging, fifty-seven state Offices on Aging, and over 229 tribal governments. This network reaches the older population in all areas of this country, connecting them to a variety of social and supportive services. In much the same way, the U.S. Public Health Service maintains an effective network of disease prevention and health promotion services through federal and state initiatives directed through local public health departments. With these systems in place, there is little need to reinvent the wheel. There is little or no need for public health departments to establish special clinical settings for elderly persons, or for area agencies on aging to establish a public health outreach program of their own when they can do so together, saving on resources and building on common strengths and interests.

After breaking traditional jurisdictional boundaries, our fourth challenge will be to build coalitions with other affected groups, such as those representing disabled individuals, AIDS victims, and the families of Alzheimer's victims. Ultimately, much of the success of our efforts to address the health needs of an aging society will be based on the political and fiscal support we can obtain for the establishment of programs and services.

A fifth challenge will be to accept the reality of increased scrutiny by those political bodies and decision makers who will determine our ability to obtain resources for addressing the needs of an aging society. There will be high levels of expectation, and how we deliver and evaluate the effectiveness of our programs will be scrutinized closely. Commonly used terms like "measurable outcomes" and "performance indicators" will be applied to the collaborative efforts of the public health and aging networks.

As we plan for the future, it is clear that public health and aging have an important role to play in our society. We share common values. We are committed to service. We are a compassionate group of professional individuals who are committed to social change. Thus, we cannot afford to engage in competition or conflict, especially in an era of diminishing resources.

Public health and aging professionals will have to work together more than ever before—not just because we have a common objective, but to survive and prosper in a more difficult and challenging time in our history. We face the need to provide a national response to the aging of our population and its impact on society at large. At the same time, the public and political mood of these times is not about gov-

ernment obtaining additional resources, nor about expanding agencies and bureaucracies. It is about responding more efficiently, effectively, and compassionately. The
public health and aging networks have tremendous opportunities to do so in the
years to come. I believe that even in an era of declining government resources, we
can more than double our capacity to respond to an aging society by working together.

Fernando Torres-Gil, Ph.D.
Assistant Secretary for Aging
Administration on Aging
U.S. Department of Health and Human Services
Washington, DC

Preface

This book represents an important outcome of a national conference held in September 1994 that brought together professionals in research and practice interested in the public health implications of a rapidly expanding older population. The agenda of the conference was to link professionals who are engaged in the practice of public health with those who provide health-related services to older people in the United States.

The conference was also a priority in the legislatively authorized mission of three federal agencies: the Administration on Aging, the Centers for Disease Control and Prevention, and the National Institute on Aging. Two additional groups in the private sector—the Gerontological Society of America and the American Association of Retired Persons—joined in cosponsoring the conference and in planning this book. From the outset, identifying avenues for and enhancing communication between researchers and practitioners in public health and aging was the central organizing theme.

A public health approach to the study of aging requires an epidemiological understanding of health and illness in later years, the inclusion of the quality of life as an important measure of health status, and a consideration of the extent of society's commitment and capacity to respond to the significant health needs of the older population. The process of aging and the experiences of old age reflect the confidence of biological inheritance and lifelong interactions between individuals and their physical and social environments. Age-related mortality and chronically disabling disease underscore the importance of factors other than age in the health dependencies of older adults. The wide array of biological, physical, environmental, and social influences on the aging process suggests the special relevance of a public health perspective on health status in late life. The need for a national agenda in aging for public health is clearly evident to public health professionals in research and practice settings who are challenged by a growing number of at-risk and chronically impaired older adults. Gaps remain between the epidemiology of aging and strategies for translating what we know into effective interventions. Building on the discussions of the conference, this book is designed to provide a basis for continuing exchange between researchers and practitioners that will contribute to the development of a national agenda to address scientific and public health policy issues.

In his 1981 Lewis A. Conner Memorial Lecture to the American Heart Association, the late Richard Remington had the following advice regarding continued scientific progress and application of findings to the treatment of disease: "Research must continue. But at an appropriate time, we must make recommendations for public programming and action . . . by doing the necessary research, by translating research into improved practice, by implementing community programs, by speaking directly to the victims of these diseases, the general public".

At the request of the National Academy of Sciences, Dr. Remington later chaired the Committee for the Study of the Future of Public Health, which undertook a comprehensive assessment of the public health infrastructure. The National Academy of Sciences committee reviewed the public health mission and its implications for federal, state, and local government agencies. The report of the committee identified the states as the central force, bearing the primary public-sector responsibility, while the localities are the "frontline" for making services available and accessible to those at risk. Beyond technical assistance and provision of funds to the states, the federal government has the obligation for "support of knowledge and the development and dissemination through data gathering, research and information exchange".

As this book was being prepared following the conference, Remington's evident concern and vision regarding continuous support of research and its application to public health practice had an even more somber ring in the growing context of limited public resources. We are reminded that he also said, "There are choices that we must never be led to make: the choice between basic and applied research, the choice between targeted and investigator-initiated research, the choice between prevention and treatment of disease, and the choice between the need to know and the need to act". Added to this list of troubling false choices is that of intergenerational equity in the distribution of resources. Focusing on an aging society is not intended to foster an unhealthy competition between the needs of young people and those of elderly people.

Thus, our experiences from the dialogue at the conference and in the preparation of this book require a fresh examination of the implications of an aging population for public health policy, for the training of professionals for public health practice, and for meeting the requirements of state and local public health and aging agencies. This book is a product of the dialogue and linkages formed between public health researchers and practitioners in aging, and is designed to bridge the gap between research and practice. The chapters are organized into four basic content areas that address the integration of research and practice within public health and aging.

The first area is the Role of Public Health in an Aging Society. The chapters in Part I address the current status of the fields of public health and of the aging service network. The authors discuss the lack of integration between public health and aging, especially in relation to health and social services for older populations. The authors vary in the degree to which they address the consequences of this lack of integration. However, they agree on the need for continued efforts to integrate public health and aging research with practice.

The chapter by Robert Kane provides an excellent overview of the major factors that have led to the current status of public health and aging. He provides specific examples to demonstrate where integration is possible between public health and the health and social service networks that serve older people. Balsam and Bottum provide a detailed overview of the aging and public health networks including their respective missions, funding sources, array of services, and target populations. This chapter also includes a thoughtful discussion of areas of common ground between the two networks, and the authors highlight advantages brought about by an integration and collaboration between public health and the aging service sector. Kaplan examines epidemiological evidence for the potential role of primary and secondary prevention with the older population. He cites evidence of the association between behavioral risk factors such as smoking and exercise on morbidity and mortality in older populations. He extends the list of health risk factors in older adults to include not only behavioral practices but also social, psychological, and socioenvironmental factors as well. He is consistent with other contributors to this book in stressing the need to focus on risk factors associated with chronic disease. While Kaplan focuses primarily on individual and immediate health risk factors, Binstock's chapter addresses macroeconomic, policy, and structural influences on the health and well-being of older populations. He provides numerous examples of how health care policy decisions affecting the financing and delivery of long-term care for older adults influence health services and, in turn, the health status of the older individual.

Part II, Aging and Chronic Illness, provides extensive epidemiological support for the impact of behavioral, social, and environmental risk factors on the morbidity and mortality of older populations. The body of evidence in these chapters provides clear examples of how gerontological epidemiology can help determine how to best target community-based health promotion interventions for older populations. Robert Wallace begins by stressing the distinction between normal aging, disease, and dysfunction. He notes that age-associated physiological changes, disease progression, and related dysfunction are often interactive and complex, leading to considerable heterogeneity in health and functional status in older populations. He cautions that public health prevention programs and health surveillance for older populations need to address the complex issue of heterogeneity.

As stated throughout this book, public health research and practice focus on a broad array of health outcomes in older populations. The chapter by Salive and Guralnik addresses the nature and extent of disability as health outcomes. The authors concentrate primarily on disabilities and limitations in basic and instrumental activities of daily living (ADL/IADL), including self-care activities that determine whether individuals can live independently in the community. They report findings on the prevalence of ADL/IADL disability associated with specific chronic diseases and comorbidities. The importance of understanding disability health outcomes in older populations is highlighted in their discussion of the role of modifiable risk factors on disability as well as the consequences of disability on the need for informal care and the use of formal health care services. Omenn and colleagues conclude this part by providing examples to reinforce Kaplan's views regarding the association between the health status of older populations and the behavioral, social, and environmental health risk factors that contribute to them. Omenn also provides supporting data for modifying health risks in older populations through comprehensive community-based health promotion programs. This chapter presents a useful discussion of how health promotion interventions can be applied to hard-to-reach older populations.

Part III of this book, Program Planning and Development for Older Populations, reviews the application of public health research to community-based health intervention programs for older populations. The contributors discuss many of the underlying factors of successful programs, including an understanding of the community, a well-designed intervention strategy based on empirical research, and a program evaluation with meaningful outcomes and health indicators sensitive to the intervention. This part also includes a discussion of methodological and measurement issues that are particularly important in assessing health outcomes in programs with older populations.

Wetle describes two case examples of how community-based public health and aging research can be integrated with day-to-day planning and practice in public health programs and services. The Hartford Puerto Rican Alzheimer's Education Program and the Educational Demonstration of Urinary Continence Assessment and Treatment for the Elderly are excellent models for translating epidemiological research, theory, and applied experimental interventions into practical community-based health programs for older populations. Wetle's chapter also demonstrates the value of a strong working partnership between public health research and practice. The chapter by Hughes provides an extensive review of surveillance measures that are useful with older populations. Stewart and Hays emphasize the importance of taking a broader view of health status in older populations. They suggest the importance of the World Health Organization's definition of health, which goes beyond the absence of disease to include physical functioning and mental and emotional well-being as important parameters of health status. They also identify common problems in health measurement with older adults, including the need to establish sensitive, reliable, and valid health outcome measures, and the problems associated with missing data, proxy respondents, and conducting health assessments. All are critical issues in deciding how to evaluate health programs and the utility of surveillance of health status in older populations.

German and Shapiro discuss the earlier theme of heterogeneity in the older population in the context of public health theory, research, intervention, and evaluation. They focus on the diversity among older groups in the prevalence of disability, disease, and death, and how this diversity should be included in public health objectives for an aging society. The complexity of diversity is emphasized with their review of the role of cohort influences, historical and cultural factors, cumulative risk, and mutable and immutable health risks on the heterogeneity observed in older populations. Ozminkowski and Branch discuss the role of program evaluation in health interventions with older populations. They stress that economic analyses of interventions, especially in programs for older populations, need to go beyond simple comparisons of dollar costs. Using several examples of evaluation programs in aging, they review many of the basic components of the evaluation process and its application to health interventions with older people.

Part IV, Challenges for Intervention and Services, discusses considerations, barriers, and limitations when implementing public health programs and goals in an aging society. Ethical issues such as freedom of choice and quality of life, as well as limits on potential health gains, are examples of these challenges. There are also challenges inherent in the health care environment, including the education and training requirements to meet the health needs of the aging population, and the organizational barriers to implementing public health goals that are appropriate to an aging society.

The chapter by Olshansky and Rudberg provides insight regarding the potential limits of health interventions in older populations brought on by biological and evolutionary factors. They caution that some nonfatal conditions common in older populations may not be modifiable. They provide useful recommendations for targeting different levels of prevention programs to health problems in older populations. The chapter by Rosalie Kane is an insightful discussion of ethical issues applied to public health practice with older people. Kane notes that there are ethical issues and value judgments inherent in public health research priorities, in the way that problems are framed, and in the outcome measures that are used. Ethical issues are also present in public health practice with older populations, including priorities for prevention and health promotion efforts, population screening, and treatment.

Prohaska and Wallace discuss the development and current status of gerontological public health training in the United States. Despite considerable growth in public health training dedicated to the issues of aging and the special health care needs of older populations, they caution that this growth may not be sufficient to meet the demands of a growing aging population. They also note that current levels of education and training are based on an unstable foundation: Academic training programs are not closely linked to the job market. In the past, the lack of professionals trained in this area has led state and local agencies to hire people trained in other areas. To encourage the growth and success of academic training programs, public health and aging service agencies will need to demand staff trained to meet their objectives for addressing the public health goals in an aging society.

The chapter by Kutza examines environmental and organizational barriers to implementing public health goals for older populations. She agrees with Balsam and Bottum that an impediment to reaching these goals is a lack of program integration between aging services and health services, which are both funded by public resources. She identifies methods to address these interorganizational barriers including more public education on the health needs and goals of an aging society.

Finally, Andersen and Pourat summarize and interpret the chapters in this book as contributing to the emergence of a new paradigm—that of an integration between research and practice in public health and aging. This paradigm has elements of both public health and aging, and emphasizes older populations, chronic disease and disability, secondary and tertiary prevention, a community orientation, and population-based interventions. This paradigm is dependent on the connection and communication among those who are engaged in the practice of public health and those who provide services to older populations.

This book is designed to appeal to researchers, practitioners, and students who are interested in the health care of older people in our society. Priorities have been identified for public health research and practice for both disease prevention and health promotion for the growing older population. The contributors and editors hope that this book will also serve as a catalyst to identify additional linkages between public health research and practice applied to the issues of aging and the health needs of the older population. Only through continued dialogue can we hope to develop and refine a public health agenda for an aging society.

Tom Hickey, Dr.P.H.
Marjorie A. Speers, Ph.D.
Samuel P. Korper, Ph.D.
Thomas R. Prohaska, Ph.D.

Contributors

Ronald Andersen, Ph.D., Professor, Department of Health Services, School of Public Health, University of California, Los Angeles, California

Alan L. Balsam, Ph.D., M.P.H., Director, Public Health and Human Services, Brookline, Massachusetts Department of Public Health, and Assistant Adjunct Professor, Boston University School of Public Health, Harvard Medical School, and Tufts School of Nutrition, Boston, Massachusetts

Shirley A. A. Beresford, Ph.D., Associate Professor, Department of Epidemiology, University of Washington School of Public Health and Community Medicine, Seattle, Washington

Robert H. Binstock, Ph.D., Professor of Aging, Health, and Society, Department of Epidemiology and Biostatistics, School of Medicine, Case Western Reserve University, Cleveland, Ohio

Carolyn L. Bottum, M.P.H., Director, Bedford Council on Aging, Bedford, Massachusetts

Laurence G. Branch, Ph.D., Professor, Center for the Study of Aging and Human Development, Duke University Medical School, Durham, North Carolina

David M. Buchner, M.D., Ph.D., Professor, Department of Health Service, University of Washington School of Public Health and Community Medicine, Seattle, Washington

Pearl S. German, Sc.D., Professor Emerita, Department of Health Policy and Management, School of Hygiene and Public Health, Johns Hopkins University, Baltimore, Maryland

Jack M. Guralnik, M.D., Ph.D., Chief, Office of Epidemiology and Demography, National Institute on Aging, Bethesda, Maryland

Ron D. Hays, Ph.D., Research Scientist, RAND Corporation, Santa Monica, California

Tom Hickey, Dr.P.H., Professor, Department of Health Behavior/Health Education, School of Public Health; Faculty Associate, Institute of Gerontology, University of Michigan, Ann Arbor, Michigan

Susan L. Hughes, D.S.W., Professor and Director, Program in Long-Term Care, Institute for Health Service Research and Policy Studies, Northwestern University, Evanston, Illinois

Robert L. Kane, M.D., Professor and Minnesota Chair in Long-Term Care and Aging, Institute for Health Services Research, School of Public Health, University of Minnesota, Minneapolis, Minnesota

Rosalie A. Kane, D.S.W., Professor, Institute for Health Services Research, School of Public Health, University of Minnesota, Minneapolis, Minnesota

George A. Kaplan, Ph.D., Professor and Chair of Epidemiology, School of Public Health, University of Michigan, Ann Arbor, Michigan

Samuel P. Korper, Ph.D., Senior Scholar, Medical Technology and Practice Patterns Institute, Washington, D.C.

Elizabeth A. Kutza, Ph.D., Professor, Institute on Aging, School of Urban and Public Affairs, Portland State University, Portland, Oregon

Andrea LaCroix, Ph.D., M.P.H., Associate Professor, Center for Health Promotion in Older Adults, University of Washington School of Public Health and Community Medicine, Seattle, Washington

Mona Martin, M.P.A., B.S.N., Research Coordinator, Northwest Prevention Effectiveness Center, Seattle, Washington

S. Jay Olshansky, Ph.D., Associate Professor, Department of Internal Medicine, University of Chicago, Chicago, Illinois

Gilbert S. Omenn, M.D., Ph.D., Professor and Dean, School of Public Health and Community Medicine, University of Washington, Seattle, Washington

Ronald J. Ozminkowski, Ph.D., Senior Health Economist, The MEDSTAT Group, Inc., Ann Arbor, Michigan

Donald L. Patrick, Ph.D., Professor, University of Washington School of Public Health and Community Medicine, Seattle, Washington

Nadereh Pourat, Ph.D., Research Associate, Center for Health Services Research, University of California, Los Angeles, California

Thomas R. Prohaska, Ph.D., Associate Professor of Community Health Sciences and Director, Center for Health Interventions with Minority Elderly, School of Public Health, University of Illinois, Chicago, Illinois

Mark A. Rudberg, M.D., M.P.H., Associate Professor, Department of Internal Medicine, University of Chicago, Chicago, Illinois

Marcel E. Salive, M.D., M.P.H., Senior Research Investigator, Epidemiology Branch, U.S. Food and Drug Administration, Rockville, Maryland

Sam Shapiro, B.S., Professor Emeritus, Health Services Research and Development Center, School of Hygiene and Public Health, Johns Hopkins University, Baltimore, Maryland

Marjorie A. Speers, Ph.D., Deputy Associate Director for Science, Office of the Associate Director for Science, Centers for Disease Control and Prevention, Atlanta, Georgia

Anita L. Stewart, Ph.D., Associate Professor in Residence, Department of Social and Behavioral Science, University of California, San Francisco, California

Edward H. Wagner, M.D., M.P.H., Director, Center of Health Studies, Group Health Cooperative, Seattle, Washington

Jeffrey I. Wallace, M.D., Assistant Professor, University of Washington School of Public Health and Community Medicine, Seattle, Washington

Robert B. Wallace, M.D., M.S., Professor and Head, Department of Preventive Medicine and Environmental Health, University of Iowa College of Medicine, Iowa City, Iowa

Steven P. Wallace, Ph.D., Associate Professor, Department of Community Health Sciences, School of Public Health, University of California, Los Angeles, California

Terrie Wetle, Ph.D., Deputy Director, National Institute on Aging, Bethesda, Maryland

Part

I

The Role of
Public Health in an
Aging Society

Chapter

1

The Public Health Paradigm

Robert L. Kane, M.D.

The work of the public health system has historically been defined by reference to population groups. The defining characteristic may be the presence of a disease or of risk factors for a disease within a group, and the index of vulnerability has focused on different groups over time. At the beginning of this century, the emphasis was placed on children. Thus, maternal and child health was a core part of public health practice and public health education. Special training funds were established to encourage the preparation of public health professionals in this area.

The demographic revolution seems to have crept up quietly. The preoccupation with children gradually gave way to a focus on the plight of older persons, who seemed especially disadvantaged in the socially active period of the mid-1960s. Somehow, however, public health never became a part of that focus. Public health was not entirely excluded; it was simply peripheral. Programs like home health care, organized around public health nursing, shifted their emphasis to include an active role in the care of frail older persons, but this change was primarily in response to a new market with designated funding. Public health was not visible in a social leadership position. Even the American Public Health Association did not form a Gerontological Health section until 1978.

Older persons are now seen as advantaged, especially in their access to health insurance (Hayward et al., 1988). Ironically, as the policy debate now questions whether the elderly segment of our society, which some view as a strong and organized political constituency, is getting too much attention (Preston, 1984), the public health system is beginning to address the needs of older citizens. To be fair, while organized public health and public health education have been relatively dormant,

TABLE 1.1. Traditional Public Health Activities Focused on the Older Population

Public Health Activity	Aging Aspects of Public Health
Assessment	
Surveillance of health status	Disease rates
	Disability rates
	Utilization rates
Identifying needs	Underservice: potential for improvement
Analyzing causes of disease and disability	Causes of death, morbidity, disability role of social factors
Collecting and interpreting data	LSOA, National LTC Survey, Current Beneficiaries Survey
Case finding	Case management
Monitoring and forecasting trends	Projections
Research on determinants of health	Natural variation effectiveness of care
Outcome evaluation	Epidemiological method: testing the role of treatment by deduction
Policy development	
Planning	Special service configurations, complex relationships, eligibility
Priority setting	Age-based rationing
Policy leadership/advocacy	Defining goals (autonomy, safety, choice) Recognizing barriers
Convening, negotiating, brokering	Service coordination—especially acute and long-term care, case management
Mobilizing resources	Coordinating multiple funding streams
Training/constituency building	Networking, consciousness raising
Public information	Facts on aging, age stereotypes
Encouraging private and public sector action through incentives and persuasion	Regulating, purchasing
Assurance	
Monitoring	Quality-of-care measures, regulation
Encouraging private sector	Regulating, purchasing
Providing services	Community care, coordinating acute and long-term care
Regulating	Changing provider behavior

many of the skills of the public health profession have been gainfully employed in understanding more about the health and related social problems of older persons. Large-scale epidemiological studies have been mounted (Coroni-Huntley et al., 1986). More often, population panels that were developed for other purposes (often heart disease studies) have been adapted to examine risk factors involved in aging (Jette and Branch, 1981; Kaplan et al., 1987). In contrast to epidemiological research with children, much of the epidemiological study of older persons addresses the onset and course of disability (Guralnik, 1994; Manton, 1988; Seeman et al., 1989) and the relationship between morbidity and the use of services (Guralnik et al., 1991; Manton, Corder, and Stallard, 1993). Specific texts addressing epidemiological issues in studying problems of older persons have appeared (Brody and Maddox, 1988; Wallace and Woolson, 1992). Programs that historically trained hospital administrators have been broadened to address issues around long-term care.

The Theoretical Basis for the Juncture of Public Health and Aging

Although its practice and academic bases are not always closely aligned, public health can be described as largely a pragmatic series of programs that have arisen from a largely theoretical base. The report by the Institute of Medicine provides at least a structure by which to examine public health and, in turn, to look for ways in which its activities and interests coincide with the needs of an aging society (Institute of Medicine, 1988). That report defines the mission of public health as "the fulfillment of society's interest in assuring the conditions under which people can be healthy." It identifies the substance of public health as "organized community efforts aimed at the prevention of disease and promotion of health." Such work requires the active participation of many disciplines, but it is built on methodology of epidemiology.

Table 1.1 summarizes the public health activities identified by the Institute of Medicine report and attempts to illustrate how many of these can have an aging focus. Most of these are self-explanatory, but a few deserve some comment. The traditional assessment activities change their shape slightly for older persons, in that they encompass a broader spectrum. Because older persons are frail, they are more sensitive to their environment. Expressions of health must emphasize even more than usual the World Health Organization (WHO) triad of physical, mental, and social well-being. The essence of geriatrics lies in the regular presence of problems in several domains, whose interaction creates special challenges. Thus, functional assessment, beyond simple morbidity measures, becomes a key to identifying population needs and the impacts of programs on disability and the quality of life.

Some have viewed the establishment of programs for older persons as putting them in an advantaged position over other neglected groups in society (Hayward et al., 1988). Some have gone so far as to decry the disproportionately high investment in health care for older persons as a threat to society and to suggest that older persons have an ethical responsibility to forgo such care (Callahan, 1987). Needless to say, the ethics of age-based rationing have been actively debated (Binstock and Post, 1991), but the issue of allocation continues to creep into policy discussions in sometimes subtle ways. For example, the prevalent use of economic measures such as quality-adjusted life years (QALYs) in various types of cost-effectiveness and cost-benefit calculations may directly disadvantage older persons (Avorn, 1984).

Because so much of health care has been shaped by payment policies rather than client needs, the service boundaries often emerge as arbitrary (and, some would add, capricious). A good example is the change in the definition of hospital care that followed the introduction of prospective payment under Medicare. Services that were formerly delivered in a hospital setting have now been moved to the community and to other sites that come under the aegis of public health. There is a great need to oversee and coordinate the transitions of frail older persons from one site of care to another. The often artificial distinction between acute care and long-term care should be countered with a focus on the individual receiving the care and the ultimate effect of such care on that person's functioning and well-being.

Agism is still rampant (Butler, 1975). Stereotypes about older persons, their problems, and their services are still pervasive (Palmore, 1988). Public health education must address the information needs of both the elderly population, who may not be aware of the help that is available to them, and the general population, who may view such programs of help as siphoning resources into a helpless cause.

Regulation has been an active theme in the health care of older persons, especially in long-term care. While the combination of public funding and private entrepreneurial provision of care for vulnerable people would be enough to trigger an active regulatory effort, the history of scandals that accompanied the broad public coverage of long-term care under Medicaid created an atmosphere of distrust that led to active regulatory efforts (Vladeck, 1980; Mendelson, 1974; Moss and Halamandaris, 1977). The issue today is not whether to regulate, but how. Regulatory efforts might be better directed toward using epidemiological and statistical control methods to emphasize the outcomes achieved by such care rather than its adherence to established orthodoxies (Kane and Kane, 1988). This would permit more creativity in the context of better accountability.

The convergence of epidemiology and aging has been quite fruitful. The intersection of these two fields has come a long way since the early meetings on this subject (Haynes and Feinleib, 1980; Ostfeld and Gibson, 1975). The importance of the field has been underscored by the development of specific methods for approaching the issues (Brody and Maddox, 1988; Wallace and Woolson, 1992). More traditional epidemiological approaches have provided valuable insights into a number of areas. For example, epidemiological studies have shown strong relationships between years of schooling and the risk of developing dementia (inverse) (Hill et al., 1993) and general well-being (positive) (Guralnik et al., 1993). Large-scale epidemiological projects in defined catchment areas have been used to better understand the natural history of aging (Coroni-Huntley et al., 1986). Cohorts previously recruited for longitudinal studies of specific diseases, such as the Framingham Study and the

Alameda Health County Study, have been converted to aging studies as their samples age (Jette and Branch, 1981; Kaplan et al., 1987).

National datasets have been established using epidemiological methods. For example, the National Long-Term Care Survey collects information on disabled older people to trace their status over time and to examine the relationship between disability and the use of services. Data from this study have been important in showing that becoming disabled in old age is not necessarily an irreversible event. Manton demonstrated that even persons with substantial disability can improve their status. Among persons living in the community with impairments in five or six activities of daily living (ADLs), he found that 42 percent had improved over a period of two years (Manton, 1988). A parallel observation was made by Rogers, who expanded the concept of "active life expectancy," which essentially measured the time until a person became disabled (Katz et al., 1983), to recognize the dynamic nature of functional incapacity whereby an older person could move in and out of states of dependency (Rogers, Rogers, and Branch, 1989).

Implications of a Chronic Disease Model

The aging of the population has been associated with a shift from a time when the most prevalent and dangerous diseases were infectious to a time of chronic disease. The strategies that worked in one era need to be reevaluated in the new context. The causal models that served us well for infectious diseases need to be reexamined (Evans, 1976). Chronic disease is less likely to have a single cause; rather, it is the result of the interactions of multiple factors. Even the assumption of single causation for infectious disease risks being labeled overly simplistic. More sophisticated techniques show different levels of infection and multiple factors that influence the presentation of frank disease. At a minimum, we recognize the importance of host factors, both genetic and social. Thus, efforts to address these problems, in terms of both treatment and prevention, require more comprehensive strategies.

Many of the necessary changes lie in the area of behavioral modification. Such changes are often difficult to induce. Moreover, they must often occur well in advance of the onset of disease if they are to alter the disease's natural history. One could argue, for example, that funds such as Medicare, which are specifically targeted for older persons, might be better used to change destructive behaviors in younger persons. However, not all behavioral prevention with older persons is inefficient. For example, smoking cessation, even at late ages, has been shown to positively affect the incidence of disease (Hermanson et al., 1988). Likewise, exercise seems to have a wide range of benefits, even among disabled older persons (LaCroix, 1987).

To some degree, older persons have been the victims of the prejudices of earlier researchers. Having systematically excluded older participants from many of the

large trials designed to test the effectiveness of broad preventive efforts, it is ironic
to argue that they should be denied preventive services because there is insufficient
evidence of their effectiveness for this population group. Preventive activities are not
entirely wasted on the old, as indicated elsewhere (cf., Omenn et al., Chapter 7). In
addition to those that confer almost immediate benefits, such as immunizations for
influenza and pneumococcal infection, there are increasing good reasons to argue
on behalf of targeting some preventive activities on an older population. As just indicated, smoking cessation among elderly persons has shown beneficial effects in a
sufficiently short time to justify its active promulgation (Jaijich, Ostfeld, and
Freeman, 1984; Omenn, 1987). Exercise is being used effectively to address a multitude of problems associated with aging for older persons at various levels of frailty
(Larson, 1991; Fiatarone et al., 1994).

The more difficult question is how to motivate older persons to become actively involved. Although there is a growing body of clinical trials demonstrating the
value of exercise, the participants in these studies are usually highly selected volunteers culled from a much larger target group. As with other age groups, the challenge to public health is not limited to testing the efficacy of preventive interventions. It must seek more effective ways to motivate older persons into sustained
participation in meaningful behavior change. This is no small task.

As with other age groups, it is generally easier to identify risk factors than to
change the risks to a point where one can demonstrate a concomitant reduction in
the disease or problem to be prevented. A good example of this dilemma is the work
on falls. A substantial body of risk factors has been accumulated (Grisso et al., 1991;
Lipsitz et al., 1991; Sobel and McCart, 1983; Tinetti and Spechley, 1989). There is
much less evidence of studies that show how to reduce the frequency of falls (Inouye
et al., 1993; Rubenstein et al., 1990; Tinetti et al., 1994).

Prevention in the context of aging must go beyond the typical focus on individual diseases, or even disease complexes associated with specific risk factors, to examine the rest of the spectrum identified in an important WHO framework, which
describes the transitions along the continuum of disease-impairment-disability-
handicap (World Health Organization, 1980). Much of the preventive attention
needed by frail older persons addresses the avoidance of unnecessary disability. The
effectiveness of activities like geriatric evaluation and management teams is directed
specifically at reducing the consequences of this transition (Stuck et al., 1993).

Implementing Change

If its perspective is truly community-wide, public health would have to gasp at
the bureaucratic maze that has grown up around multiple overlapping, poorly coordinated programs for older persons, each with its own requirements for eligibil-

ity and definitions of services. Making change will require first an understanding of this morass, and then a commitment to finding ways to increase the level of coordination and reduce the redundancy in order to use the available resources more efficiently. This is, also, no small task. Administrative and political skills will be taxed to achieve even a dent.

The first step is to understand the territory. Insufficient numbers of public health professionals speaking the jargon of aging are familiar with the labyrinthine organization of the agencies that serve older persons. To quote Meredith's *The Music Man*, "You gotta know the territory."

Public health professionals also need to appreciate the differences in approach and philosophy between them and the aging network. The latter has historically been driven by external pressures to establish programs for older persons with more concern to outreach and the establishment of political opportunities and less attention to questions of effectiveness. Indeed, the map of older services and the activities of aging network organizations varies a great deal from one area to another. In some places, area agencies on aging are active participants in delivering services and directing care, while in other places they are more marginalized, operating programs that emphasize services to relatively well, functional older persons. Indeed, much of the direct care action for older persons (and the large service dollars that go with it) is controlled by programs that may be independent of both the aging network and public health—namely, Medicare and Medicaid. Creative solutions are needed to find ways to integrate these efforts with the larger aging agenda.

The Changing Nature of Public Health

Public health itself may be on the verge of a major revolution. Traditionally, public health has had responsibility for guarding the health commons and caring for those who are without other resources (Hiatt, 1975). Its view of a population at risk has stood in sharp contrast to the client-focused approach of service providers, who recognized service needs only when they presented for care and dismissed them when the client left. Although recent political events have dampened the enthusiasm of many about the likelihood of establishing some form of universal coverage (thus removing, or at least mitigating, one of the principal burdens of public health), other changes in health care structure will dramatically influence the practice of public health.

Perhaps the most significant change in health care organization is the rise of managed care. This new form of care, in effect, combines the insurance and delivery functions. It collects a fixed fee that is intended to cover the actuarial costs of care for an individual. The fee can be levied on a community-rated basis, the most common approach, or a risk-adjusted basis. Because managed care shifts attention from encounters to people, it reinforces the principles of public health. It represents a denominator-based approach to looking at health care, with an accountability for defined groups of persons whether or not they actually use health care services.

In its purest form, managed care offers a mechanism to redistribute resources rationally. In lieu of individual actions by health care providers to maximize the investments in each case, some overarching restriction is recognized and steps are implemented to establish consistent (and hopefully fair) processes for allocation. Whereas the traditional entrepreneurial individual provider model encouraged individuality, managed care opens the way for consistency and the establishment of rules and procedures. Systematic and systemic procedures, driven by an information management system, can provide both guidance and accountability at levels not possible before.

However, managed care can also be a vehicle for simply redistributing resources. Whereas under the former fee-for-service system, physicians and others could become wealthy, managed care places more controls on physicians and hospitals, and centralizes wealth in the hands of a few administrators.

This shift to health status accountability and the definition of populations of persons at risk (i.e., enrollees) create an environment that replicates many of the traditional functions of public health. To the extent that they are effective, investments in prevention should be actively pursued. The challenge to public health is to establish the cost-effectiveness of such interventions with older persons (Omenn et al., 1994). Thus, while the role of formal public health will be altered, the principles can still be actively pursued. Some of its activities may be usurped, but its knowledge and skills should be in greater demand.

Managed care, however, even in a situation of complete market penetration, will not prove to be the complete substitute for public health. Not only will there remain broader societal functions such as sanitation and water quality, the time lines for managed care may not lead to the hoped for investment in prevention. If managed care is administered on the basis of return on investment, certain preventive actions may have too slow a payoff to be attractive. Given a choice between a concern about showing a quick offsetting savings and the practical problems of discounting delayed benefits, the attractive preventive programs will be those that promise quick results. Alas, many of the most important preventive activities require sustained commitment for long periods, a formula that is both expensive to maintain and slow to pay off.

Managed care has thus far been less than it promised with regard to the care of older persons. It does not appear to have been the effective vehicle to achieve the savings that many hoped. Instead, once adjustments are made for case mix differences, Medicare actually seems to cost more than fee-for-service care (Brown et al., 1993). Although managed care offers the potential to apply many of the fundamental geriatric principles of investment in activities like comprehensive assessment—in the expectation that such actions will lead to reduced subsequent utilization (Stuck et al., 1993)—the promise has not been achieved. Although there are some examples of innovative approaches to caring for frail older persons (Kramer, Fox, and Morgenstern, 1992), the majority of Medicare risk-based HMOs have not embraced geriatric principles (Friedman and Kane, 1993).

One example of a public health practice that should be appealing to managed care is health promotion, but the story is more complicated than it seems at first blush. Given an opportunity to establish a program that could reduce subsequent care costs, a rational firm should be willing to invest in prevention. However, for this arrangement to make fiscal sense, two conditions must be met beyond the effectiveness of the preventive intervention. First, the lag between the prevention action and the payoff must be short enough to be financially attractive, not only in terms of discounting the value of the resources saved but also to be incorporated in a fiscal planning cycle. Second, there must be some assurance that the clients in whom the prevention investment was made will still belong to the same program when the benefits are harvested. The longer the lag time, the less likely that condition will be met. In programs like Medicare's risk-based HMO option, beneficiaries retain the right to disenroll at any time, and many do change plans.

As a result, health promotion may not make as much financial sense to a managed care organization as one might hope. In contrast, the motivation for pursuing health promotion activities aggressively is likely to have more to do with marketing. A managed care program that offers a generous preventive program and a modest treatment program (especially around benefits like prescription drugs) is likely to be more attractive to well clients than sick ones. As a result, it will enjoy favorable selection. If the payment is roughly equivalent for each enrollee regardless of the person's risk status, a managed care program can profit handsomely from a preventive attitude.

Implications for Academic Public Health

Academic public health has an important contribution to make to aging in the areas of both education and research. Public health education has a model derived from experience with maternal and child health efforts, which offers both positive and negative lessons. Stimulated by training funds dedicated to preparing public health professionals, major areas of concentration and specific training programs have been established in this area. Curricula have been developed and refined that offer courses in germane fields and adapt the core areas of public health education to focus on their implications for a specific population group. In addition to educational programs for professional students, postgraduate training in various forms has been offered. Similar efforts could readily be mounted for aging. Indeed, in several schools of public health such courses of study have already been developed.

The experience with maternal and child health also offers some lessons about how the emphasis should be changed. Until recently, training grants have funded only educational and training activities. Their use in support of research efforts was prohibited. This prohibition stultified the academic development of maternal and child health (MCH). As other areas of public health became more sophisticated, maternal and child health trailed in its development of innovative approaches and failed to expand the empirical base of information that could encourage new approaches to achieving its goals. While targeted support for aging education in public health would undoubtedly catalyze development in this important area, it should include resources to encourage a strong research base.

Academic efforts in aging must contend with the perennial distinction between gerontology and geriatrics—a difference that is more than semantics. At its heart, it implies a difference in emphasis between theories of aging and applied research. Although it is not appropriate to strive to develop clinicians under a public health banner, education in aging for public health should emphasize applications to the same degree that public health's mission is fundamentally one of applied science. This position does not imply that public health education should ignore gerontological theory. Rather, the theory should be linked to specific applications.

Ideally, this theory would be linked conceptually to general public health skills and knowledge in the core areas of epidemiology, biostatistics, administration, behavioral science, health services research, demography, and ethics. For example, research design for aging activities requires some special adaptations of traditional approaches (especially intercohort and longitudinal models). While many of the models for behavior change may be appropriate for older persons, knowledge of gerontological findings may suggest ways to alter the approach to best fit the needs and receptivity of an older target group. The principles of medical care organization are not different for programs serving an older population, but they may be much more complex. Integration of health and social services (including a working knowledge of the latter) is a more prominent feature of these programs for older persons than with a younger population. Principles of evaluation are no different for programs serving older persons, but the nature of the disease processes and the choice of outcome measures may be. A whole new set of measures around disability and function in many dimensions may need to be covered. New ethical ground may be broken with regard to issues around potential trade-offs of safety for control and autonomy. Traditional concerns over paternalism may be exacerbated in situations of extreme frailty, especially cognitive frailty.

There is also some special content beyond the application of each of these areas to aging populations. For example, students need to know about the specific data bases that are available for secondary analyses. They will need to be familiar with the organization of long-term care services. They should understand the limitations and potential biases of certain approaches (e.g., cost-benefit analysis). They must know at least enough about normal aging to be able to anticipate the expected course of events and to recognize deviations (a special challenge when one of the hallmarks of aging is an increase in natural variation). Also, measures capable of addressing the end results of multiple interactive problems and a vocabulary that emphasizes function will be needed.

The challenge to public health curriculum building in aging lies in achieving the right balance between aging-specific material and general public health principles. This dilemma is common to virtually all public health educational endeavors. There is always a tension between preparing students for their first job and for a lifetime career.

Several alternative structures are available. One might offer a specific aging major along with other areas of emphasis. Some schools emphasize a strong core curriculum to which specific aging courses could be appended. These might include such topics as the epidemiology of aging, the politics of aging, aging services, long-term care administration, health care policy for older persons, long-term care policy, the economics of aging, prevention and health promotion for older persons, and special issues in research on older persons. Some courses might preferably address cross-generational topics such as disability (management, programs, policies), functional measurement, and ethical issues (e.g., rationing).

A less-favored alternative would be to introduce aging content into regular courses. This choice is more precarious because the aging content may be so subtle that it gets lost. In other venues, this strategy has sometimes become diluted to the point of simply using older individuals as patients. The very essence of geriatrics—the differences in clinical presentation, the interaction of multiple domains—may be overlooked in such an approach.

Several important issues must be faced in developing an aging content for public health. Like any similar enterprise, an aging program will need a critical mass of students and faculty to be successful. Tokenism will not suffice, although it may satisfy. At the same time, one should avoid unnecessary and unproductive duplication of effort. Many programs that feature a series of majors often attempt to take responsibility for a disproportionate share of the curriculum in an effort to assure that their area gets adequate emphasis. Core areas may thus be taught by persons who are less expert because these instructors can imbue them with applications in the major area. The task of synthesizing specific content with general principles may be better accomplished with a separate exercise that occurs once the fundamentals are mastered.

As in any educational endeavor, the quality of coverage is important. Those instructing need to be active scholars, preferably with practical experience as well. Model curricula are now available to serve as departure points for the faculty entrusted with conveying the aging related information (Bureau of Health Professions, 1992). One way to assure that the aging content will continue to be timely is to encourage faculty to become actively involved in research. Such activity includes both primary data collection and secondary analyses. Students educated in such an environment have a much greater likelihood of acquiring firsthand experience with the fundamental methods of gerontological inquiry.

The time for making aging a fundamental part of public health education and practice has come. The current and anticipated pressures on our society created by an aging population, and the attendant shift to an era of chronic disease, demand a public health response. The social and ethical challenges of such a transition cannot go unnoticed. The public health profession has an important contribution to make. Many of its skills are already being actively employed. It is time they were properly recognized.

References

Avorn, J. 1984. Benefit and cost analysis in geriatric care: Turning age discrimination into health policy. *New England Journal of Medicine* 310:1294–1301.

Binstock, R. H., and Post, S. G. 1991. *Too Old for Health Care?: Controversies in Medicine, Law, Economics, and Ethics.* Baltimore: Johns Hopkins University Press.

Brody, J. A., and Maddox, G. L., eds. 1988. *Epidemiology and Aging: An International Perspective.* New York: Springer Publishing Company.

Brown, R. S., Clement, D. G., Hill, J. W., Retchin, S. M., and Bergeron, J. W. 1993. Do health maintenance organizations work for Medicare? *Health Care Financing Review* 15(1):7–23.

Bureau of Health Professions. 1992. *Geriatric Training Curriculum for Public Health Professionals.* U.S. Dept. of Health and Human Services, Public Health Service, Resources and Services Administration.

Butler, R. 1975. *Why Survive? Being Old In America.* New York: Harper & Row.

Callahan, D. 1987. *Setting Limits: Medical Goals in an Aging Society.* New York: Simon & Schuster.

Coroni-Huntley, J., Brock, D., Ostfeld, A., Taylor, J., and Wallace, R., eds. 1986. *Established Populations for Epidemiologic Studies of the Elderly: Resource Data Book* (NIH Publication No. 86-2443). Bethesda, MD: National Institute on Aging.

Evans, A. S. 1976. Causation and disease: The Henle-Koch postulates revisited. *Yale Journal of Biology and Medicine* 49:175–95.

Fiatarone, M. A., O'Neill, E. F., Ryan, N. D., Clements, K. M., Solares, G. R., Nelson, M. E., Roberts, S. B., Kehayias, J. J., Lipsitz, L. A., and Evans, W. J. 1994. Exercise training and nutritional supplementation for physical frailty in very elderly people. *New England Journal of Medicine* 330(25):1769–75.

Friedman, B., and Kane, R. L. 1993. HMO medical directors' perceptions of geriatric practice in Medicare HMOs. *Journal of the American Geriatrics Society* 41:1144–49.

Grisso, J. A., Kelsey, J. L., Strom, B. L., O'Brien, L. A., Maislin, G., LaPann, K., Samuelson, L., and Hoffman, S. 1991. Risk factors for falls as a cause of hip fracture in women. *New England Journal of Medicine* 324:1326–31.

Guralnik, J. M. 1994. Understanding the relationship between disease and disability. *Journal of the American Geriatrics Society* 42:1128–29.

Guralnik, J. M., LaCroix, A. Z., Branch, L. G., Kasl, S. V., and Wallace, R. B. 1991. Morbidity and disability in older persons in the years prior to death. *American Journal of Public Health* 81:443–47.

Guralnik, J. M., Land, K. C., Blazer, D., Fillenbaum, G. G., and Branch, L. G. 1993. Educational status and active life expectancy among older blacks and whites. *New England Journal of Medicine* 329(2):110–16.

Haynes, S. G., and Feinleib, M., eds. 1980. *Second Conference on the Epidemiology of Aging.* Bethesda, MD: National Institutes of Health.

Hayward, R. A., Shapiro, M. F., Freeman, H. E., and Corey, C. R. 1988. Inequities in health services among insured Americans: Do working-age adults have less access to medical care than the elderly? *New England Journal of Medicine* 318:1507–11.

Hermanson, B., Omenn, G. S., Kronmal, R. A., and Gersh, B. J. 1988. Beneficial six-year outcome of smoking cessation in older men and women with coronary artery disease. *New England Journal of Medicine* 319:1365–69.

Hiatt, H. H. 1975. Protecting the medical commons: Who is responsible? *New England Journal of Medicine.* 293(5):235–41.

Hill, L., Klauber, M., Salmon, D., Yu, E., Liu, W., Zhang, M., and Katzman, R. 1993. Functional status, education, and the diagnosis of dementia in the Shanghai survey. *Neurology* 43(1):138–45.

Inouye, S. K., Wagner, D. R., Acampora, D., Horwitz, R. I., Cooney, L. M., and Tinetti, M. E. 1993. A controlled trial of a nursing-centered intervention in hospitalized elderly medical patients: The Yale geriatric care program. *Journal of the American Geriatrics Society* 41(12), 1353–60.

Institute of Medicine. 1988. *The Future of Public Health.* Washington, DC: National Academy Press.

Jaijich, C. L., Ostfeld, A. M., and Freeman, D. H. 1984. Smoking and coronary heart disease mortality in the elderly. *Journal of American Medical Association* 252:2831–34.

Jette, A. M., and Branch, L. G. 1981. The Framingham disability study: II. Physical disability among the aging. *American Journal of Public Health* 71(11):1211–16.

Kane, R.A., and Kane, R. L. 1988. Long-term care: Variations on a quality assurance theme. *Inquiry* 25:132–46.

Kaplan, G., Seeman, T., Cohen, R., Knudsen, L., and Guralnik, J. 1987. Mortality among the elderly in the Alameda County Study: Behavioral and demographic risk factors. *American Journal of Public Health* 77(3), 307–12.

Katz, K., Branch, L. G., Branson, M. H., Papsidero, J. A., Beck, J. C., and Greer, D. S. 1983. Active life expectancy. *New England Journal of Medicine* 309:1218–24.

Kramer, A. M., Fox, P. D., and Morgenstern, N. 1992. Geriatric care approaches in health maintenance organizations. *Journal of the American Geriatrics Society* 40(10):1055–67.

LaCroix, A. Z. 1987. Determinants of health: Exercise and activities of daily living. In Havlik, R. J., Liu, B. M., and Kovar, M. G., eds. *Health Statistics on Older Persons, United States, 1986.* Vital and Health Statistics, Series 3, no. 25. DHHS Pub. No. (PHS) 87-1409. Washington, DC: U.S. Government Printing Office.

Larson, E. B. 1991. Exercise, functional decline, and frailty. *Journal of the American Geriatrics Society* 39(6):635–36.

Lipsitz, L. A., Jonsson, P. V., Kelley, M. M., and Koestner, J. S. 1991. Causes and correlates of recurrent falls in ambulatory frail elderly. *Journal of Gerontology* 46(4):M114–22.

Manton, K. G. 1988. A longitudinal study of functional change and mortality in the United States. *Journal of Gerontology* 43(5):S153–61.

Manton, K. G., Corder, L. S., and Stallard, E. 1993. Estimates of change in chronic disability and institutional incidence and prevalence rates in the U.S. elderly population from the 1982, 1984, and 1989 national long term care survey. *Journal of Gerontology: Social Sciences* 48(4):S153–66.

Mendelson, M. A. 1974. *Tender Loving Greed.* New York: Alfred A. Knopf.

Moss, F. E., and Halamandaris, V. J. 1977. *Too Old, Too Sick, Too Bad: Nursing Homes in America.* Germantown, MD: Aspen Systems Corp.

Omenn, G. S. 1987. Lessons from a fourteen-state study of Medicaid. *Health Affairs* Spring: 118–22.

Omenn, G. S., Beresford, S. M., Buchner, D. M., LaCroix, A., Martin, M., Patrick, D. L., Wallace, J. I., and Wagner, E. H. 1994. *Evidence of Modifiable Risk Factors in Older Adults as a Basis for Health Promotion/Disease Prevention Programs.* Center for Health Promotion in Older Adults, University of Washington School of Public Health and Community Medicine, presented at CDC meeting, September 22.

Ostfeld, A. M., and Gibson, D. C., eds. 1975. *Epidemiology of Aging.* Bethesda, MD: U.S. Department of Health, Education, and Welfare.

Palmore, E. B. 1988. *The Facts of Aging Quiz: A Handbook of Uses and Results.* Vol. 21. New York: Springer Publishing Company.

Preston, S. H. 1984. Children and the elderly in the U.S. *Scientific American* 251(6):44–49.

Rogers, A., Rogers, R. G., and Branch, L. G. 1989. A multistage analysis of active life expectancy. *Public Health Reports* 104:222–26.

Rubenstein, L. Z., Robbins, A. S., Josephson, K. R., Schulman, B. L., and Osterweil, D. 1990. The value of assessing falls in an elderly population. *Annals of Internal Medicine* 113:308–16.

Seeman, T. E., Guralnik, J. M., Kaplan, G. A., Knudsen, L., and Cohen, R. 1989. The health consequences of multiple morbidity in the elderly. *Journal of Aging and Health* 1:50–66.

Sobel, K. G., and McCart, G. M. 1983. Drug use and accidental falls in an intermediate care facility. *Drug Intelligence and Clinical Pharmacy* 17(7-8):539–42.

Stuck, A. E., Siu, A. L., Wieland, G. D., Adams, J., and Rubenstein, L. Z. 1993. Comprehensive geriatric assessment: A meta-analysis of controlled trials. *Lancet* 342:1032–36.

Tinetti, M. E., and Spechley, M. 1989. Prevention of falls among the elderly. *Medical Intelligence* 320(16):1055–59.

Tinetti, M. E., Baker, D., McAvay, G., Claus, E., Garrett, P., Gottschalk, M., Koch, M., Trainor, K., and Hurwitz, R. 1994. A multifactorial intervention to reduce the risk of falling among elderly people living in the community. *New England Journal of Medicine* 331(13):821–27.

Vladeck, B. G. 1980. *Unloving Care: The Nursing Home Tragedy.* New York: Basic Books.

Wallace, R. B., and Woolson, R. F., eds. 1992. *The Epidemiologic Study of the Elderly.* New York: Oxford University Press.

World Health Organization. 1980. *International Classification of Impairments, Disabilities, and Handicaps: A Manual of Classification Relating to the Consequences of Disease.* Geneva: World Health Organization.

Chapter

2

Understanding the Aging and Public Health Networks

Alan L. Balsam, Ph.D., M.P.H., and Carolyn L. Bottum, M.P.H.

As more attention of the acute and long-term care health systems focuses on older adults, the public health profession will be increasingly called on to provide services to elders to prevent and manage the health conditions that rob them of independence and drain the nation's health care resources. Fortunately, a comprehensive system of community-based services that both directly and indirectly affect health already exists. In fact, in 1990, older adults received over a billion dollars' worth of home care, disease prevention, and related services through the Administration on Aging alone (O'Shaugnessy, 1990). This network of aging services has almost thirty years of experience serving older adults and is acutely aware of their special physical and emotional needs, as well as of the most effective means to reach and care for them.

The public health network, meanwhile, possesses expertise in offering health promotion and disease prevention programs, providing health services to identify and intervene with both infectious and noninfectious diseases. It also has expertise in organizing and administering large-scale community health programs.

A coordinated continuum of services formed by the integration of the two networks is already needed—and will be increasingly essential—to meet the needs of older adults. The first step toward such cooperative efforts is a greater understanding by each of the two networks of the history, philosophy, services and resources of the other.

The Aging-Services Network

Mission and Funding

In 1965, as part of the program for Lyndon Johnson's "Great Society," Congress passed The Older Americans Act, creating the Administration on Aging and funding senior center demonstration programs. Among the goals of The Older Americans Act, as amended in 1988, is assisting older people to "secure equal opportunity to the full and free enjoyment of . . . the best possible physical and mental health which science can make available and without regard to economic status" (The Older Americans Act, 1988). This and other aims have been pursued by funding an array of services that are the backbone of the aging services network. The overall philosophy of these services is to give older adults the support they need to maintain independence in the community. Not only does this reduce institutionalization costs, but also it enhances the physical and mental well-being of the older adults.

Funding is provided by the Administration on Aging to the fifty-seven state and territorial units on aging (National Association of Area Agencies on Aging, undated) on a formula basis that targets services to those in "greatest economic" and "greatest social" need, especially low-income, minority, older adults. These state government agencies are mandated by The Older Americans Act to oversee all aging services in their state or territory. The state agencies coordinate services, create plans, provide technical assistance to agencies providing services, and serve as an advocate for older adults in the state (The Older Americans Act, 1988).

Different titles within The Older Americans Act fund various services, including nutrition, transportation, in-home services, preventive health services, employment programs, research, and ombudsman programs. Of particular interest is Title III-B, which provides funds for the establishment and maintenance of senior centers, and through which older adults may receive transportation, health education, health screenings, fitness programs, recreation, counseling, information and referral services, housing assistance and home repair, chore services, shopping services, legal assistance, aged abuse prevention programs, and other services (The Older Americans Act, 1988).

As part of their function, the state units on aging designate area agencies on aging. For some states, the state unit on aging may be the area agency on aging. In general, however, the state unit on aging divides the state into regions and names a nonprofit organization, a municipal or county government agency, a regional planning and development commission, or other organization to be the area agency on aging for that region. Area agencies on aging that are administered by municipal governments are sometimes called councils on aging (J. Englund, personal communication, 1994).

The nation's 670 area agencies on aging develop plans for and administer funding for nutritional, home care, and other supportive services, as well as the establishment of senior centers, among other activities (National Association of Area Agencies on Aging, undated).

Finally, the funds are distributed by the state unit on aging to local agencies that provide services. Some agencies, which can include nonprofit organizations, churches and synagogues, municipal agencies, and councils on aging specifically created to provide senior programming, offer only minimal services to a few seniors, whereas others are multiple-service agencies serving thousands of seniors.

For virtually all services, federal funds are joined with state and local funding and private contributions. State units on aging must provide a minimum of 15 percent of the funds for the federally funded programs (The Older Americans Act, 1988). Private nonprofit organizations also support senior services, either by contributions or by establishing their own services. Finally, while no seniors are required to contribute to the services they receive, they are encouraged to make a small donation.

Health-Related Programs

The aging network serves older adults in the community, those who are homebound and, less frequently, those in institutions. When an aged person is referred to an aging-service agency, one or more services are often packaged into a care plan by a case manager, usually a social worker. The services offered are designed to facilitate older adults' independence and/or enhance their health, whether directly or through increased mental and social well-being.

Participants in almost every community gather at senior centers or other public sites for hot lunches. Meals are most often served on weekdays and may include breakfast and dinner. In 1993, about 127 million meals were served at congregate sites (Administration on Aging, July 13, 1994). Not only nutritionally beneficial, these meals also give older adults a chance to socialize and attend educational and recreational programs.

Homebound older adults receive hot or cold home-delivered meals five days a week. (Weekend home-delivered meal programs are also available in some locations.) More than 103 million home-delivered meals were served in 1993 (Administration on Aging, July 13, 1994). The home deliverer can use the meal delivery as an opportunity to check on the health of the older person, as well as provide a little conversation and human contact. The Older Americans Act requires that home-delivered meals programs also offer nutritional education (O'Shaugnessy, 1990).

Meal programs are sometimes geared toward people who, because of cultural, religious, or language differences, might not feel comfortable or welcome at a local senior center, or otherwise might not wish to attend the center. With this in mind, centers may offer one meal a week from a particular culture's cuisine or bring the meals to a more convenient location (Balsam and Rogers, 1987).

Mandated by The Older Americans Act (1988), nutrition education may include printed materials distributed at congregate meal sites or handed to homebound meal program participants by their meal deliverers.

Health Promotion and Disease Prevention Programs

Beginning in 1992, the Administration on Aging began funding health promotion and disease prevention programs under The Older Americans Act Title III-F. In fiscal year 1992, state units on aging received a total of $17 million, and the same amount was distributed in 1993 (National Association of State Units on Aging, 1993). State units on aging may use funds for statewide programing or distribute these funds for local programing to organizations that include councils on aging and senior centers, health departments, colleges and universities, hospitals and other medical facilities, home health agencies, and visiting nurse associations, among others (Hooker, 1994).

All programs must, by law, be targeted to areas that are considered to be "medically underserved" and "with large numbers of individuals who have the greatest economic and social need of such services" (The Older Americans Act, 1988). About half of state units on aging use the same funding formulas for distributing III-F funds to local agencies as they do for distributing funds for nutrition and other Older Americans Act programs. Programs may be in one of a number of priority areas designated in The Older Americans Act.

The overwhelming majority of health promotion and disease prevention programming includes the categories of health screening (93%), physical activity (89%) and programs on chronic disabling conditions (85%). Other programs include nutritional screening and educational services (76%), health risk assessments and information about age-related diseases and chronic disabling conditions (75%), mental health screening, education, and referral (69%), home injury control services (65%), counseling about social services and follow-up health services (51%), and gerontological counseling (35%) (Administration on Aging, 1994).

State units on aging are developing innovative services that meet the unique needs of the older adults in their state (National Association of State Units on Aging, 1993). Some states are expanding or maintaining programs that have already proven to be effective. Others are encouraging local areas to initiate new programs. Many states are planning statewide efforts for some of their funding, including statewide conferences, workshops and training sessions, statewide special events, and the distribution of health promotion technical assistance kits to senior center personnel. Some states are mandating each area agency on aging to carry out well-defined programming, while others are allowing each area agency on aging to choose from among programs or develop their own.

Seventy-eight percent of the programs reported that they collaborate with their state health department. These efforts include, in descending order of mention, program collaboration; membership on state health department committees, task forces, and other groups; cross-training and consultation; and obtaining materials from the state health department (Administration on Aging, 1994).

Violence and Aged Abuse Prevention

To prevent the physical, emotional, and financial abuse and neglect of older adults by professional or family caregivers and others, The Older Americans Act authorized special funds for states to use to:

■ educate the public and professionals, especially those most likely to come into contact with abused older adults, about abuse and how to detect it.

■ operate programs that receive and investigate complaints and provide protective services. However, few safehouses or shelters exist, and most older adults do not have the physical or financial resources to live alone. Therefore, most are faced with staying in the home with their abuser.

■ refer cases to law enforcement agencies and other agencies responsible for protecting older adults.

In addition, most states have now enacted laws initiating programs to assist victims, as well as requiring reporting of suspected abuse cases by such professionals as doctors, nurses, and social workers. These programs can be administered by state, county, or local agencies (AARP, 1987). Many area agencies on aging now also operate victim assistance and crime and violence prevention programs. Services include advocating for aged crime victims, including accompanying them through court proceedings, community organizing, and education about preventing victimization.

Title III and Title V Programs

The Older Americans Act also funds, under its Titles III and V, a number of programs that enhance the health of older adults. These are administered through area agencies on aging and include programs for those living in the community, those who are homebound, those in institutions, and caregivers of older adults. Among the services provided for community-residing older adults are recreational and social events, health education and health promotion programs, and transportation services, as well as volunteer programs and employment services (The Older Americans Act, 1988).

Services provided to homebound older adults include shopping assistance for food, home and personal care assistance to individuals with impairments with activities of daily living (e.g., bathing, dressing), cleaning and chore services, and friendly visiting and telephone reassurance.

The services needed by Alzheimer disease patients residing in the community are similar to those of other frail older adults in that they also receive in-home care through the aging network. However, in view of their special needs, and the increased level of their needs, The Older Americans Act specifically targets funds for demonstration grants that develop and evaluate community service programs for Alzheimer patients and their families (The Older Americans Act, 1988).

Services for institutionalized elderly include ombudsman programs. These services assign trained volunteers to nursing homes to ensure the residents' physical and mental health by meeting with them and acting as a channel through which disputes with the facility are resolved.

Services are also provided to aid the caregivers of the frail older population. For example, respite care services are designed to help unpaid family caregivers, most often women, who provide more than 50 percent of long-term care for older adults (U.S. Department of Labor, 1986). Respite care by nurses or home care workers can temporarily relieve the burden of caregiving and provide caregivers time to attend to personal, medical, or household matters, or take a vacation.

Although not of direct benefit to the health of the older population, legal services and the home repair program provide assistance to the older individual. Free legal services are usually offered through nonprofit legal services corporations and assist older adults in receiving health benefits, such as Medicare and Medicaid as well as with other legal problems. Home repair programs provide free or at-cost basic repairs on the older adults' residences and allow them to remain safely in their homes.

Research Grants (Title IV)

Besides their service programs, the Administration on Aging operates a research program under Title IV. The purpose of the program is "knowledge building, program innovation and development, information dissemination, training, technical assistance, and related capacity-building efforts" (Administration on Aging, 1994a). The program funds state units on aging, state health departments, universities and other institutions, and community-based agencies, among others, for projects in areas designated by the Secretary for Health and Human Services within the mandate of The Older Americans Act. In 1994, for example, major initiatives were funded in home and community-based long-term care, older women, nutrition and malnutrition, planning for the retirement of future generations, multigenerational and intergenerational programs, volunteerism, and minority aging.

Trends in Services for the Aged

Services for older adults are rapidly changing to address the increasing heterogeneity of the population. The age distribution of older adults has changed in recent years, with a higher percentage of people living past 80. It is not uncommon for a 40-year age difference to exist between older adults. Considerable variation in physical functioning and mental health among the older population is becoming increasingly common.

Aging services are finding that they are serving two very different groups. One is younger older adults, 65 to 80 years old who tend to be in relatively good physical condition and require services that fit their active lifestyles (e.g., senior centers, Senior Olympics, adult education programs). On the other end of the age spectrum are the oldest old, those over about 85 who tend to be more frail and may require more hours of intensive home medical services.

Another trend in services for the older population are those offered by the corporate sector. As more and more workers become caregivers of older relatives, corporations are finding that it is profitable for them to offer some services, such as referral to services and adult day health programs, to employees. These services are provided by employees of the corporation or outside consulting firms. Some aging-services networks have established subsidiaries to provide this consultation to corporations.

The Public Health Network

History and Mission

In contrast to the relatively recent development of the aging-services network, the public health network draws on a much longer history. From ancient times, those with infectious diseases have been outcast, to protect the community as a whole. A new dimension was added when the diseases of the poor began to be treated in public facilities, including hospitals, insane asylums, and poorhouses. Community-based health interventions can be traced to 1678, when the first colonial health education campaign was launched in the form of a Boston broadsheet about the care of smallpox victims (Murphy, 1988). The first large-scale vaccination program in the English-speaking world also took place in Boston, against smallpox, in 1721 (Murphy, 1988). These two missions of public health—to protect and create health of community at large; and to provide care, no matter how rudimentary, for those who cannot afford private care—are still pursued by the public health network today.

The federal public health effort began in 1798, with the establishment of hospitals to provide for the medical needs of "sick and disabled seamen" (Mullen, 1989). A loosely managed system of hospitals with a corps of career physicians was created over the next century, until a "Supervising Surgeon," forerunner to the Surgeon General, was appointed in 1871. In 1879, a National Board of Health was formed as an independent government agency that oversaw military medical care, conducted public health surveillance, granted funds to states for sanitary work, and published a monthly bulletin on disease outbreaks. Though called the Marine Hospital Service, the service provided public health services throughout the nation to immigrants, during outbreaks of infectious disease, and in many other instances, performing the functions of the Public Health Service. In 1902, the name was changed to The Public Health and Marine Hospital Service, and it was led by the Surgeon General.

Local boards of health were established in the eighteenth century, and the first state agency for health, the State Board of Health for Massachusetts, later called the Massachusetts Department of Public Health, was established in 1869 (Murphy, 1988). By the mid-nineteenth century, almost all the elements of modern public health were being proposed. Public infirmaries and hospitals had already been established throughout the United States.

With the discovery of bacteriology and immunology in the late nineteenth century, public health strengthened its focus on infectious diseases through quarantine, monitoring of water supplies, and other means. Whereas earlier public health was orchestrated by social reformers concerned about the living conditions of the poor, with more emphasis on infection control, public health became firmly grounded in the medical model, driven by physicians and medical science (Murphy, 1988).

In recent years there has been a counterbalance to the medicalization of the public health system. An ecological, socially driven public health model is emerging that is reconsidering the environmental conditions related to disparities in health status as well as identifying social conditions that, when altered by public health strategies, can influence health-enhancing behaviors. These avenues have expanded the public health system to include diverse networks of groups, organizations, professionals, and volunteers within communities.

Each of these historical factors contributes to the "mission" of the public health network. This mission is expressed by what public health professionals call "core functions" that public health agencies should, at a minimum, address. These core functions have been redefined as (IOM, 1988):

■ Assessment/surveillance, including assessing health care needs and barriers to health care use of large and small populations; surveillance of disease trends, health care utilization, vital statistics, and other information necessary for program planners to create programs responsive to the needs of the public; and program monitoring and evaluation to ensure that goals of health care programs are being met and that effective models are available for replication.

■ Policy development, including leadership and advocacy for public health; planning to make sure that the health care needs of both the current and future populations are served; collaborative partnerships with community-based agencies, other state, local, and federal agencies serving the agency's population, and consumers of health programs; ensuring financing so that those most vulnerable have access to essential care; and innovations, to meet changing public health needs.

■ Assurance, including health promotion and disease-prevention programs; education and training of those providing care; early identification of those needing special care; care coordination; direct services to those who have no other resource for care; information and referral to ensure that the complete needs of the public are met; licensing and regulation to control the quality of professional care and facilities; and quality improvement, to enhance the care of the future.

■ Capacity-building/infrastructure development so that the health care needs of our communities can be met with locally based, high-quality services.

Structure and Funding

Federal public health agencies.   Like the aging network, the structure of the public health network is three-tiered, with federal, state, and local agencies. The Public Health Service, part of the U.S. Department of Health and Human Services, is comprised of the U.S. Centers for Disease Control and Prevention, the National Institutes of Health, the World Health Organization, the Indian Health Service, the Health Resources and Services Administration, and the Alcohol, Drug Abuse and Mental Health Administration, among others. The Public Health Service funds state public health programs through block grants, including the Alcohol, Drug Abuse and Mental Health Block Grant, Maternal and Child Health Block Grant, and the Prevention Health and Health Services Block Grant and discretionary funding programs. Some programs are initiated by the agency and others by Congress (Mullen, 1989).

Other federal agencies' policies and programs significantly affect the health of older adults. Three of those most directly having an impact on the health of older adults include:

■ The Health Care Financing Administration, an agency of the Department of Health and Human Services, administers Medicare, an insurance program that covers over 90% of older adults (Lauderdale et al., 1993). Its policies on reimbursement have been shown to influence utilization of both private practitioners and health care facilities like hospitals. In addition, it oversees a research program that funds projects dealing with various aspects of reimbursement. Increasingly it has begun to cover preventive care, including immunizations and cancer screenings.

■ The Food and Drug Administration, another agency of the Department of Health and Human Services, regulates the millions of doses of prescription and nonprescription drugs taken by older adults every day. Decisions that affect drug availability and price have a direct effect on the health of almost all the nation's older adults.

■ The Veterans Administration, whose hospitals and health services are a major source of care to millions of older adults, mainly men who are veterans.

State public health agencies. State-level activities are carried out by state health departments. According to the Centers for Disease Control's *Profile of State and Territorial Public Health Systems, 1990* (U.S. Centers for Disease Control and Prevention, 1994), each of the fifty states and eight territories had state-level agencies designated to carry out public health functions. In thirty-seven states and territories, the agency is freestanding, reporting directly to the governor or state board of health, and in twenty it is part of a larger department such as human or social services. Not all public health programs are carried out in these agencies, however. Many important functions, including health care financing and access programs, environmental protection, and mental health services may be located in other agencies, depending on the state.

Budgets of some state health agencies are substantial. In three states, the annual budget is more than $400 million. However, the budget of twenty-five state agencies was $100 million or less, and less than $200 million in another fifteen states. These funds are used to administer direct service programs, and for program grants to local health agencies and community-based agencies for local programing.

Local public health agencies. Closest to the community level are local public health agencies. Almost 3,000 of these local public health agencies nationwide develop health policy, implement programs, and monitor health of local citizens. In 72 percent of states these are counties, in 11 percent they are towns or townships, in 6 percent city/counties, and in 4 percent multiple-county. The budgets of local public health agencies range from a low of $57,000 in New Hampshire to a high of $439 million in California. In the majority, thirty states, expenditures are about $100 million. Supporting these agencies are state funds, local funds, federal grants, and fees.

Staff varies as a function of the size of the agency from basic clerical, administrative, public health nursing, and environmental health staff in small agencies to larger agencies that employ physicians, health educators, nutritionists/dieticians, and epidemiologists. Almost all agencies provide immunizations, health information materials, child health service, tuberculosis control, sexually transmitted disease control, and HIV testing. Some provide, additionally, education and chronic disease prevention programs. Thirty-five to 50 percent provide services to disabled people including laboratory and dental services. Less than one-quarter offer occupational safety and health, primary care, and emergency medical services.

Other locally based organizations that serve older adults are hospitals and clinics receiving public health funds, and visiting nurse associations and home health agencies, among others. These agencies and organizations sometimes serve large numbers of older adults, including the most poor and frail, and must be included in successful collaborations. Community and neighborhood health centers have the capacity to serve older adults, and some do have special programing for older adults or large adult patient populations. In general, however, the patient population of many community health centers is younger, reflecting both an emphasis on maternal and child health and a reluctance of older adults to use clinics when private practitioners are available. However, when activities, such as regional seminars, are undertaken to encourage collaboration between state agencies on aging and community health centers, progress toward increasing aged utilization of community health centers has been achieved (Madden and Campbell, 1990).

Elder Health Programs in Public Health Agencies

Historically, the elderly have not been a primary target population for public health services, except as they happen to be part of the general target population in the community. In recent years, however, in response to the growing numbers of older adults and the shift of focus to the chronic diseases, some health departments have begun programs to determine the health needs of older adults and respond to them.

This new direction is taking place at federal, state, and local levels. Increasingly, funds for research and programing grants from the Centers for Disease Control and Prevention and National Institutes of Health target older adults with breast and cervical cancer, prostate cancer, osteoporosis, diabetes, and urinary incontinence. In some cases these programs are mandated by Congress.

On the state level, a 1993 survey by the Public Health Foundation found that forty-one states had staff designated to work on public health of elders (Public Health Foundation, 1993). Of these, only eleven had words in the person's title referring to older adults. Others had placed older adults under chronic disease, long-term care, and home health care programs. This indicates a focus on aging as a deterioration process, and on older adults as frail and dependent, rather than on healthy aging leading to an active and independent old age.

The Massachusetts Department of Public Health in 1994 conducted a survey of these state health agency liaisons and discovered that seventeen states had an established program for older adults. Staff who lead the aged health programs generally have master's degrees or higher (social work, public health, health services), with several having R.N. degrees. Twelve programs have more than one staff person.

Elder health programs provide the following key services:

- Surveillance. Currently states collect the following data from the following sources: census data, vital records, uniform hospital discharge data sets, Behavioral Risk Factor Surveilance System, cancer registries, and aged abuse data, among others.

- Regulation. State health agencies regulate the following facilities for elder care: nursing homes, assisted living facilities, adult day care centers, visiting nurse services, and others.

- Health promotion/disease prevention programs. Services include education of field workers and administrators in aging and health, health education for seniors, fitness programs, injury prevention programs, immunizations, smoking cessation programs, mammography and breast examination, other cancer screening, and hypertension screening.

- Contracted services, including nursing and medical services.

Trends in Public Health

Perhaps the most important trend for older adults is the emphasis toward health promotion and elimination of behavioral risk factors. As the role of behavioral factors such as diet and exercise on mobility and mortality in older adults is determined, more and more effort is being placed on health education and health promotion programs. This can be seen most clearly in the change of name of the U.S. Centers for Disease Control to U.S. Centers for Disease Control and Prevention. Unfortunately, older adults have not, in the past, been prime targets for prevention programing. This is disconcerting, given that these health risk behaviors contribute to many of the chronic diseases experienced by older adults and, further, that they are as receptive as younger adults to health promotion interventions (Lavizzo-Mourey and Diserens, 1989).

Older adults also have characteristics that ensure that they will fit into an emerging paradigm of prevention that emphasizes community responses to health conditions as well as individual behavior change. Public health programs that acknowledge and address the role of social inequities in health and that develop communities and build on community strengths are well matched to an older population for which poverty and social isolation are significant risk factors and which views community participation as a civic duty and has a well-developed voluntary organization network already in place. Strategies that have been developed using this paradigm include coalition-building, training and skill-building, and increasing access to primary and tertiary care. Of course, such public health programing must also take into account that the most vulnerable, old, and frail older adults are the least able to participate in community activities.

As our understanding of the complexity of factors that influence health grows, the population becomes more diverse, and consumers begin to demand more comprehensive care responsive to their personal needs, the health care delivery system is beginning to change. Programing that was once categorical, disease-specific, program-oriented, medically based, professionally driven, and with separate spheres for public and private care, is now becoming more focused on the total health of the person, community-based, consumer-driven, with integrated public and private efforts, and supports for individuals who wish to enhance their own health.

As a result, the mission of public health agencies is also changing. Increasingly, public health agencies—especially state agencies encouraged by federal agencies—are building capacity for community-based care, improving health care systems within their state, distributing funds for direct services to community-based agencies, and planning services that meet the medical, social and financial needs of the individual. Because most older adults are well connected to their community and present a complexity of problems as they age, these new models of service should be especially effective.

Seeking Common Ground

As comprehensive as these networks are, each has problems with fragmentation, lack of data for program planning, and the need to train professionals to meet fast-emerging needs. Many of the functions of the two networks are parallel, and significant enhancements in quality could be achieved through coordination and sharing of resources.

Surveillance is a major function of both systems. Coordinating and sharing information on a regular basis would increase the quality of planning and program implementation for each network. Following are discussions of four data sources that are prime candidates for such efforts.

The Aging Network

To better determine levels of service provided by state units on aging and to ensure that those in greatest social and economic need are receiving the services, the

Administration on Aging has instituted the National Aging Program Information System. Through this system, the state units on aging provide detailed information about units of service provided and data on clients, including minority status, age, gender, functional status, rural status, whether living alone, income, self-declared disabilities, and cognitive status. In addition, the states are directed to conduct needs assessments of service gaps. This information is to be reported to the Administration on Aging annually (The Older Americans Act, 1992).

The Public Health Network

Each state, as well as the U.S. Centers for Disease Control and Prevention, collects morbidity and mortality data by population and over time. These give valuable information about the changing health needs of older adults.

Each state health agency conducts a Behavioral Risk Factor Surveillance Survey, which asks a random selection of individuals about their behavior as it relates to health risks, their use of early detection and screening, and their functional status. Stratification by age can render important information about those behaviors to be targeted in public education campaigns and health promotion programs. The state health agency, frequently the agency that licenses health care facilities, can also provide information on the level and type of facilities in the state, the age, gender, functional level and other demographic characteristics of the residents, reimbursement sources, lengths of stay, staffing, and other data, both currently and over time.

Professional associations, like the American Medical Association and American Academy of Nurse Practitioners, provide information about practitioners, by geographic region and type of practice, that yields valuable data about health care access. The U.S. Department of Health and Human Services has data about levels of Medicare participation by physicians by region. The Health Resources and Services Administration can offer information about federally funded health care facilities like community health centers.

The Health Resources and Services Administration has information about what populations are underserved by various practitioners, including physicians, psychiatrists, and dentists, as well as utilization rates of various health care facilities such as community health centers. In addition, the Health Care Financing Administration has information on use of health care services that are reimbursed by Medicare (Lauderdale et al., 1993).

In many cases, elder service and public health network agencies provide similar and, frequently, the same services. A health promotion/disease prevention clinic that offers high blood pressure screening, immunization, or blood glucose testing is the same to the aged individual whether the services are offered in senior housing, a council on aging, a community health center, or a board of health. The differences are apparent only to those arranging and staffing the clinic who must find funding and who are implementing programing to fulfill a particular agency's goals. However, these services tend to be in the intersection of what could be visualized as the two networks' continuums of programing going from community to individual practitioner-based services.

Regulation

Both networks perform licensing, certification, and monitoring of professionals and facilities providing care to older adults. The state public health agencies license health care facilities and agencies and those who work in them, such as nursing home nurses aides. The state units on aging oversee social and nonmedical in-home programs in councils on aging, senior centers, and other sites. In many cases, a third agency, a Board of Registration, may license individual professionals.

The more vulnerable the aged person, the more necessary is coordination between the two networks. Older adults in nursing homes should be protected by both agencies, by the state health agency in overseeing the health care facility and professionals who work in it, and by the state unit on aging through their ombudsman program. Older adults who are abused and those who wish to assist them may discover a dangerous lack of coordination. A state that mandates reporting of suspected aged abuse may have two separate systems—one for older adults abused at home, reports about whom need to be submitted to the state unit on aging, and one for older adults abused in a health care facility, whose plight is the responsibility of the state health agency.

Research

Each of the networks conducts research on innovative programing, social and behavioral aspects of health-seeking behavior of individuals and communities, the social factors that affect health, and the physiological process of aging. These programs are conducted by a number of different agencies and some tend to be driven by categorical mandates rather than attempting to coordinate with research already being conducted.

Collaborative Activities of Public Health and Aging Agencies

Some state health departments are already collaborating with state units on aging. The Massachusetts Department of Public Health survey showed that five responding state health departments had memoranda of agreement with their state units on aging. A survey of eight health departments done by Centers for Disease

Control and Prevention (Spriggs, 1993) showed other collaborative activities include participating in each other's boards and task force teams, consultation for developing health promotion and disease prevention materials, and joint applications for grants. While most discussions of collaborative activities are concerned with efforts of professionals and managers at the highest levels, those actually providing services must also have opportunities to coordinate programs at the local level.

Collaboration can take place in each of three spheres: needs assessment and planning, implementation, and evaluation. Program coordination must begin where the programs themselves begin, which is often with funding. Thus, planning must take place among funding agencies, which are usually federal and state-level agencies. Sharing plans for issuing requests for proposals, joining grant programs so that agencies can respond to similar funding programs with coordinated proposals, and ensuring that new requests for proposals do not duplicate—but rather enhance and build on previous programs—would all provide for more coordinated services.

All program planners need data, and while data do exist that would be of value to both networks, they are not generally shared, are not standardized so that the data generated can be compared, and are not always easily available. Linking the data systems, standardizing reporting forms, and providing access over data networks or other means will greatly enhance federal, state, and local efforts.

Cooperative services can take the form of community-based programing using both aging network and public health network resources and personnel. Conducting public health programs in aged service sites and senior housing, where older adults are comfortable and available, is one way to join forces to increase use of services. Conversely, ensuring that existing public health facilities serve older adults is an important way to enhance the accessibility of care. Research has shown, for example, that community health centers do not generally serve large numbers of older adults. In addition, they are increasingly facing financial shortfalls. By making community health centers welcoming to older adults through such means as aged health clinics and separate waiting rooms, the needs of both older adults who may not have good primary care and centers who need patients with insurance can be met (Keehn, Madden, and Campbell, 1990).

Perhaps the most important cooperation is coordination of individual care plans of older adults. Communication among those who care for an individual aged—through either team meetings of care providers of one aged person or opportunities for numbers of providers from the two networks to meet and form professional relationships—enhances referrals for services and prevents loss of information vital to an aged person's health. For example, a personal care attendant may notice a lump in an older woman's breast that should be communicated to the aged person's nurse, who may work for another agency. Also, reducing the number of contacts an aged person must make to arrange for a plan of services increases the chance that an aged person will actually receive all the services necessary, no matter how many agencies may be involved. Single intake forms and assessments that result in eligibility for a number of programs are a particularly important way of coordinating services.

Joint research can yield important results for both networks. Sharing results of research can provide valuable data for increasing effectiveness of similar programs from either network, as well as providing program models for replication by both networks. Joint conferences and professional meetings, as well as publishing articles about research in journals read by professionals in both networks, can disseminate information widely.

In addition, institutional barriers exist that will need to be overcome and eventually dismantled. Funding streams, whether public or private, that have traditionally served one network or the other may be reluctant or unable to provide funds across networks. For example, some funds provided by the Administration on Aging are sometimes available only to state units on aging, while some provided by the Public Health Service specify that only state health departments can apply. This bureaucratic isolation of networks extends beyond funding to data collection and dissemination, professional education and training through conferences and other means, and other areas. Of course, while it can be a challenge for one network to access the resources of another, this can also be a spur to collaboration inasmuch as one agency needs the cooperation of another to gain access to funds, information, and training.

Collaborations can be implemented by a number of mechanisms ranging from formal memoranda of agreement or understanding to informal task forces to provide technical consultation. Formal memoranda can define roles and responsibilities to reduce gaps and duplication, designate staff from each agency to lead aged health and liaison activities, direct agency staff to coordinate services and set up the mechanisms to do so, and initiate such efforts.

Creating offices in each agency to serve as a locus of activity for aged health programs helps ensure coordination and collaboration to the extent that the offices communicate regularly, provide information about programs as early in the planning process as possible, collaborate when appropriate, and provide evidence of success to encourage enhanced programing dollars from common sources of funds, such as legislatures and private funders.

Joint professional training, workshops, and conferences enhance the knowledge and skill level of each network in serving older adults, offer opportunities for communication and cross-referrals, and provide the means of disseminating information resulting from research and data collection systems to both networks. These can take the form of one-time conferences, a series of workshops, or formal certificate or professional education programs, such as the Geriatric Education Centers.

Throughout the collaborative process, agencies will want to provide technical information and consultation through serving on each other's agency's task forces and committees, having regular communication meetings, assisting in the preparation of proposals, and jointly organizing professional education.

Summary and Practical Implications

As the public health system increasingly targets older adults with programing and specialized health care, and costs are of increasing concern to policy makers, it is vital that the public health and aging systems enhance collaboration. However, the aging services network and the public health network, though they are concerned with many of the same health problems, have significant differences. One is young, one is old; one is historically on a medical model (though this is changing), one a social model; one has traditionally served the younger age spectrum, while the other by definition serves older adults. These barriers, though sometimes difficult to overcome, are not insurmountable, and collaborations are being forged between health and aging agencies at all levels of government.

Thus, public health and aging service agencies at all levels need to:

■ Initiate communication with their counterparts in the other network.

■ Determine areas of common need and service delivery and explore how services can be enhanced by collaboration.

■ Coordinate data collection and dissemination, when appropriate.

■ Ensure that regulatory efforts are responsive to the needs of older adults for both health and safety—historically of great concern to public health—and for quality of life and independence—high priorities for aging services.

■ Integrate research in such a way that results will be of practical use by practitioners in both networks.

■ Design and test new strategies for cooperation and collaboration.

By finding ways to cooperate, to coordinate, and to meet the challenge of an increasingly aging population, both networks will better serve older adults, ensure that resources are used most cost-effectively, find new practice models and increase flexibility of thinking, and provide a model of inter-network collaboration and cooperation that will prove valuable for increasing the integration of services for all populations.

References

Administration on Aging. 1994a. Program Announcement No. AoA-94-2, Title V.
Administration on Aging. 1994b. Title III Elderly Nutrition Program Data US AoA (OPCA) 94-63, July 13, 1994.

American Association of Retired Persons (AARP). 1987. *Domestic Mistreatment of the Elderly: Towards Prevention.* Washington, DC: Author.

American Association of Retired Persons (AARP). 1990. *A Profile of Older Americans, 1990.* Washington, DC: Author.

Balsam, A., and Osteraas, G. 1987. Developing a continuum of community nutrition services: Massachusetts elderly nutrition programs. *Journal of Nutrition for the Elderly* 6(4):51–67.

Balsam, A., and Rogers, B. 1987. *Service Innovations in the Elderly Nutrition Program: Strategies for Meeting Unmet Needs.* Medford, MA: Tufts University School of Nutrition.

Balsam, A., Hoopes, M., Daniels, R., and Tepstitch, J. 1992. Patients in time: VA and aged services. *VA Practitioner* 9(3):79–81.

Balsam, A., Webber, D., and Oehlke, B. 1994. The farmers' market coupon program for low-income elders. *Journal of Nutrition for the Elderly* 13(4):35–42.

Hadidian, P. 1990. *Health Promotion and Health Education Activities in Massachusetts Senior Centers.* Boston: Division of Elderly Health, Massachusetts Department of Public Health.

Hooker, T. 1994. *AOA RO Letter 94-34.* Boston: Administration on Aging.

Keehn, A., Madden, S. K., and Campbell, P. 1990. *Evaluating the Collaboration of State Agencies on Aging and State Primary Care Association on Health Service Development for the Elderly in Community and Migrant Health Centers and Area Agencies on Aging.* Boston: John Snow, Inc.

Lauderdale, D., Furner, S., Miles, T., and Goldberg, J. 1993. Epidemiologic uses of Medicare data. *American Journal of Epidemiology* 15(2):319–27.

Lavizzo-Mourey, R., and Diserens, D. 1989. Preventive care for the elderly. In Lavizzo-Mourey, R., Day, S. C., Diserens, D., and Grisso, J. A., eds., *Practicing Prevention for the Elderly,* 1–7. Philadelphia: Hanley and Belfus, Inc.

Madden, S. K., and Campbell, P. 1990. *Evaluating the Collaboration of State Agencies on Aging and State Primary Care Associations on Health Service Development for the Elderly in Community and Migrant Health Centers and Area Agencies on Aging.* Boston: John Snow, Inc.

Mullen, F. 1989. *Plagues and Politics: The Story of the United States Health Service.* New York: Basic Books.

Murphy, R. 1988. *Public Health Trails in Massachusetts: A History and Guide.* Boston: Massachusetts Public Health Association.

National Association of Area Agencies on Aging. undated. *Area Agencies on Aging.* Washington, DC: Author.

National Association of State Units on Aging. 1993. *Disease Prevention and Health Promotion Services: Summary of Proceedings, Teleconferences on Title III-F of The Older Americans Act.* Minority Issues Subcommittee, National Association of State Units on Aging, January 13–14.

The Older Americans Act. 1988. Washington, DC: Government Printing Office.

The Older Americans Act. 1992. Washington, DC: Government Printing Office; Amendments.

O'Shaugnessy, C. 1990. *The Older Americans Act Nutrition Program.* Washington, DC: Congressional Research Service, Library of Congress.

Public Health Foundation. 1993. *Wearing Well: Public Health Aged Care Challenges and Resources.* Washington, DC: Author.

Public Policy Institute, American Association of Retired Persons. 1994. *Elderly Out-of-Pocket Health Care Expenditures.* Washington, DC: Author.

Spriggs, M. C. 1993. *Interagency Communication Patterns and Strategies to Increase Collaborative Efforts between State Health Agencies.* Atlanta: U.S. Centers for Disease Control and Prevention.

U.S. Centers for Disease Control and Prevention. 1994. *National Profile of Local Health Departments*. Atlanta: Author.

U.S. Department of Labor. 1986. *Facts on U.S. Working Women: Caring for Elderly Family Members*. Washington, DC: U.S. Department of Labor, Women's Bureau.

U.S. Public Health Service. 1990. *Health People 2000: National Health Promotion and Disease Prevention Objectives* (DHHS Publication No. PHS 91-50212). Washington, DC: Government Printing Office.

Chapter

3

Behavioral, Social, and Socioenvironmental Factors Adding Years to Life and Life to Years

George A. Kaplan, Ph.D.

Though it has been recognized for some time that the U.S. population is aging, responses by many public health agencies have been muted by competing new threats to public health, by inadequate resources, by a lack of appreciation of the magnitude of the demographic changes, and by the specter of intergenerational warfare over diminishing resources. Indeed, there is even considerable controversy about what these population changes portend, ranging from optimistic forecasts of increasing numbers of hale and hearty older Americans to dire projections of pandemics of disease, disability, and dementia.

Our knowledge base concerning the potential role for primary and secondary prevention with aged people is still relatively small, and numerous conceptual and methodological problems beset those who study health promotion and disease prevention (Kaplan, Haan, and Cohen, 1992; Wallace and Woolson, 1992). Nevertheless, a rapidly increasing literature in public health disciplines points to the importance of such preventive efforts. Behavioral, social, psychological, and socioenvironmental factors appear to play an important role in the health of aged persons; indeed, they may become increasingly important in older age, and may represent critical areas of intervention in public health practice.

Before reviewing the evidence that buttresses this strong claim, it is important to highlight the plasticity of the relationship between age and health. Between 1950 and 1991 there were large declines in age-specific mortality rates from all causes among older populations (National Center for Health Statistics, 1994). For example, for those between 65 and 74 years of age, death rates fell by 35.6 percent during those four decades. For those 75 to 84 years of age the decrease was 36.9 percent, and for those 85 or older it was 25.5 percent. Thus, while being older conveys increased risk and death, the magnitude of this increased risk associated with a particular age varies over time. It has been noted that, in recent years, much of this decline in risk and death has been due to declines in risk of cardiovascular mortality (Kochanek, Maurer, and Rosenberg, 1994). The impact of these declines in mortality rates is, of course, reflected in increased life expectancy. During the same period, life expectancy at age 65 increased 3.6 years, or 26 percent. This increase of 3.6 years in life expectancy at age 65 represents 49 percent of the increase in life expectancy at birth between 1950 and 1991. These declines in age-specific mortality, the resultant increases in life expectancy at the older ages, and declines in birth rates since the "baby boom" have led to the aging of the population.

Primary and Secondary Prevention in Older Populations

What is to be prevented in older populations? In many respects the agenda is no different from that in younger populations. However, the increasing burden of subclinical and diagnosed disease and comorbidity which often, but not always, accompany aging, and the increased potential for impaired function, loss of independence, and decreased quality of life lead to a somewhat broader approach to prevention among the aged.

Figure 3.1 schematically presents some of the key points of intervention in preventive efforts in the aged. Clearly, the imperative to prevent the development of disease and to lengthen the healthy period (Part A) does not disappear when applying preventive approaches to the aged. It is well to remember that coronary heart disease used to be considered a disease of senescence, but we now have a considerable armamentarium for its prevention and no longer see it as irrevocably tied to aging. As subclinical disease begins to develop (Part B), preventive approaches can be applied to slowing the rate of deterioration, thus decreasing the slope of the line and delaying the next transition. The threshold at which subclinical disease is detected will be dependent on screening, technology, and other nondisease factors. It is significant primarily because early detection will often trigger focused approaches, both clinical and behavioral, to slowing down the rate of disease progression. Slowing down the rate of disease progression (Part C) will help to delay any number of com-

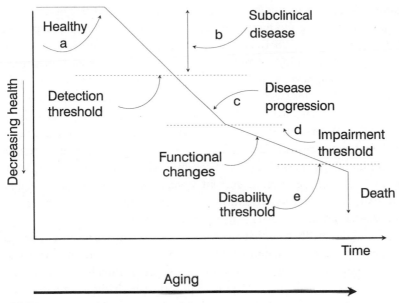

FIGURE 3.1 Opportunities for prevention.

plications, the most important of which, in the present discussion, is the development of declines in function—physical, cognitive, social, or psychological. If the transition to functional impairment is crossed (Part D), the next target for prevention is to slow down the rate of decline in impairment, to prevent or delay the development of disability (Part E). Finally, attempts can be made to slow the progression of disability.

Thus, there is a broad spectrum across which both primary and secondary prevention efforts can be applied in older populations. Following is some of the evidence that behavioral, social, and socioenvironmental factors could be effective in influencing the stages and transitions in Figure 3.1. While many other examples could be chosen, the intent is to present illustrative examples of the association between these factors and longevity and disability.

Behavioral Factors

Current evidence suggests that smoking and physical activity are strongly tied to health status and quality of life among aged persons. While other factors are important, the strength of the evidence and the potential for public health intervention justify a focus on these two.

Smoking. A number of studies have indicated an increased risk of death associated with smoking in aged populations (Barrett-Connor et al., 1984; Kaplan et al., 1987; LaCroix et al., 1991; U.S. Department of Health and Human Services, 1990; Schoenfeld et al., 1994). A typical example of such findings comes from a seventeen-year follow-up of current, former, and never smokers in the Alameda County Study (Kaplan et al., 1987). For those who were 60 to 90 years of age, current smokers had almost 50 percent higher rates of death (RR = 1.46, 95% C.I. = 1.21-1.78) than those who never smoked. When only those over 70 years of age were considered, there was still a 1.4-fold increased risk (RR = 1.43, 95% C.I. = 1.08-1.89). Similar results from three studies of aged persons are reported by LaCroix and associates (1991). Among those 65 years of age or more, current smokers were consistently at higher risk of death than never smokers, with former smokers at intermediate risk. Again, there is a substantial impact of current smoking on mortality.

While it is undoubtedly true that smoking exerts its impact on mortality via the development of numerous pathophysiological changes affecting multiple systems, there is an impact of smoking on mortality even in healthy, high-functioning older Americans. In a study of 70- to 79-year-old people who had no disabilities, no cognitive defects, and one or no chronic conditions, comprising the top 30 percent of those in this age group, current versus never smoking was associated with a twofold increased 3-year risk of death (Schoenfeld et al., 1994).

In most of these studies, former smokers have considerably lower mortality risk than current smokers. This suggests that smoking cessation, even at older ages, may be protective. There is some evidence that this is true. For example, Kaplan and Haan (1989), using the Alameda County Study, examined mortality risks as a function of nine-year smoking histories. Those who continued to smoke, compared to those who never smoked, had a 76 percent increased risk of death (RR = 1.76, 95% C.I. = 1.33-2.31), while those who quit smoking during this nine-year period had only a 33 percent increased risk (RR = 1.33, 95% C.I. = 0.98-1.82). A reduction in all cause mortality risk associated with quitting smoking was also found by Hermanson, Omenn, Kronmal, and Gersh (1988) in their study of the survival of patients with angiographically documented coronary artery disease. This latter finding is particularly interesting because it suggests considerable benefit from smoking cessation in this high-risk group.

Evidence is also accumulating that suggests that smoking may exact a considerable burden with respect to level of physical functioning (Guralnik and Kaplan, 1989; Mor et al., 1989; Pinsky, Leaverton, and Stokes, 1987; Branch, 1985; Kaplan, 1992; Kaplan et al., 1993; LaCroix et al., 1993). For example, Guralnik and Kaplan (1989), in a nineteen-year follow-up of the participants in the Alameda County Study, found that those who were current smokers in 1965, and who survived to 1984, were twice as likely to show reduced levels of physical functioning and ability to complete basic and instrumental activities of daily living (IDL and

IADLs) as were those who never smoked. LaCroix et al. (1993) examined loss of mobility over four years in the three cohorts from the Established Populations for Epidemiologic Studies of the Elderly. Loss of mobility was defined as becoming unable to walk half a mile or walk up and down stairs without help. Figure 3.2 shows the relationship between smoking status and four-year loss of mobility for men and women in these three community studies. In all groups who were mobile at baseline, those who were current smokers at baseline had the highest rate of losing mobility. Former smokers were intermediate, and never smokers were at lowest risk. Using a more comprehensive measure of physical functioning, Kaplan et al. (1993) found that six-year changes in physical function were related to smoking status, with current smokers showing greater declines in functioning than former and never smokers.

Although it has not been well studied, there is also some indication that those who smoke show higher rates of functional problems related to chronic conditions. For example, Kaplan (1992) found twice the risk of incident mobility problems among smokers, compared to nonsmokers, who reported incident stroke, arthritis, or heart trouble. Clearly this is an area where more work is necessary in order to tease out the causal pathways. For example, patients who smoke may have poorer functional outcomes because they suffer more severe disease, because they have more comorbidities that exert an impact on function, or for other reasons.

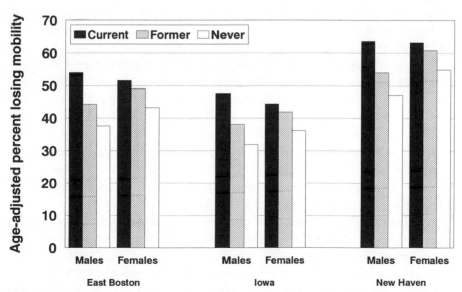

FIGURE 3.2 Four-year loss of mobility by smoking status in persons 65+ years of age: Three communities in Established Populations for Epidemiologic Studies of the Elderly.
Source: Data from LaCroix et al., 1993.

Physical activity. Considerable evidence also indicates that being physically active may prolong life, even at older ages (Kaplan et al., 1987; Foley et al., 1990; Blair et al., 1989; Paffenbarger et al., 1993; Boult et al., 1994). For example, the impact of a sedentary lifestyle on seventeen-year mortality risk among older persons was found in the Alameda County Study (Kaplan et al., 1987). A physical activity score based on the frequency with which a variety of leisure-time physical activities were performed was strongly associated with mortality risk. Among those who were 60 years of age or older, those who reported low levels of leisure-time physical activity had 40 percent higher mortality risk than those who reported higher levels of activity (RR = 1.41, 95% C.I. = 1.20-1.66). This pattern was found even when there was adjustment for other behavioral risk factors, and for presence of chronic conditions, symptoms, and disabilities. When the results were examined for different age groups, there was little change in the magnitude of the association after age 50. Indeed, those who were 70 years of age or older who were sedentary were at 37 percent increased risk of death over the next seventeen years.

Studies with more precise measurement of physical activity and fitness also show similar results. Paffenbarger et al. (1993) found in a 12- to 16-year follow-up of men 60 to 74 years of age that energy expenditure from walking, climbing stairs, and sports was monotonically related to risk of death. Among those 60 to 69 years of age, those with weekly energy expenditures less than 500 kcal had approximately twice the risk of death of those expending at least 2000 kcal. Similarly, Blair et al. (1989) found a linear relationship between fitness quintile, based on exercise test findings, and risk of death among those age 60 or older. Interestingly, the impact of fitness on risk of death was greater for those above 60 years of age than for those below.

Increases in physical activity also seem to benefit older populations. Kaplan and Haan (1989) found that those who increased their levels of physical activity over a nine-year period had subsequently decreased mortality risk compared to those who stayed the same or to those who decreased. These results persisted even when the analyses were restricted to those who were healthy at baseline, or when there was extensive adjustment for risk factors and for prevalent and incident chronic conditions and disabilities. Similarly, analyses by Paffenbarger et al. (1993) indicate that older men who began moderately vigorous sports activities had decreased mortality risk compared to those who remained less active.

An increasing number of studies indicate that low levels of physical activity are involved in the development of problems in physical functioning (Mor et al., 1989; LaCroix et al., 1993; Kaplan, 1992; Kaplan et al., 1993; Camacho et al., 1993). Analyzing the Longitudinal Study on Aging two- and four-year follow-up data, both Mor et al. (1989) and Boult et al. (1994) found associations between no activity and development of problems in functioning. In the Boult et al. (1994) analyses, having no regular exercise was associated with a 37 percent increased risk of developing a functional limitation over four years. In the analyses of factors associated with loss of mobility by LaCroix et al. (1993), a summary index of physical activity based on the frequency of walking, gardening, and performing vigorous exercise was strongly associated with loss of function. Those who engaged in such activities three or more times per week had 60 percent the risk of losing mobility of those who did not so engage. Some of the largest effects were seen by Kaplan (1992) in examining nine-year incidence of self-care and mobility problems in the Alameda County Study. Those who were sedentary were at 5.2-fold and 3.0-fold risk of developing self-care or mobility problems, respectively.

Levels of physical activity also seem to be associated with overall declines in physical functioning. A scale based on the frequency with which five leisure-time physical activities were performed was inversely associated with changes in six-year physical functioning—lower levels of physical activity predicted greater declines in function, even after adjustment for baseline level of physical functioning and chronic conditions related to changes in function (Kaplan et al., 1993). Finally, in one of the first studies to look at long-term patterns of physical activity and physical functioning, Camacho et al. (1993) examined the relationship between levels of physical activity assessed on three occasions over almost 20 years and level of physical functioning in a group who had reached age 80 or older. Their findings showed a strong relationship between the number of previous waves of data collection in which they reported some physical activity and level of functioning. Level of physical functioning rose monotonically with the practice of physical activity over the previous two decades, even though the participants were 61 years of age or older at baseline and had survived two to three decades longer than their life expectancy at birth.

While we do not know precisely what it is about physical activity that is important, a growing number of studies suggest that conditioning and strengthening interventions might improve the functioning of older persons, particularly those who already have compromised function (Buchner et al., 1992; Fiatarone et al., 1994). Exercise interventions may have broad effects in community populations, influencing overall health, role functioning, and physical functioning (Stewart, King, and Haskell, 1993). Extrapolating from one small study (Hu and Woollacott, 1994), increased physical functioning may even improve postural stability, thereby decreasing falls and fractures. Finally, there are some indications that exercise interventions may improve some aspects of cognitive function (Stones and Dawe, 1993).

Social Factors

Over the last fifteen years, a substantial literature has appeared linking mortality risk to aspects of social functioning reflected in measures of social networks and social support (House, Landis, and Umberson, 1988). A number of these studies indicate that the increased risk of death associated with social isolation is also found among the aged (Seeman et al., 1987; Orth-Gomer and Johnson, 1987; Welin et al., 1985; Steinbach, 1992; Blazer, 1979; Boult et al., 1994; Sugisawa, Liang, and Liu, 1994; Seeman et al., 1993). Seeman et al. (1987), analyzing the experience of the Alameda County Study cohort, found a strong relationship between social network participation, as indexed by the Berkman and Syme (1979) social network index and risk of death. The social network index is a composite measure of social network participation that combines information about marital status, numbers of close friends and relatives, frequency of seeing close friends and relatives, and group participation. Low compared to high levels of this index were associated with a 50 to 70 percent increased risk of death in various age groups over 50 years of age. Examining the component items of the index, in those age 70 or older, marital status and membership in nonreligious groups has only weak, and marginally statistically significant, association with seventeen-year risk of death, but both low contacts with friends and relatives and nonmembership in religious groups were associated with approximately 30 percent increased risk of death. Analyzing mortality experience of participants in the Longitudinal Study on Aging, both Steinbach (1992) and Boult et al. (1994) found that low levels of contacts with others were associated with increased risk of death. In the Boult et al. (1994) study, the report of no social contacts was associated with a 2.3-fold increased risk of death over the next four years. In a national sample of elderly persons in Japan, Sugisawa, Liang, and Liu (1994) found that those who reported no social participation were at 1.5-fold increased three-year risk of death.

The extent of social networks and support also appears to be related to levels of functional status, although there are fewer studies than those examining social functioning and mortality. Several of these studies are based on analyses of the Alameda County Study cohort. For example, being socially isolated was associated with 1.7-fold increased nine-year risk of developing self-care problems (Kaplan, 1992). Examining the functional status of those 80 years of age or older, Camacho et al. (1993) found that those who were consistently involved with others over the previous two decades had higher levels of functioning. Also using data from the Alameda County Study, Kaplan et al. (1993) observed an association between low social network participation and decreases in physical functioning over a six-year period. Similar findings were reported by Boult et al. (1994) in participants in the Longitudinal Study on Aging. Those who reported no recent social contacts were at 2.3-fold increased risk of developing impaired physical function.

A larger number of studies report an important effect of social functioning on the health of persons diagnosed with specific conditions (Cummings et al., 1988; Verbrugge, Gates, and Ike, 1991; Nickel and Chirikos, 1990; Kaplan, 1992; Magaziner et al., 1990; Marottoli, Berkman, and Cooney, 1992; Berkman, Leo-Summers, and Horwitz, 1992; Ruberman et al., 1984; Williams et al., 1992; Colantonio et al., 1993). In the Cummings et al. (1988) study of recovery of function in hip fracture patients, greater numbers of social supports were associated with increased probability of regaining the ability to walk unaided six months after the fracture. Magaziner et al. (1990), also studying recovery of function in hip fracture patients, found that greater contact with social networks was associated with better walking ability, less physical dependence, and less instrumental dependence at one year post stroke. Higher social network participation is also associated with better survival in patients with angiographically documented coronary artery diseases (Williams et al., 1992). Among stroke patients, Colantonio et al. (1993) found that larger social networks prior to the stroke were associated with fewer limitations in physical functioning and lower risk of institutionalization.

Socioeconomic Factors

Low socioeconomic level has been found to be associated with increased risk of death in numerous studies of older persons (Lew and Garfinkel, 1990; Branch and Ku, 1989; Sugisawa, Liang, and Liu, 1994; Schoenfeld et al., 1994; Feldman et al., 1989). While the increased risks associated with lower socioeconomic level are often not as great as those found in younger groups, it is important to keep in mind that measures like assets and home ownership may be better indices of current economic resources in older populations than income or education. Nevertheless, socioeconomic level does appear to be related to mortality risk among older persons. For example, in analyses that were based on almost 50,000 persons over age 75 years who participated in the Cancer Prevention Study-I (Lew and Garfinkel, 1990) there was an inverse association between level of education and death rates.

Socioeconomic level is also strongly associated with level of physical functioning and disability in the elderly (Guralnik and Kaplan, 1989; Lammi et al., 1989; Mor et al., 1989; Pinsky, Leaverton, and Stokes, 1987; Kaplan, 1992; Harris et al., 1989; Kaplan et al., 1993; Camacho et al., 1993; Maddox and Clark, 1992; Guralnik et al., 1993; Rogers, Rogers, and Belanger, 1992; Clark and Maddox, 1992; Keil et al., 1989; Seeman et al., 1994; Boult et al., 1994). Examining seventeen-year predictors of mortality and physical function in individuals ages 65 to 89, Guralnik and Kaplan (1989) found that those at low levels of income, who survived, were one-third as likely to have high levels of function as those who had high levels of income. Also in the Alameda County Study, low income was associated with an almost threefold elevation in the nine-year risk of developing mobility limitations (Kaplan, 1992), and with six-year declines in physical functioning (Kaplan et al., 1993). The fact that different measures of socioeconomic level may show different associations in different groups is highlighted in the Guralnik, LaCroix et al. (1993) study of factors associated with loss of mobility. For men and women, low income was associated with a 50 percent increased risk of losing mobility. However, low education was only associated with increased risk for men.

Finally, Guralnik, Land et al. (1993), putting together the impact of education on mortality and mobility by calculating active life expectancy at age 65, found differences in active life expectancy at age 65 related to education level. Black and white men and women who had less than a high school education, compared to those with at least that level of education, had 2.4 to 3.9 years less of life expectancy.

Socioenvironmental Factors

It is intuitively obvious that properties of the physical environment should have some impact on the health of aged persons, but there have been few attempts to examine such efforts. What little evidence there is provides some support. Figure 3.3 schematically presents the dilemma that faces many older pedestrians when they attempt to cross a street. According to data from the EPESE (J. Guralnik, personal communication) and allowing a one-second interval from light change to the beginning of crossing, most older pedestrians would not be able to cross the street. Hoxie and Rubenstein (1994) studied this problem at one intersection in an area of Los Angeles with a high density of older persons. They found that while all pedestrians estimated to be under 65 years of age were able to cross in the allocated time,

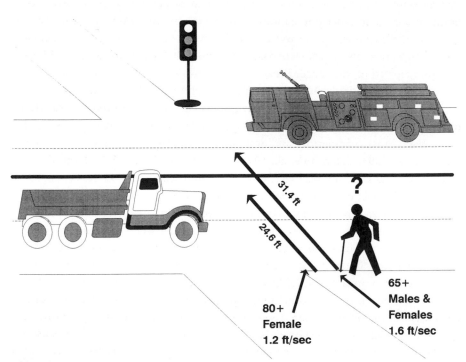

FIGURE 3.3 Problems in crossing streets for elderly persons.
Source: Kaplan and Strawbridge, 1994. Reprinted with permission.

27 percent of all pedestrians judged to be 65 years of age or older were unable to do so. As they point out, this surely underestimates the problem, for many older persons probably do not attempt to cross a street if they feel they cannot cross in the time available. One attempt to intervene in order to increase the safety of older pedestrians was successful in lowering traffic-related mortality (MMWR, 1989). The intervention involved several environmental adjustments including lengthening crossing times, placing signals on median strips, and other modifications, in addition to increased traffic law enforcement and an educational campaign. Because of insufficient study, one can only speculate as to the impact of such environmental barriers on the health of aged persons.

Environmental factors can also have an indirect effect on health through their influence on health promotion behaviors. It is not too speculative to assume that the perception of a neighborhood as unsafe leads to a reduction of physical activity and resultant decreased fitness, as well as an increase in social isolation, depression, and other factors that would result in poorer health and function. Reductions in physical activity may then lead to poorer balance, further mobility problems, and a downward cascade.

The impact of environmental hazards on risk of falls in older persons has been examined in a number of studies. It has been estimated that environmental hazards, in the context of intrinsic limitations, play a role in one-third to one-half of all home falls (Hornbrook et al., 1994). For example, Studenski et al. (1994) conducted an audit of homes and calculated an environmental hazard score based on their observations. The probability of recurrent falls was significantly related to this index of environmental hazards in the home. Given that 60 percent of aged home owners have lived in the same house for twenty years or longer, and the relatively higher costs of housing for the aged (Newman, Zais, and Struyk, 1984), it would not be surprising to determine that many older persons live in houses with features that could be environmental hazards. One attempt to intervene regarding rates of accidental falls in the aged actually provided technical and financial assistance to correct hazards in the home (Hornbrook et al., 1994). This intervention, which also included education and modification of behavioral and physical risk factors, resulted in a 16 percent reduction in total falls in the intervention group compared to a normal group. While there were no significant declines in the average number of falls, fractures, or fall-related hospitalizations, the decline in total falls provides some initial support for this type of intervention.

There are many other socioenvironmental factors that might be important in prolonging life and maintaining function, but they have not been studied. For example, the design of housing and neighborhoods, outdoor lighting and safety, the age-mix of areas, and many other factors could easily affect levels of physical activity, social networks and social support, and depression. Each of these might then influence the slope and transitions present in Figure 3.1.

Implications

While the evidence cited in this chapter suggests an important role for be-havioral, social, and socioeconomic factors in prolonging both life and indepen-dent functioning, this area is in need of considerable additional study. We know little of the natural history of risk factors, risk factor change, morbidity, func-tional problems, and health transitions in the aged. The relative role of long-term patterns of exposure to risk factors versus changes in them at older ages has been virtually unstudied; the specific ways in which behavioral, social, and socioenvi-ronmental factors interact with diagnosed and preclinical disease in the determi-nation of functional health status is only beginning to be studied. Likewise, issues related to comorbidities and their synergistic effect on longevity and quality of life need to be further examined within the context of the biology of disease and function. Despite the plausibility of socioenvironmental effects on the health of the aged, there is little information. Finally, we need much more information on the complex, recursive interactions between health status and behavioral, social, psy-chological and socioenvironmental factors in the aged (Kaplan and Strawbridge, 1994).

With all these gaps in our knowledge, what are the implications for public health practice? It is clear that preventive activities related to the health of the aged are relatively underrepresented in most state and local health departments. In ad-dition, there is a virtual absence of data at the state and local level on morbidity and disability levels among the aged. Such information is critical for the efficient targeting of preventive interventions for the aged. But, the information reviewed in this chapter does have implications for public health practice, even in the pres-ence of unfilled research needs and lack of local data. With an aging population and increased demands on limited resources, prevention—ranging from primary to tertiary—looms more and more important. Based on the available evidence, preventive activities hold great promise in retarding the downward transitions rep-resented in Figure 3.1. This evidence suggests that such activities may well be im-portant in promoting independent functioning in the aged and reducing costly in-stitutionalization. A growing body of evidence indicates that interventions to reduce smoking and increase physical activity in the aged are feasible, but we know little of the impact of interventions directed at social isolation, poverty, or so-cioenvironmental hazards on the health of the aged. It is reasonable to think that such interventions could have a major public health impact, and the time is ripe for public health professionals to take on such efforts. Together with an active cadre of researchers investigating the role of preventive factors in the aged, pub-lic health professionals can—and should—increase their efforts not only to add years to life, but also to add life to years.

References

Barrett-Connor, E., Suarez, L., Khaw, K., Criqui, M., and Wingard, D. 1984. Ischemic heart disease risk factors after age 50. *Journal of Chronic Diseases* 37:903–8.

Berkman, L., and Syme, S. 1979. Social networks, host residence, and mortality: A nine-year follow-up study of Alameda County residents. *American Journal of Epidemiology* 109:186–204.

Berkman, L., Leo-Summers, L., and Horwitz, R. 1992. Emotional support and survival after myocardial infarction: A prospective, population-based study of the elderly. *Annals of Internal Medicine* 117:1003–9.

Blair, S., Kohl, H. I., Paffenbarger, R., Clark, D., Cooper, K., and Gibbons, L. 1989. Physical fitness and all-cause mortality: A prospective study of healthy men and women. *Journal of the American Medical Association* 262:2395–2401.

Blazer, D. 1979. Social support and mortality in an elderly community population. *American Journal of Epidemiology* 115:684–94.

Boult, C., Kane, R., Louis, T., Boult, L., and McCaffrey, D. 1994. Chronic conditions that lead to functional limitations in the elderly. *Journals of Gerontology* 49(1):M28–36.

Branch, L. 1985. Health practices and incident disability among the elderly. *American Journal of Public Health* 75:1436–9.

Branch, L., and Ku, L. 1989. Transition probabilities to dependency, institutionalization, and death among the elderly over a decade. *Journal of Aging and Health*, 1:370–408.

Buchner, D., Beresford, S., Larson, E., LaCroix, A., and Wagner, E. 1992. Effects of physical activity on health status in older adults. II. Intervention studies. *Annual Review of Public Health* 13:469–88.

Camacho, T., Strawbridge, W., Cohen, R., and Kaplan, G. 1993. Functional ability in the oldest old: Cumulative impact of risk factors from the preceding two decades. *Journal of Aging and Health* 5(4):439–54.

Clark, D., and Maddox, G. 1992. Racial and social correlates of age-related changes in functioning. *Journals of Gerontology* 47:S222–32.

Colantonio, A., Kasl, S., Ostfeld, A., and Berkman, L. 1993. Psychosocial predictors of stroke outcomes in an elderly population. *Journals of Gerontology* 48:S261–8.

Cummings, S., Phillips, S., Wheat, M., Black, D., Goosby, E., Wlodarczyk, D., Trafton, P., Jergesen, H., Winograd, C., and Hulley, S. 1988. Recovery of function after hip fracture: The role of social supports. *Journal of the American Geriatrics Society* 36:801–6.

Feldman, J., Makuc, D., Kleinman, J., and Cornoni-Huntley, J. 1989. National trends in educational differentials in mortality. *American Journal of Epidemiology* 129:919–33.

Fiatarone, M., O'Neill, E., Ryan, N., Clements, K., Solares, G., Nelson, M., Roberts, S., Kehayias, J., Lipsitz, L., and Evans, W. 1994. Exercise training and nutritional supplementation for physical frailty in very elderly people. *New England Journal of Medicine* 330(25):1769–75.

Foley, D., Branch, L., Madans, J., Brock, D., Guralnik, J., and Williams, T. 1990. Physical function. In J. Cornoni-Huntley, R. Huntley, and J. Feldman, eds., *Health Status and Well-Being of the Elderly: National Health and Nutrition Examination Survey—I Epidemiologic Follow-up Study.* 221–36. New York: Oxford University Press.

Guralnik, J., and Kaplan, G. 1989. Predictors of healthy aging: Prospective evidence from the Alameda County Study. *American Journal of Public Health* 79:703–8.

Guralnik, J., LaCroix, A., Abbott, R., Berkman, L., Satterfield, S., Evans, D., and Wallace, R.

1993. Maintaining mobility in late life: Part I. *American Journal of Epidemiology* 137:845–57.

Guralnik, J., Land, K., Blazer, D., Fillenbaum, G., and Branch, L. 1993. Educational status and active life expectancy among older blacks and whites. *New England Journal of Medicine* 329(2):110–16.

Harris, T., Kovar, M., Suzman, R., Kleinman, J., and Feldman, J. 1989. Longitudinal study of physical ability in the oldest-old. *American Journal of Public Health* 79:698–702.

Hermanson, B., Omenn, G., Kronmal, R., and Gersh, B. (Participants in the Coronary Artery Surgical Study). 1988. Beneficial six-year outcome of smoking cessation in older men and women with coronary artery disease. *New England Journal of Medicine* 319:1365–69.

Hornbrook, M., Stevens, V., Wingfield, D., Hollis, J., Greenlick, M., and Ory, M. 1994. Preventing falls among community-dwelling older persons: Results from a randomized trial. *The Gerontological Society of America* 34(1):16–23.

House, J., Landis, K., and Umberson, D. 1988. Social relationships and health. *Science* 241:540–45.

Hoxie, R., and Rubenstein, L. 1994. Are older pedestrians allowed enough time to cross intersections safely? *Journal of the American Geriatrics Society* 42:241–44.

Hu, M-H., and Woollacott, M. H. 1994. Multisensory training of standing balance in older adults: I. Postural stability and one-leg stance balance. *Journals of Gerontology* 49:M53–61.

Kaplan, G. 1992. Maintenance of functioning in the elderly. *Annals of Epidemiology* 2:823–34.

Kaplan, G., and Haan, M. 1989. Is there a role for prevention among the elderly? Epidemiological evidence from the Alameda County Study. In M. Ory and K. Bond, eds., *Aging and Health Care: Social Science and Policy Perspectives,* 27–51. London: Routledge.

Kaplan, G., and Strawbridge, W. 1994. Behavioral and social factors in healthy aging. In R. Abeles, H. Gift, and M. Ory, eds., *Aging and Quality of Life,* 57–78. New York: Springer Publishing Company.

Kaplan, G., Haan, M., and Cohen, R. 1992. Risk factors and the study of prevention in the elderly: Methodological issues. In R. Wallace and R. Woolson, eds., *The Epidemiologic Study of the Elderly,* 20–36. New York: Oxford University Press.

Kaplan, G., Seeman, T., Cohen, R., Knudsen, L., and Guralnik, J. 1987. Mortality among the elderly in the Alameda County Study: Behavioral and demographic risk factors. *American Journal of Public Health* 77:307–12.

Kaplan, G., Strawbridge, W., Camacho, T., and Cohen, R. 1993. Factors associated with change in physical functioning in the elderly: A six-year prospective study. *Journal of Aging and Health* 5:140–53.

Keil, J., Gazes, P., Sutherland, S., Rust, P., Branch, L., and Tyroler, H. 1989. Predictors of physical disability in elderly blacks and whites of the Charleston Heart Study. *Journal of Clinical Epidemiology* 42:521–29.

Kochanek, K., Maurer, J., and Rosenberg, H. 1994. Causes of death contributing to changes in life expectancy: United States, 1984–89. National Center for Health Statistics. Vital Health Stat 20(23).

LaCroix, A., Lang, J., Scherr, P., Wallace, R., Cornoni-Huntley, J., Berkman, L., Curb, J., Evans, D., and Hennekens, C. 1991. Smoking and mortality among older men and women in three communities. *New England Journal of Medicine* 324:1619–25.

LaCroix, A., Guralnik, J., Berkman, L., Wallace, R., and Satterfield, S. 1993. Maintaining mobility in late life. II. Smoking, alcohol consumption, physical activity, and body mass index. *American Journal of Epidemiology* 137:858–69.

Lammi, U., Kivela, S., Nissinen, A., Punsar, S., Puska, P., and Karvonen, M. 1989. Predictors of disability in elderly Finnish men: A longitudinal study. *Journal of Clinical Epidemiology* 42:1215–25.

Lew, E., and Garfinkel, L. 1990. Mortality at ages 75 and older in the Cancer Prevention Study (CPS-I). *CA: A Cancer Journal for Clinicians* 40:210–24.

Maddox, G., and Clark, D. 1992. Trajectories of functional impairment in later life. *Journal of Health and Social Behavior* 33:114–25.

Magaziner, J., Simonsick, E., Kashner, T., Hebel, J., and Kenzora, J. 1990. Predictors of functional recovery one year following hospital discharge for hip fracture: A prospective study. *Journals of Gerontology* 45:M101–7.

Marottoli, R., Berkman, L., and Cooney, L. 1992. Decline in physical function following hip fracture. *Journal of the American Geriatrics Society* 40:861–66.

MMWR 61–64. 1989. Queens Boulevard pedestrian safety project, New York City.

Mor, V., Murphy, J., Masterson-Allen, S., Willey, C., Razmpour, A., Jackson, M., Greer, D., Katz, S. 1989. Risk of functional decline among well elders. *Journal of Clinical Epidemiology* 42:895–904.

National Center for Health Statistics. 1994. *Health, United States, 1993*. Hyattsville, MD: Public Health Service.

Newman, S., Zais, J., and Struyk, R. 1984. Housing older America. In I. Altman, M. Powell Lawton, and J. Wohlwill, eds., *Elderly People and the Environment*, 17–55. New York: Plenum Press.

Nickel, J., and Chirikos, T. 1990. Functional disability of elderly patients with long-term coronary heart disease: A sex-stratified analysis. *Journals of Gerontology* 45:S60–8.

Orth-Gomer, K., and Johnson, J. 1987. Social network interaction and mortality: A six year follow-up study of a random sample of the Swedish population. *Journal of Chronic Diseases* 40:949–58.

Paffenbarger, R. Jr., Hyde, R., Wing, A., Lee, I., Jung, D., and Kampert, J. 1993. The association of changes in physical-activity level and other lifestyle characteristics with mortality among men. *New England Journal of Medicine* 328:538–45.

Pinsky, J., Leaverton, P., and Stokes, J. III. 1987. Predictors of good function: The Framingham Study. *Journal of Chronic Diseases* 40 (Suppl. 1):15S–67S.

Rogers, R., Rogers, A., and Belanger, A. 1992. Disability-free life among the elderly in the United States. *Journal of Aging and Health* 4:19–42.

Ruberman, W., Weinblatt, E., Goldberg, J., and Chaudhary, B. 1984. Psychosocial influences on mortality after myocardial infarction. *New England Journal of Medicine* 311:552–59.

Schoenfeld, D., Malmrose, L., Blazer, D., Gold, D., and Seeman, T. 1994. Self-rated health and mortality in the high-functioning elderly—A closer look at healthy individuals: MacArthur field study of successful aging. *Journals of Gerontology* 49:M109–15.

Seeman, T., Kaplan, G., Knudsen, L., Cohen, R., and Guralnik, J. 1987. Social network ties and mortality among the elderly in the Alameda County Study. *American Journal of Epidemiology* 126:714–23.

Seeman, T., Berkman, L., Kohout, F., LaCroix, A., Glynn, R., and Blazer, D. 1993. Intercommunity variations in the association between social ties and mortality in the elderly: A comparative analysis of three communities. *Annals of Epidemiology* 3:325–35.

Seeman, T., Charpentier, P., Berkman, L., Tinetti, M., Guralnik, J., Albert, M., Blazer, D., and Rowe, J. 1994. Predicting changes in physical performance in a high-functioning elderly cohort: MacArthur studies of successful aging. *Journals of Gerontology* 49:M97–108.

Steinbach, U. 1992. Social networks, institutionalization, and mortality among elderly people in the United States. *Journals of Gerontology* 47:S183–90.

Stewart, A., King, A., and Haskell, W. 1993. Endurance exercise and health-related quality of life in 50–65-year-old adults. *The Gerontological Society of America* 33(6):782–89.

Stones, M., and Dawe, D. 1993. Acute exercise facilitates semantically cued memory in nursing home residents. *American Geriatrics Society* 41:531–34.

Studenski, S., Duncan, P., Chandler, J., Samsa, G., Prescott, B., Hogue, C., and Bearon, L. 1994. Predicting falls: The role of mobility and nonphysical factors. *Journal of the American Geriatrics Society* 42(3):297–302.

Sugisawa, H., Liang, J., and Liu, X. 1994. Social networks, social support, and mortality among older people in Japan. *Journals of Gerontology* 49:S3–13.

U.S. Department of Health and Human Services. 1990. The health benefits of smoking cessation. Rockville, MD: USDHHS, Public Health Service, Centers for Disease Control, Office on Smoking and Health.

Verbrugge, L., Gates, D., and Ike, R. 1991. Risk factors for disability among U.S. adults with arthritis. *Journal of Clinical Epidemiology* 44:167–82.

Vogt, T., Mullooly, J., Ernst, D., Pope, C., and Hollis, J. 1992. Social networks as predictors of ischemic heart disease, cancer, stroke, and hypertension: Incidence, survival and mortality. *Journal of Clinical Epidemiology* 45:659–66.

Wallace, R., and Woolson, R., eds. 1992. *The Epidemiologic Study of the Elderly.* New York: Oxford University Press.

Welin, L., Tibblin, G., Tibblin, B., Svardsudd, K., Ander-Peciva, S., Larsson, B., and Wilhelmsen, L. 1985. Prospective study of social influences on mortality. *Lancet* 1:915–18.

Williams, R., Barefoot, J., Califf, R., Haney, T. L., Saunders, W. B., Pryor, D. B., Hlatkey, M. A., Siegler, I. C., Mark, D. B. 1992. Prognostic importance of social and economic resources among medically treated patients with angiographically documented coronary heart disease. *Journal of the American Medical Association* 267:520–24.

Chapter

4

■ Issues of Resource Allocation in an Aging Society

Robert H. Binstock, Ph.D.

The financing of health care in the United States is undergoing continuous and major revisions. Such changes are largely due to attempts by governmental and corporate entities, which pay for an overwhelming proportion of American health care, to limit their payments in an era when health care prices are inflating at a high rate. Some changes, however, are also a result of efforts by reformers to create new mechanisms for providing more effective care on a cost-efficient basis.

A central ingredient in these changes is the allocation of health care resources spent on older persons, and it will remain so for many years ahead. One reason is that persons aged sixty-five and older account for roughly one-third of annual U.S. health care costs (U.S. Senate, 1994); in 1994 this amounted to about $300 billion out of $900 billion. Per capita expenditures on older persons are four times greater than on younger persons (Waldo et al., 1989). In addition, a substantial amount of health care for older persons is financed through in-kind services from relatives and friends that are not readily quantifiable as expenditures. Governments finance nearly two-thirds of health care for older Americans. The federal Medicare program, which provides a basic package of health insurance for most Americans who are aged sixty-five and older (as well as persons who receive federal disability insurance, and those with end-stage renal disease), accounts for 45 percent of the total. Medicaid, jointly funded by the federal and state governments to pay the costs of care for poor people, provides another 12 percent, principally for long-term care in nursing homes and residential environments. Care financed through the Department of Veterans Affairs, Department of Defense,

Indian Health Services, and a variety of other federal, state, and local government programs constitutes about 6 percent of the total. An additional 8 percent is funded through private insurance, largely from so-called Medigap supplemental policies, and less than 1 percent comes from philanthropy (U.S. Senate, 1991).

Older persons pay 28 percent of the costs of their care out-of-pocket. Much of this outlay is to pay for skilled nursing which, along with mental health services, is only minimally covered by Medicare. Nearly two-thirds of prescription drug expenses, not covered at all by Medicare, are paid for out-of-pocket (U.S. Senate, 1994). Persons who can afford Medigap policies have their deductibles and co-payments covered reasonably well through insurance. Poor older persons can have their deductibles and co-payments under Medicare (as well as their Medicare Part B Supplemental Medical Insurance premiums) paid for by Medicaid through a Qualified Medicare Beneficiary program enacted in 1988.

Two fundamental factors have brought to the fore as major issues in American society the resources allocated for health care for older people and the ways in which those resources are financed. One factor is the growth of the older population needing health care, a growth that will accelerate sharply in the early decades of the twenty-first century. The other is the ongoing struggles of federal and state officials to keep their budgets in balance, struggles that are considerably exacerbated by rapidly growing expenditures on health care for older people, principally through the Medicare and Medicaid programs.

This chapter presents an overview of contemporary issues affecting resource allocation and financing. First, it considers whether the growth of the older population, in itself, will force the United States to spend an even larger share of its wealth on health care than it presently does. Second, it examines various pressures to slow the growth of Medicare spending, and the implications of various responses to those pressures. Third, it lays out the complex dilemmas involved in paying for long-term care, presents some possible consequences of changes that are contemplated in Medicaid, and describes a series of experimental models for financing and delivering long-term care. Finally, it suggests that the most important pathway for achieving a reasonable balance between resources for health care of older people and the need for such care is greater investment in biomedical research and technological developments that can maintain and restore the health and functional independence of older people. The promise of this kind of investment is that demands for care of older persons will be substantially reduced in the years ahead.

Population Aging and National Health Care Spending

Because the U.S. older population is growing, absolutely and proportionally—from 31 million persons in 1990 to an estimated 65 million in the year 2030 (Taeuber,

1992)—health care costs for older persons have frequently been depicted as an unsustainable burden, or, as one observer put it, "a great fiscal black hole" that will absorb an unlimited amount of national resources (Callahan, 1987). A particular cause for concern is that the population conventionally termed "old" is becoming older, on average, within itself, and rates of morbidity and disability are markedly higher at advanced old ages.

The number of persons aged 75 and older will grow from 13 million to 30 million between 1990 and 2030, and those aged 85 and older will have increased from 3 million to 8 million. One reflection of increased prevalence of disability as cohorts reach more advanced old age can be found in the present rates of nursing home use in different age categories. At present, about 1 percent of Americans aged 65 to 74 years are in nursing homes; this compares with 6.1 percent of persons ages 75 to 84, and 24 percent of persons aged 85 and older (U.S. Bureau of the Census, 1993). Similarly, disability rates increase in older old-age categories among older persons who are not in nursing homes, from nearly 23 percent of those aged 65 to 74, to 45 percent of those aged 85 and older (Cassel, Rudberg, and Olshansky, 1992).

But demography is not destiny with respect to national health care expenditures. U.S. health care spending increased from less than 6 percent of the gross domestic product (GDP) in 1965 (when Medicare and Medicaid were established) to over 14 percent of GDP in 1993 (U.S. Senate Special Committee on Aging, 1994). However, neither increases in the number and proportions of older persons nor the aging of the older population have been major factors in this growth. Demographic factors have been negligible contributors to spiraling health care costs, compared with increases in per capita use of services; intensity of services per day or per visit; health-sector specific price inflation; and general inflation (Sonnenfeld et al., 1991).

A study by Mendelson and Schwartz (1993), for instance, indicated that while population aging (growth in the number and proportion of older people) accounted for 22 percent of the annualized rise in real expenditures for long-term care from 1987 through 1990, it was a relatively negligible factor in the rise of spending on hospitals, physicians, and other forms of health care. Moreover, this analysis found a steady reduction in the contribution of population aging to overall health care costs between 1975 and 1990, and projected little impact of aging on costs through 2005. Earlier analyses (Arnett et al., 1986; Sonnenfeld et al., 1991) yielded similar findings regarding the minimal impact of aging and other demographic changes on increases in overall health care expenditures through the end of this century. If population aging has a major impact on U.S. health care costs, it will not be felt strongly until after 2015, when the baby boomers—a cohort of 74 million Americans born between 1946 and 1964—begin to join the ranks of persons aged 65 and older; and even this is far from certain.

In fact, cross-national comparisons of health care expenditures and population aging provide no evidence that substantial and/or rapid population aging causes high levels of national economic burden from expenditures on health care. As can be seen in Figures 4.1 and 4.2, health care costs are far from "out of control" or even "high" in many nations that have comparatively large proportions of people aged 65 and older or have experienced more rapid rates of population aging than the United States. Even when such comparisons are made with respect to proportions of na-tional populations at more advanced old ages, such as age 80 and over, there is no apparent relationship with the amount of national wealth spent on health care (Binstock, 1993). The public and private structural features of health care systems (e.g., whether they have relatively fixed or open-ended health care budgets)—and behavioral responses to them by citizens and health care providers—are far more important determinants of a nation's level of health care expenditures than popu-lation aging and other demographic trends.

However, a distinctive feature of American health care—in contrast with the other industrialized nations—is that it is funded largely on an open-ended basis. This is the primary reason why the percentage of national wealth spent on health care is far higher in the United States than in any other nation in the world.

But, as indicated at the outset, the structural features of American health care that nourished open-ended funding are undergoing substantial change as the twen-tieth century comes to a close. Prominent on the policy agendas of federal and state governments are attempts to curb public spending on the care of older people.

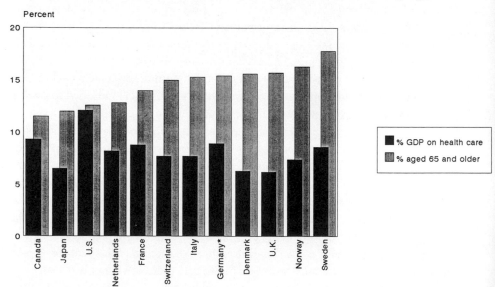

FIGURE 4.1 Selected nations ranked by the percentage of the population aged 65 years or older, com-pared with the percentage of the gross domestic product (GDP) spent on health care, 1990.
*Both percentages are for the Federal Republic of Germany, 1988.
Source: Binstock, 1993; assembled from data in Schieber, Poullier, and Greenwald, 1992.

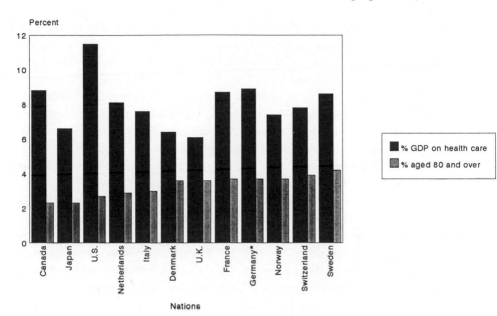

FIGURE 4.2 Selected nations ranked by the percentage of the population aged 80 years or older, compared with the percentage of the gross domestic product (GDP) spent on health care, 1989.
*Both percentages are for the Federal Republic of Germany, 1988.
Source: Binstock, 1993; assembled from data in Schieber, Poullier, and Greenwald, 1992.

Pressures to Curb Medicare Expenditures

Most of the specific public policy actions and proposals to contain health care costs in recent years have focused on Medicare. To date, there has been no evidence that changes in the program have adversely affected the health care or health status of older persons. But efforts to curb federal Medicare expenditures are ongoing, and could ultimately have a negative impact on older people.

There are a number of fundamental reasons why Medicare has been a major target in governmental efforts to slow the growth of national health care costs. First, it is the biggest single source of payment for health care in America. Its large aggregate national costs, as well as its rapid inflation, are easily determined and highly visible. In 1994 the program paid $159 billion for personal health care services. Medicare expenditures are projected to grow at an annual rate of 7.5 percent (in inflation-adjusted dollars), and reach $220 billion in fiscal year 1999 (U.S. Congress, 1994).

Second, because the federal government pays the bills for Medicare patients, Medicare costs are more directly responsive to government action than those paid for through private insurance and out-of-pocket. The most far reaching cost-containment measures undertaken to date have been changes in reimbursement procedures under Medicare, such as prospective payment on the basis of diagnosis-related groups (DRGs) to control expenditures on the services of hospitals (Coulam and Gaumer, 1991), the introduction of a "resource based relative-value scale" (RBRVS) for reimbursing physicians, and the introduction of Medicare Health Maintenance Organizations (HMOs) (Brown et al., 1993).

Third, changes in Medicare approaches to paying for care are a plausible strategy for implementing the more general goal of cost-containment. This nationwide governmental program affects the financial incentives of most American hospitals, nursing homes, physicians, and other health care providers and suppliers. Consequently, changes in Medicare have impacts on the overall health care arena that extend beyond the provision of services to Medicare patients.

Fourth, the issue of how to pay for Medicare is rather immediate. Recent annual reports of the Trustees of the Social Security Trust Funds have consistently estimated that, in the latter half of the 1990s, Medicare's Part A Hospital Insurance (HI) costs will substantially exceed revenues from the payroll tax that finances it. Shortly after the turn of the century the HI trust fund reserves will be exhausted. Moreover, the financing of Medicare's Part B (nonhospital) Supplementary Medical Insurance (SMI) has moved from being principally financed by premiums from Medicare enrollees, in the early years of the program, to being 75 percent financed from general revenues, today. As SMI expenditures increase, so does the amount of general revenues needed to support them. The Omnibus Budget Reconciliation Act (OBRA) of 1993 partially responded to these immediate issues by enacting Medicare spending reductions and revenue increases totaling an estimated $85 billion over the five-year period 1994 to 1998 (U.S. Congress, 1993). But these measures have not been sufficient to eliminate the near-term financing problems.

Finally, as implied by spending projections, Medicare could contribute substantially to increases in the federal deficit in the years to come unless significant changes are made in the program (U.S. Congress, 1995). Consequently, as national policymakers become increasingly serious about balancing the budget, their attention is inevitably drawn to limiting the growth of government financing for Medicare. For example, Congress passed a budget resolution in 1995 that called for a $270 billion reduction in projected Medicare spending by 2002 (Eaton and Diemer, 1995).

One of the strategies contemplated for achieving this goal was to require individuals enrolled in Medicare to bear an increased portion of payment for their health care. Among the measures considered were larger deductibles; the introduction of co-payments for services that did not previously require them, such as home health services, medical laboratory tests, and skilled nursing facilities; and larger premiums for Part B SMI insurance. Also contemplated was the establishment of a series of incentives and constraints for encouraging Medicare enrollees to abandon the open-ended fee-for-service approach to paying for care by joining HMOs and similar arrangements in which health care financing is limited through flat per capita enrollment charges (Pear, 1995).

These types of Medicare reforms could engender adverse consequences for older persons. A possible effect of a strategy requiring older persons to pay more is that those who are relatively poor—but not poor enough to qualify for Medicaid—will be unable or less inclined to seek appropriate health care. A possible difficulty with the strategy of encouraging participation in HMOs is that the financial incentives of such managed care organizations foster undertreatment of patients. Nothing in the decade-long experience of Medicare HMOs launched by the federal Health Care Financing Administration (HCFA) is reassuring on this score because enrollees in these programs tended to be relatively healthy older persons (Brown et al., 1993).

Parallel to these contemplated measures for reducing the growth of Medicare have been propositions to deny acute care for older people. Public suggestions that health care should be rationed on the basis of old age began to emerge in the early 1980s and have continued into the 1990s. The most prominent of such proposals has been that of a biomedical ethicist, Daniel Callahan, who urged that Medicare payments for life-saving care of people aged in their late 70s or older be categorically denied (Callahan, 1987). His proposal provoked widespread and ongoing discussion in the media and public forums and directly inspired a number of books (e.g., Binstock and Post, 1991) and scores of journal articles dealing with the topic of old age and health care rationing.

Although Callahan and other proponents of rationing care for very old people imply that their suggestions would be of great significance in curbing the growth of U.S. health care costs, in fact they would not. Medicare payments associated with additional years of life at advanced old ages decrease as the age of death increases. For instance, lifetime Medicare outlays for persons who die at age 101 or older average only $9,500 higher (in adjusted dollars) than for those who die at 80 (Lubitz, Beebe, and Baker, 1995). And high-tech medical care for persons of advanced old age does not have much bearing on Medicare's rising costs; the intensity of care declines at older old ages (Scitovsky, 1994).

Moreover, various rationing scenarios even at younger old ages would not have a substantial financial impact. For example, suppose it were ethically and morally possible to deny high-cost care to patients aged 65 and older who are going to die within a year even with such care (although, clinically, it is rarely possible to make reliable prospective distinctions between high-cost survivors and decedents). In 1994, implementing a policy of this kind would have reduced national health care expenditures by about one-half of 1 percent (Binstock, 1994a).

Such facts about the economic insignificance of futile care are not widely known or appreciated. Yet, even if they come to be understood, it seems very likely that issues of high cost acute care for those older persons who *survive*, as well as those who die, will continue to be debated in the years immediately ahead. A substantial agenda of research needs to be implemented to inform such debates about specific types of aggressive care—coronary artery bypass operations, kidney and liver transplants, and so on—for patients of advanced age.

The Dilemmas of Financing Long-Term Care

Although the contemporary policy agenda with respect to Medicare is essentially one of cutting government costs, the issues of resource allocation for long-term care are more complex. Out-of-pocket payments are large and unaffordable for many. Private insurance is expensive and limited in coverage. Medicaid plays a key role in financing long-term care for poor people and those who become poor through paying for their care out-of-pocket, but the program is both a big and an increasing cost for federal and state governments. A few years ago it seemed that the federal government might expand public funding for long-term care by creating a new insurance program. Now, however, policy makers are attempting to cut back on Medicaid spending and to find new models for delivering care within the context of fixed budgets.

Overall Costs

Expenditures for long-term care of older people are substantial, and are very likely to increase in the decades immediately ahead. The total bill in 1993 was $75.5 billion; 72 percent was spent on nursing home care, and 28 percent on home and community-based care (Wiener, Illston, and Hanley, 1994). Out-of-pocket payments by individuals and their families account for 44 percent of the total. Only 1 percent is paid for with private insurance benefits. The remainder is financed by federal, state, and local governments.

The demand for long-term care of older people will increase considerably in the twenty-first century. As noted earlier, the number of people aged 65 and older will have more than doubled between 1990 and 2030 (Taeuber, 1992). Moreover, in the same time period, the number of persons in advanced old-age ranges will also more than double.

Experts disagree as to whether rates of disability in old age will increase or decline in the future. But even those who report a decline in recent years in the prevalence of disability at older ages emphasize that there will be large absolute increases in the number of older Americans needing long-term care in the decades ahead (see, e.g., Manton, Corder, and Stallard, 1993). Accordingly, the Congressional Budget Office (U.S. Congress, 1991), using 1990 as a baseline year, projects that total national costs of long-term care will almost double by 2010 and more than triple by 2030.

The Role of Individuals and Their Families

Many persons needing formal, paid, long-term care services have no way to pay for them. In one study, for example, about 75 percent of unpaid, informal caregivers of dementia patients said that they did not use paid services because they could not afford them (Eckert and Smyth, 1988). Although dozens of governmental programs provide funding for long-term care services (U.S. General Accounting Office, 1995), many persons needing long-term care are ineligible for these programs and are unable to pay out-of-pocket for services.

Although nearly half of the national bill for long-term care is paid for out-of-pocket, such payments are a significant financial burden for many individuals and their families. The annual cost of a year's care in a nursing home averages $37,000 (Wiener and Illston, 1996) and ranges higher than $100,000. While the use of a limited number of services in a home or other community-based setting is less expensive, noninstitutional care for patients who would otherwise be appropriately placed in a nursing home is not less expensive, and is often more expensive (Weissert, 1990).

A number of research efforts have documented that about 80 percent of the long-term care provided to older persons outside of nursing homes is presently provided by family members—spouses, siblings, adult children, and broader kin networks. About 74 percent of dependent community-based older persons receive all their care from family members or other unpaid sources; about 21 percent receive both formal and informal services, and only about 5 percent use just formal services (Liu, Manton, and Liu, 1985). The vast majority of family caregivers are women (Brody, 1990; Stone, Cafferata, and Sangl, 1987). The family also plays an important role in obtaining and managing services from paid service providers.

The capacities and willingness of family members to care for disabled older persons may decline, however, when the baby boom cohort reaches old age because of a broad social trend. The family, as a fundamental unit of social organization, has been undergoing profound transformations that will become more fully manifest over the next few decades as baby boomers reach old age. The striking growth of single-parent households, the growing participation of women in the labor force, and the high incidence of divorce and remarriage (differentially higher for men) all entail complicated changes in the structure of household and kinship roles and relationships. There will be an increasing number of "blended families," reflecting multiple lines of descent through multiple marriages and the birth of children outside of wedlock through other partners. This growth in the incidence of step- and half-relatives will make for a dramatic new turn in family structure in the coming decades. Already, such blended families constitute about half of all households with children (National Academy on Aging, 1994).

One possible implication of these changes is that kinship networks in the near future will become more complex, attenuated, and diffuse (Bengtson, Rosenthal, and

Burton, 1990), perhaps with a weakened sense of filial obligation. If changes in the intensity of kinship relations significantly erode the capacity and sense of obligation to care for older family members when the baby boom cohort is in the ranks of old age and disability, demands for governmental support to pay long-term care may increase accordingly.

The Role of Private Insurance

Although Medicare pays for short-term, subacute nursing care, it does not reimburse patients for long-term care, either in nursing homes or at home. Private long-term care insurance, a relatively new product, is very expensive for the majority of older persons, and its benefits are limited in scope and duration. The best-quality policies—providing substantial benefits over a reasonable period of time—charged premiums in 1991 that averaged $2,525 for persons aged 65 and $7,675 for those aged 79 (Wiener and Illston, 1996). Only about 4 percent to 5 percent of older persons have any private long-term care insurance, and only about 1 percent of nursing home costs are paid for by private insurance (Wiener, Illston, and Hanley, 1994). A number of analyses have suggested that even when the product becomes more refined, no more than 20 percent of older Americans will be able to afford it (Crown, Capitman, and Leutz, 1992; Friedland, 1990; Rivlin and Wiener, 1988; Wiener, Illston, and Hanley, 1994). Although some studies suggest a potential for a higher percentage of customers, they assume relatively limited packages of benefit coverage (e.g., Cohen et al., 1987).

A variation on the private insurance policy approach to financing long-term care is continuing care retirement communities (CCRCs), which promise comprehensive health care services—including long-term care—to all members (Chellis and Grayson, 1990). CCRC customers tend to be middle- and upper-income persons who are relatively healthy when they become residents and pay a substantial entrance charge and monthly fee in return for a promise of "care for life." It has been estimated that about 10 percent of older people could afford to join such communities (Cohen, 1988). Most of the 1,000 CCRCs in the United States, however, do not provide complete benefit coverage in their contracts, and those that do have faced financial difficulties (Williams and Temkin-Greener, 1996). Because most older people prefer to remain in their own homes rather than join age-segregated communities, an alternative product termed "life care at home" (LCAH) was developed in the late 1980s and marketed to middle-income customers with lower entry and monthly fees than those of CCRCs (Tell, Cohen, and Wallack, 1987). There are, however, only about 500 LCAH policies in effect (Williams and Temkin-Greener, 1996).

A relatively new approach for providing long-term care in residential settings is the "assisted living" facility. It has been created for moderately disabled persons—

including those with dementia—who are not ready for a nursing home, and provides them with limited forms of personal care, supervision of medications and other daily routines, and congregate meal and housekeeping services (Kane and Wilson, 1993). Assisted living has yet to be tried out with a private insurance approach. The monthly rent in a first-class nonprofit facility averages about $2,400 for a one-bedroom apartment; the rent is higher in for-profit facilities.

The Role of Medicaid

For those who cannot pay for long-term care out-of-pocket or through various insurance arrangements, and who are not eligible for care through programs of the Department of Veterans Affairs, the available sources of payment are Medicaid and other means-tested government programs funded by the Older Americans Act, Social Service Block Grants (Title XX of the Social Security Act), and state and local governments. The bulk of such financing is through Medicaid, which paid an estimated 52 percent of the total national nursing home expenditures in 1993, accounting for one-quarter of all Medicaid spending (Burner, Waldo, and McKusick, 1992).

Medicaid, the federal-state program for the poor, finances the care—at least in part—of about three-fifths of nursing home patients (Wiener and Illston, 1996). However, Medicaid does not pay for the full range of home care services that are needed for most clients who are functionally dependent. Most state Medicaid programs provide reimbursement only for the most "medicalized" services that are necessary to maintain a long-term care patient in a home environment; rarely reimbursed are essential supports such as chore services, assistance with food shopping and meal preparation, transportation, companionship, periodic monitoring, and respite programs for family and other unpaid caregivers.

Medicaid does include a special waiver program that allows states to offer a wider range of nonmedical home care services, if limited to those patients whose services will be less costly than Medicaid-financed nursing home care. But the volume of services in these waiver programs—which in some states combine Medicaid with funds from the Older Americans Act, the Social Services Block Grant program, and other state and local government sources—is small in relation to the overall demand (Miller, 1992).

Although many patients are poor enough to qualify for Medicaid when they enter a nursing home, a substantial number become poor after they are institutionalized (Adams, Meiners, and Burwell, 1993). Persons in this latter group deplete their assets in order to meet their bills and eventually "spend down" and become poor enough to qualify for Medicaid.

On the other hand, asset sheltering has become a source of considerable concern to the federal and state governments as Medicaid expenditures on nursing homes are increasing rapidly—projected to triple from 1990 to 2000 (Burner, Waldo, and McKusick, 1992). An analysis in Virginia estimated that the aggregate of assets sheltered through the use of legal loopholes in 1991 was equal to more than 10 percent of what the state spent on nursing home care through Medicaid in that year (Burwell, 1993).

Efforts to Expand and Contract Public Funding

From the mid-1980s until the mid-1990s a number of national policy makers were sympathetic to these various dilemmas—the inability of individuals and their families to pay for services, the limitations of private insurance, and the anxieties of spending down. Since then, however, the main concern in Washington, as well as in the states, has been to limit Medicaid expenditures. In this new context, the most likely prospect is that public resources for long-term care will be even less available, in relation to the need, than they have been to date.

In the early 1990s advocates for the elderly, as well as younger disabled persons, were optimistic that the federal government would establish a new program for public long-term care insurance that would not be means-tested as is Medicaid. A number of bills introduced from 1989 to 1994 included some version of such program, including President Clinton's failed proposal for health care reform (see Binstock, 1994b). None became law. The major reason was that any substantial version of such a program would cost tens of billions of dollars each year just at the outset, and far more as the baby boom reaches old age.

By 1995, however, legislative focus had shifted from creating a new program to curbing the costs of public expenditures for long-term care. As part of its overall effort to achieve a balanced budget by 2002, Congress proposed to cap the rate of growth in Medicaid expenditures to achieve savings of $175 billion, and to turn over administration of the program to state governments through block grants (Rosenbaum, 1995).

Medicaid's expenditures on long-term care had been growing at an annualized rate of 13.2 percent since 1989 (U.S. General Accounting Office, 1995). According to one analysis (Kassner, 1995), congressional proposals for limiting Medicaid's growth would trim long-term care funding by as much as 11.4 percent by 2000, and would mean that 1.74 million Medicaid beneficiaries would lose or be unable to secure coverage. In addition, this analysis assumed that states would make their initial reductions in home and community-based care services (because nursing home residents have nowhere else to go), and concluded that such services would be substantially reduced from their current levels. Five states were projected to completely eliminate home and community-based services by the end of the century, and another 19 to cut services by more than half. Although this proposal did not become law during the 104th Congress, it is expected to surface again before the end of the century.

Experimental Programs

Both during the periods when national policy makers were focused on expanding federal resources for long-term care and when they began contracting them, a number of experiments in new ways to finance and deliver care have been underway. These experiments—sponsored by private foundations and state governments, as well as the federal government—have been attempting to demonstrate that appropriate long-term care can be delivered in fashions that limit out-of-pocket and governmental expenditures, and that effectively integrate acute and long-term health care.

Private Insurance/Medicaid Partnerships

The Robert Wood Johnson Foundation has undertaken experimental programs in four states intended to enable middle- and upper-income older persons to protect their assets from being spent down and yet have Medicaid pay for their long-term care (Meiners, 1996). At the same time these programs are designed to reduce the period that Medicaid needs to finance the care of individuals whose services are reduced by the program.

Through this Partnership for Long-Term Care Program, state governments agree to exempt individuals who apply for Medicaid eligibility from having to spend down assets in order to qualify for the program, if they have previously had some long-term care paid for by a state-certified private insurance policy. In California, Connecticut, and Indiana, the Medicaid agencies will allow a dollar of asset protection for each dollar that has been paid by insurance. In New York, after three years of private insurance coverage for nursing home services or six months of home health care, protection is granted for all assets, although the individual's income, along with Medicaid, must be devoted to the cost of care. This experiment is in its early stages and cannot yet be evaluated.

Financing through Integration with Acute Care

Experimental models have also been developed for financing long-term care services by integrating them with acute care. These models are being refined through field demonstrations. Each involves mechanisms of managed care. Their differences illustrate some of the issues and challenges generated by various sources of funding and different types of older patient populations.

A model initially tested at several sites in the 1980s is the Social/Health Maintenance Organization (S/HMO), financed by the federal government. The S/HMO offers customers a limited package of home and community-based long-term care benefits on a capitated basis as a supplement to Medicare HMO benefits, and attempts to enroll primarily healthy older customers (Leutz et al., 1985). Results from these early experiments were equivocal with respect to the viability of financing arrangements and target populations (Newcomer, Harrington, and Friedlob, 1990). Consequently, Congress has called for a second round of S/HMO demonstrations to test refinements such as: heavy involvement of geriatricians and geriatric nurse practitioners; standard protocols for obtaining adequate medical and social histories, and for diagnosing and managing conditions frequently found in older patients; increased attention to the effects of prescription drugs on patients; and outpatient alternatives to hospitalization and nursing home placement.

While the S/HMO attempts to enroll healthy older persons to demonstrate what is feasible financially with such a population, the On Lok model, developed at a San Francisco neighborhood center in the 1970s and early 1980s, is targeted to community-based older persons who are already sufficiently dependent in daily functioning to be appropriately placed in a nursing home. In this capitated model most patients are eligible for both Medicare and Medicaid. Services are organized around an adult day care program that not only serves as a social program and as a respite for caregivers, but also functions much like a geriatric outpatient clinic with substantial medical observation and supervision (Zawadski and Eng, 1988).

The On Lok model, now being replicated at ten demonstration sites as a Program for All-Inclusive Care for the Elderly (PACE), appears to have integrated acute and long-term care fairly well under its managed care approach. Whether it can be extended beyond the very frail population it has served to date—patients who are already functionally dependent, and dually eligible for Medicare and Medicaid—remains to be seen. (To some extent, this is what is being explored in the second round of the S/HMO demonstrations.) Early evaluations of the PACE demonstrations indicate that they are experiencing problems of financial viability, of high staff turnover among physicians and adult day health center directors, and in getting the right patient mix in terms of both acuity and dementia (Kane, Illston, and Miller, 1992).

Still another model for attempting to integrate the financing and delivery of acute and long-term care for older persons is the Minnesota Long-Term Care Options Project (LTCOP). It incorporates elements of both the S/HMO and On Lok models. In contrast to the S/HMO, however, LTCOP will target Medicaid-eligible enrollees and accordingly offer a benefit package that includes nursing home care as well as home and community-based care. It will also include a less functionally dependent population than the On Lok model. Hence, it provides an opportunity to test broader approaches to integrating acute and long-term care than have been tried to date.

To the extent that any of these demonstration models seem to be effective in integrating care as they are tested in the years immediately ahead, their broader import in the American health care delivery system for older adults will still depend on further action by the federal government and in the private sector. The government would need to allow the pooling of Medicare and Medicaid funds more generally for this purpose (the various demonstration models operate under special waivers from HCFA, which administers these two programs). And to make such care integration available for those older persons not covered by Medicaid for long-term care expenses, private insurance companies will need to be satisfied that such managed care arrangements are financially viable.

Resources for Research and Development

Even as policy makers are now oriented toward cutting back on governmental obligations to pay for the health care of older people, they might well consider greater allocation of resources to research and development. To be sure, fixed budgets, managed care, and other structural changes in health care financing and organization are likely to have some effects in reducing costs for government as well as for individuals and their families. But, given the rapid population aging that the United States will experience in the early decades of the twenty-first century, the impact of such reforms in the health care system will be dwarfed by increased needs—especially for long-term care. Far more important for achieving a match between resources for health services and the need for them will be continuing progress in maintaining and restoring the health and functional independence of older people which, in turn, can reduce the need for care. Progress in this area can only be achieved through greater allocation of resources for biomedical research and technological development.

Improvements in traditional medical technology are constantly increasing our ability to improve functional status and quality of life for aging individuals. For example, progress in cardiac surgery has allowed common disorders such as coronary artery disease and aortic stenosis to be surgically treated in people well into their 80s and 90s, thereby enhancing their functional capacities. New, more targeted approaches to chemotherapy based on monoclonal antibodies and other techniques can improve the effectiveness of cancer treatments while reducing their potentially devastating side effects.

Advances in cataract surgery, and in orthopedic surgery—particularly hip replacement and knee replacement—have become more and more important in reducing functional impairments that used to be common in elderly people. Still, much can be developed in the way of treatment, prosthetics, and rehabilitative techniques to reduce functional disability brought on by losses in vision and hearing, osteoarthritis, osteoporosis (which affects up to 50 percent of people aged 65 and older), hypothyroidism, incontinence, and other nonfatal conditions that bring about dependence and overall decline.

As more and more people survive into their late 70s and 80s, degenerative brain function related to Alzheimer disease may be the single most important area of societal need for biomedical research. Current medical treatment does not produce dramatic changes in the function of people suffering from Alzheimer disease, but many experts believe that major research advances can be made that would allow us to postpone the decline caused by this disease.

Research currently being done on memory-enhancing drugs might well show significant progress within the next decade, in time to benefit baby boomers in old age. In addition, research has isolated a gene that is linked with the common variety, late-onset Alzheimer disease. As knowledge about such markers grows, it will help researchers to identify better the underlying causes of Alzheimer disease and perhaps be able more effectively to prevent their expression. Developments in this area will also allow a more targeted approach to diagnosis and care for individuals identified as being at high risk for developing Alzheimer disease.

As many advances as there have been in these and related areas, the federal government can still establish biomedical research funding and priorities that will more strongly emphasize the preservation and enhancement of functional independence in later years. Such priorities would stress research and development on causes, treatments, prosthetics, and rehabilitation techniques pertinent to a substantial range of nonfatal conditions, including those outlined above, as well as amplify the current emphasis on the causes of and treatments for Alzheimer disease.

In addition, greater resources could be allocated to harness various technological advances in the service of older (and younger) disabled persons living in the community, particularly those removed from easy access to kin and formal services. Development and application of technology in support of long-term care could have a substantial impact in maintaining and enhancing functional independence. Such applications could include, for example, so-called smart houses and networking intelligence for smart communities defined by the flow of information rather than proximity; robotic devices; programed medication sensors; voice recognition and synthesis technology with neural network processing; and so on.

The federal government could explore and assess the potential value of harnessing selected technologies in support of frail and functionally impaired persons living in the community, by drawing on expert sources inside and outside of government. An effort of this nature, however, should explicitly consider the need for ensuring strong safeguards against invasions of individual privacy and independence that could take place through such technological applications.

Summary and Implications

At present, about $300 billion—roughly one-third of U.S. annual health care expenditures—is allocated to the care of persons aged 65 and older. The number of Americans in this age group is projected to increase sharply, by about 100 percent over the next several decades, and the numbers in older old-age groups—75 and over, and 85 and over—will more than double. This growth of the older population will substantially increase the demand for health care because older people experience much higher rates of morbidity and functional disability than do younger people. Such rates are exceptionally high for people aged in more advanced old-age ranges. Extrapolation from current allocation patterns and structural features of American health care, when combined with these demographic projections, results in predictions that an enormous increase will take place in the amount of resources allocated to the health care of older people.

However, these predictions may not be accurate. Population aging, in itself, does not necessarily lead to higher levels of national spending on health care. Comparisons with other industrialized nations (including those that presently have much higher proportions of older people than the United States) indicate that it is principally the structural features of health care systems, especially their financing arrangements, that account for the proportion of national wealth that is spent on health care.

Two-thirds of the resources for health care of older Americans is financed by governments, primarily through the Medicare and Medicaid programs. Driven by budgetary concerns, federal and state policy makers are attempting to limit the growth of expenditures on these programs. If such policy efforts succeed, they may substantially reduce the public resources available for health care of older people, even as the older population grows markedly in the early part of the twenty-first century. As this happens, many older people and their families will find it financially difficult or impossible to fill the resource gap through increased out-of-pocket payments or by purchasing private insurance coverage. Adverse consequences are likely to ensue in the form of poorer health and functional status.

Perhaps the most important policy measure that could be undertaken to achieve a suitable symmetry between health care resources and the health care needs of a growing older population is greater funding priority for biomedical research and technological development. Advances in these areas could preserve and enhance the functional independence of older people and thereby reduce the demand for health care services.

Whether substantial limits will be imposed on public funding for Medicare and Medicaid will be strongly influenced by the politics of older people, themselves. Up to now, older people have not been a cohesive political force, and various advocacy groups that purport to represent them have not been an important political factor either in the creation of old-age policies or in their attempts to forestall cutbacks in such policies (Binstock and Day, 1996). But the focus of policy makers on limiting Medicare and Medicaid is relatively new. Proposals to curb significantly the growth of these programs may serve to cohere the political actions of older people (and, perhaps, their adult children) as never before because of their heavy and widespread reliance on public funds to pay for their health care. If so, they may be able to undermine the present efforts of policy makers, and resources for their health care may continue to increase in relation to the growth of the older population. By the same token, such political cohesion would be necessary to substantially elevate the priority given to research and development that might reduce the need for care of older people.

References

Adams, E. K., Meiners, M. R., and Burwell, B. O. 1993. Asset spend-down in nursing homes: Methods and insights. *Medical Care* 31:1–23.

Arnett, R. H. III, McKusick, D. R., Sonnenfeld, S. T., and Cowell, C. S. 1986. Projections of health care spending to 1990. *Health Care Financing Review* 7(3):1–36.

Bengtson, V. L., Rosenthal, C., and Burton, L. 1990. Families and aging: Diversity and heterogeneity. In R. H. Binstock and L. K. George, eds., *Handbook of Aging and the Social Sciences* (3rd ed., pp. 263–87). San Diego: Academic Press.

Binstock, R. H. 1993. Health care costs around the world: Is aging a fiscal "black hole"? *Generations* XVII(4):37–42.

Binstock, R. H. 1994a. Old-age-based rationing: From rhetoric to risk? *Generations* XVIII(4):37–41.

Binstock, R. H. 1994b. Older Americans and health care reform in the 1990s. In P. V. Rosenau, ed., *Health Care Reform in the Nineties* (pp. 213–35). Thousand Oaks, CA: Sage Publications.

Binstock, R. H., and Day, C. L. 1996. Aging and politics. In R. H. Binstock and L. K. George, eds., *Handbook of Aging and the Social Sciences* (4th ed.). San Diego: Academic Press.

Binstock, R. H., and Post, S. G., eds. 1991. *Too Old for Health Care?: Controversies in Medicine, Law, Economics, and Ethics.* Baltimore: Johns Hopkins University Press.

Brody, E. M. 1990. *Women in the Middle: Their Parent-Care Years.* New York: Springer Publishing Company.

Brown, R. S., Bergeron, J. W., Clement, D. G., Hill, J. W., and Retchin, S. M. 1993. *Does Managed Care Work for Medicare?: An Evaluation of the Medicare Risk Program for HMOs.* Princeton, NJ: Mathematica Policy Research, Inc.

Burner, S. T., Waldo, D. R., and McKusick, D. R. 1992. National health expenditures projections through 2030. *Health Care Financing Review* 14(1):1–29.

Burwell, B. 1993. *State Responses to Medicaid Estate Planning.* Cambridge, MA: SysteMetrics.

Callahan, D. 1987. *Setting Limits: Medical Goals in an Aging Society.* New York: Simon & Schuster.

Cassel, C. K., Rudberg, M. A., and Olshansky, S. J. 1992. The price of success: Health care in an aging society. *Health Affairs* 11(2):87–99.

Chellis, R. D., and Grayson, P. J. 1990. *Life Care: A Long-Term Solution?* Lexington, MA: Lexington Books.

Cohen, M. A. 1988. Life care: New options for financing and delivering long-term care. *Health Care Financing Review, Annual Supplement*, 139–43.

Cohen, M. A., Tell, E., Greenberg, J., and Wallack, S. S. 1987. The financial capacity of the elderly to insure for long-term care. *Gerontologist* 27:494–502.

Coulam, R. F., and Gaumer, G. L. 1991. Medicare's prospective payment system: A critical appraisal. *Health Care Financing Review, Annual Supplement* 45–77.

Crown, W. H., Capitman, J., and Leutz, W. N. 1992. Economic rationality, the affordability of private long-term care insurance, and the role for public policy. *Gerontologist* 32:478–85.

Eaton, S., and Diemer, T. 1995, June 30. Congress approves balanced budget plan. *Plain Dealer*, p. 1.

Eckert, S. K., and Smyth, K. 1988. *A Case Study of Methods of Locating and Arranging Health and Long-Term Care for Persons with Dementia.* Washington, DC: Office of Technology Assessment, Congress of the United States.

Friedland, R. 1990. *Facing the Costs of Long-Term Care: An EBRI-ERF Policy Study.* Washington, DC: Employee Benefits Research Institute.

Kane, R. A., and Wilson, K. B. 1993. *Assisted Living in the United States: A New Paradigm for Residential Care for Older People?* Washington, DC: American Association for Retired Persons.

Kane, R. L., Illston, L. H., and Miller, N. A. 1992. Qualitative analysis of the Program of All-Inclusive Care for the Elderly (PACE). *Gerontologist* 32:771–80.

Kassner, E. 1995. *Long-Term Care: Measuring the Impact of a Medicaid Cap.* Washington, DC: Public Policy Institute, American Association of Retired Persons.

Leutz, W., Greenberg, J. N., Abrahams, R., Prottas, J., Diamond, L. M., and Gruenberg, L. 1985. *Changing Health Care for an Aging Society: Planning for the Social/Health Maintenance Organization.* Lexington, MA: Lexington Books.

Liu, K., Manton, K. M., and Liu, B. M. 1985. Home care expenses for the disabled elderly. *Health Care Financing Review* 7(2):51–58.

Lubitz, J., Beebe, B. A., and Baker, C. 1995. Longevity and Medicare expenditures. *New England Journal of Medicine*, 332:999–1029.

Manton, K. G., Corder, L. S., and Stallard, E. 1993. Estimates of change in chronic disability and institutional incidence and prevalence rates in the U.S. elderly population from the 1982, 1984, and 1989 National Long Term Care Survey. *Journal of Gerontology: Social Sciences* 48:S153–66.

Meiners, M. R. 1996. The financing and organization of long-term care. In R. H. Binstock, L. E. Cluff, and O. von Mering, eds., *The Future of Long-Term Care: Social and Policy Issues.* Baltimore: Johns Hopkins University Press.

Mendelson, D. N., and Schwartz, W. B. 1993. The effects of aging and population growth on health care costs. *Health Affairs* 12(1):119–25.

Miller, N. A. 1992. Medicaid 2176 home and community-based care waivers: The first ten years. *Health Affairs* 11(4):162–71.

National Academy on Aging. 1994. *Old Age in the Twenty-first Century.* Washington, DC: Syracuse University.

Newcomer, R. J., Harrington, C., and Friedlob, A. 1990. Social health maintenance organizations: Assessing their initial experience. *Health Services Research* 25:425–54.

Pear, R. 1995, May 11. G.O.P. suggests smaller benefit adjustments. *New York Times*, p. A.15.

Rivlin, A. M., and Wiener, J. M. 1988. *Caring for the Disabled Elderly: Who Will Pay?* Washington, DC: The Brookings Institution.

Rosenbaum, D. E. 1995, May 10. Committee puts balanced budget on Senate table. *New York Times*, p. 1.

Schieber, G. J., Poullier, J. P., and Greenwald, L. M. 1992. U.S. health expenditure performance: An international comparison and data upate. *Health Care Financing Review* 13(4):1–15.

Scitovsky, A. A. 1994. "The high cost of dying" revisited. *Milbank Quarterly* 72:561–91.

Sonnenfeld, S. T., Waldo, D. R., Lemieux, J., and McKusick, D. R. 1991. Projections of national health expenditures through the year 2000. *Health Care Financing Review* 13(1):1–27.

Stone, R., Cafferata, G. L., and Sangl, J. 1987. Caregivers of the frail elderly: A national profile. *Gerontologist* 27:616–26.

Taeuber, C. M. 1992. *Sixty-five Plus in America.* Current Populations Reports, Special Studies, P23-178. Washington, DC: U.S. Government Printing Office.

Tell, E. J., Cohen, M. A., and Wallack, S. S. 1987. New directions in lifecare: An industry in transition. *Milbank Quarterly* 65:551–74.

U.S. Bureau of the Census. 1993. *Nursing Home Population, 1990.* CPH-L-137. Washington, DC: U.S. Government Printing Office.

U.S. Congress, Congressional Budget Office. 1991. *Policy Choices for Long-Term Care.* Washington, DC: U.S. Government Printing Office.

U.S. Congress, Congressional Budget Office. 1993. *The Economic and Budget Outlook: An Update.* Washington, DC: U.S. Government Printing Office.

U.S. Congress, Congressional Budget Office. 1994. *Reducing Entitlement Spending.* Washington, DC: U.S. Government Printing Office.

U.S. Congress, Congressional Budget Office. 1995. *The Economic and Budget Outlook, Fiscal Years 1996–2000.* Washington, DC: U.S. Government Printing Office.

U.S. General Accounting Office. 1995. *Long-Term Care: Current Issues and Future Directions.* Washington, DC: U.S. Government Printing Office.

U.S. Senate, Special Committee on Aging. 1991. *Aging America: Trends and Projections.* Washington, DC: U.S. Government Printing Office.

U.S. Senate, Special Committee on Aging. 1994. *Developments in Aging, 1993, Vol. I.* Washington, DC: U.S. Government Printing Office.

Waldo, D. R., Sonnefeld, S. T., McKusick, D. R., Arnett, R. H. III. 1989. Health expenditures by age group, 1977 and 1987. *Health Care Financing Review* 10(4):111–20.

Weissert, W. G. 1990. Strategies for reducing home care expenditures. *Generations* XIV(2):42–44.

Wiener, J. M., and Illston, L. H. 1996. Health care financing and organization for the elderly. In R. H. Binstock and L. K. George, eds., *Handbook of Aging and the Social Sciences* (4th ed.). San Diego: Academic Press.

Wiener, J. M., Illston, L. H., and Hanley, R. J. 1994. *Sharing the Burden: Strategies for Public and Private Long-Term Care Insurance.* Washington, DC: The Brookings Institution.

Williams, T. F., and Temkin-Greener, H. 1996. Older people, dependency, and trends in supportive care. In R. H. Binstock, L. E. Cluff, and O. von Mering, eds., *The Future of Long-Term Care: Social and Policy Issues.* Baltimore: Johns Hopkins University Press.

Zawadski, R. T., and Eng, C. 1988. Case management in capitated long-term care. *Health Care Financing Review, Annual Supplement,* 75–81.

Part

II

Aging and
Chronic Illness

Chapter

5

Variability in Disease Manifestations in Older Adults: Implications for Public and Community Health Programs

Robert B. Wallace, M.D., M.S.

The health literature on older persons notes the substantial variation in health status among individuals as well as populations. While much of this literature was originally based on clinical and anecdotal observations, much has been at least confirmed, with important clinical, public health, and programmatic implications. The complexity and variation of the health status of older persons has now been amply demonstrated (Minaker and Rowe, 1985), as has the challenge to capture, understand, measure, and apply this complexity in planning and evaluating health programs. This chapter has the following goals: (1) to briefly characterize the process called aging and distinguish it from disease and dysfunction, (2) to delineate some of the implications of age-related health changes for disease etiology, prevention, and clinical management, and (3) to discuss the relevance of the health status of older persons to program planning, management, and assessment.

This work was supported in part by grants AG-10127 and AG-09682 from the National Institute on Aging.

Aging, Age-Related Biological Change, and Disease

Any perspective on the health status of older persons must begin with a discussion of the nature of "aging" and how it relates to "disease." To begin, no one has yet discovered a single biological process that is called "aging." This means that there is no single chemical or metabolic activity or genetic timer that proceeds inexorably and irreversibly, dictating how long we will live. In fact, in laboratory animals, dramatic increases in longevity have been demonstrated by interventions as simple as dietary caloric restriction (Weindruch et al., 1986). Rather, aging appears to be a large series of complex, diverse, time-related and age-related biologic changes, both genetically and environmentally based, that interact with each other to determine the health and functional trajectory that we observe in the laboratory, clinic, or community. This has several immediate implications. For example, if aging is not one process, and age-related body changes differ from one organ and tissue to another in both rate and manifestations, then there will likely be no single intervention or cure for aging. Similarly, preventive or treatment interventions will themselves have to be diverse and tailored to the target organs or functions of interest.

Age-related processes that occur across the lifespan are so diverse that they are difficult to capture and precisely measure. At a crude level, we observe these processes in three general ways: (1) the pattern of survivorship in specific populations and various species, (2) the age when certain universal milestones occur, such as the age at menopause, and (3) gradual, age-related physiological and metabolic changes that generally occur in all persons. The last group might include such varied effects as changes in the way our connective tissue holds together (causing wrinkling), how good our immune system responds to influenza or other important vaccines, the graying of hair, how well our genes can chemically repair themselves if altered by an environmental exposure, and how fast we can run or how much air we can breathe in a minute. In general, all our organs and bodily functions decline with age to some extent, but there is great variation among individuals and, most importantly, in many persons these changes can be mitigated, at least to a measurable extent.

While we cannot always affect them, all age-related changes undoubtedly have causes (albeit often as yet undiscovered) as well as important consequences for health. Whatever the nature of these changes, they should be regarded as the same set of processes that lead to disease, for several reasons. First, diseases occur in the same set of body machinery as these age-related changes. Second, what might seem slow, inevitable, and universal (how aging is sometimes described) might be preventable. For example, in the past, atherosclerosis (hardening of the arteries) was thought to be an aging process because everyone seemed to have it and it was more extensive with increasing age. Third, age-related changes in organ function, whatever the causes, can progress to organ failure—whether the brain, heart, kidneys, or muscles—with serious health consequences and the need for intervention.

While the issue will not be argued here, for practical purposes the difference between aging and disease is almost totally semantic, and depends mostly on whether a health professional labels an age-related phenomenon as a clinical condition or not. Any bodily condition, whether a gradual age-related change or a sudden, localized process, is a disease or condition if it threatens the health and function of an individual. Thus, the distinction between age-related processes and diseases may not be important; rather, it is imperative only to define whatever the processes are and to devise appropriate remedies and preventives where possible. One additional example: Degenerative arthritis (osteoarthritis), an all but universal disease in western societies, most frequently causes pain and limitation of motion in weight-bearing joints, such as the knees and hips. However, if it occurs at the junction of the ribs and vertebrae, it may decrease the maximum capacity to breathe, with increasing age, and be mistaken for an "age-related physiological change." But no matter what the cause of age-related decline in breathing capacity, there may be an increased risk of acquiring lung diseases, such as pneumonia. The basic contention here is that age-related physiological change and disease pathogenesis are in fact the same large, complex set of events, differing only in the forms of response by the organism and the approach of the healing professions to them.

Regardless of the distinction between aging and disease, there is one immediate implication for health programs. Older adults perceive age-related changes in themselves and sometimes attribute remediable conditions to irreversible aging. Because of this, symptoms and problems that might be brought to medical attention may be ignored. Thus, it may be useful to screen for important symptoms that otherwise would not be spontaneously volunteered.

Age-Related Changes and the Nature and Variation of Disease in Older Persons

Whatever the causes and nature of age-related changes in bodily processes, they are nonetheless quite real and have implications for understanding the special nature, causes, prevention and management of important diseases and dysfunctions in older populations. The following are some examples to illustrate these implications and how variation in these populations can occur.

The pathogenesis of some diseases may be altered with age. Many diseases and conditions require active immune responses for either their pathogenesis (development) or control. For example, as is widely known, many infections cannot be controlled or cured unless there is an effective bodily immune response, whether for common viruses, such as influenza, or bacteria that might cause skin or urinary tract infections. Age-related declines in immune function might lead to more severe or prolonged infections in older persons, as well as possibly higher mortality rates. Also, there may be to some extent a lesser immune response in older persons, with decreased pain and inflammation, that causes some not to perceive immediately the symptoms of a perforated appendix or gall bladder as quickly as would a younger person. However, some complex conditions that occur when the immune system actually attacks the body, such as in lupus or Hashimoto thyroiditis (which causes some hypothyroidism), may not have as high an incidence among elders in part because of immune system decline. Thus, it is likely, although imperfectly understood, that age-related changes in bodily processes might both impede and promote the development of various conditions, partially explaining why the epidemiology of illness among elders is different than among younger persons.

Age-related physiological changes in certain organ systems may not cause overt clinical illness, but lead to altered susceptibility to disease in other organ systems. There is ample precedent for this. For example, the normal increase in pulse and cardiac output that occurs when a recumbent person stands up may be retarded in many older persons. This may not be clinically important in itself, but if there is a partial blockage in an artery within the brain, this inadequate response to standing up might increase the risk of a stroke (blockage or bleeding of an artery in the brain), which otherwise might not have occurred. Although somewhat speculative, there is also precedent for age-related changes that may *retard* diseases in other organ systems. For example, lactose intolerance, the inability of the intestines to tolerate and digest the sugar contained in milk and other dairy products, increases with age and causes a decrease in dairy product consumption. This may decrease the total dietary fat intake and retard atherogenesis. Similarly, loss of teeth or related dental conditions may decrease the ability to chew certain foods such as steak and also might lead to beneficial—as well as harmful—effects.

Age-related physiological changes can lead to altered disease occurrence or severity upon environmental challenge. The increased susceptibility to disease in older persons after a given environmental perturbation has been well described. For example, the modest but measurable reduction in glucose tolerance (the ability to metabolize dietary sugar) that comes with age may have no obvious disease effects in itself, but it may increase the risk of overt diabetes mellitus if a person is stressed, such as during general anesthesia. Similar adverse effects of environmental stress may occur in the presence of diminished lung or cardiac function. Other examples include the higher case-fatality rates among elders in automobile crashes and the greater risk of morbidity and mortality among frail or chronically ill elders when exposed to temperature extremes. It is this increased susceptibility to environmental stress in older persons that places a premium on avoiding these stresses as a preventive measure, such as by providing a controlled residential situation.

A similar situation may occur when age-related alterations in body composition or metabolism lead to altered risk of adverse reactions to prescription drugs, and perhaps also to other chemicals such as environmental pollutants. That is why considerable attention is given to appropriate medication prescribing and use (Chrischilles, Segar, and Wallace, 1992). However, it is also possible that these same age-related changes may decrease the risk in some instances. Some chemicals or drugs may be more poorly absorbed or metabolized to an active form in older persons, who are then in a certain sense "protected" from the harmful effects of those agents.

Some age-related physiological changes may affect the perception of clinical signs and symptoms. While it may be difficult to prove conclusively, it is apparent that elders may have a lesser ability to sense some bodily symptoms and problems, possibly due to age-related deterioration in sensory function. For example, older persons may have lesser perception of cardiac pain, resulting in more "silent" heart attacks. Similarly, decreased visual acuity may deter early self-recognition of harmful skin lesions, and decreased range of neck motion may limit the parts of the body that are visible for inspection. Also, perception, attribution, and reporting of bodily signs and symptoms may sometimes require intact and sophisticated cognitive function, and to the extent that this is compromised among older persons, there may be a progressive inability for self-recognition of clinical problems. This has two important implications: It provides an additional reason why older persons may not report signals of disease as readily as younger persons, leading to delays in coming to treatment; also, this relative lack of appreciation of various conditions may lead to undercounting of morbidity rates in public health surveillance of older populations.

Some conditions or their treatments alter the pathogenesis and progression of others. Older adults often have several simultaneous chronic conditions, so-called comorbidity, and it is likely that some alter the manifestations of others because of direct effects of diseases or their treatments, leading to altered clinical manifestations and detection. There is considerable evidence that this occurs, but how often and to what extent are not well understood. As an obvious example, if someone has limited mobility due to arthritis, there may be no opportunity to walk far enough to elicit cardiac pain, angina pectoris. Severe chronic illness associated with weight loss from various causes might lead to improvement in glucose tolerance and lower blood pressure and cholesterol. That is not to suggest that this is a desirable situation, but only that some conditions will affect the natural history of others in ways that are complex and not always predictable.

The same issues occur for disease treatments, which may have unintended effects on other conditions, both negative and positive. Many clinical examples exist. The panoply of adverse effects of many medications is well described. However, many medications may have positive, salient effects in addition to their main indications for prescribing. For example, several commonly used analgesics, such as aspirin, also have anticoagulant properties. Some medications for blood pressure control also protect against heart pain or rhythm problems. Thiazide diuretics, used in the treatment of hypertension, are associated with both increased bone density and possible protection from osteoporosis and fractures (LaCroix et al., 1990). The treatment of intestinal ulcers with some antacids in certain instances increases calcium intake. Thus, the occurrence and outcomes of certain illnesses depend to some extent on the presence of other conditions, and their presence must be detected and considered.

Aging and Disease: Behavioral, Social, and Health Care Dimensions

Until now, the discussion has focused on changing biology and its implications for variation in disease occurrence and manifestations among older populations. Yet, disease rates and manifestations may also vary in older populations due to the changing social and behavioral environment that occurs with age, including interactions with the health care system. Following are some of the important reasons that this occurs.

Decreased Exposure to the Work Environment

While the dangers of workplace exposures vary substantially, with retirement from lifetime careers there is of course less exposure to workplace hazards, including the transportation injuries that may come with commuting. Over time this is likely to decrease the risk of workplace-related conditions, including the chemical, physical, and biological environments. However, after retirement, there may be replacement exposures from recreational or alternative occupational activities, but at least some level of change in job-associated health risks can almost assuredly be anticipated.

Altered Social Activities and Residential Locations

At older ages there are clear changes in social participation and networks. This in turn has implications for illness recognition, management, and exposures. To the extent that older persons learn about illness recognition and management through informal discussion with friends and relatives, this may be altered with age. This may also be true for management of illnesses, where informal assistance and care come to bear, possibly changing the natural history of many conditions. Changing social networks and contacts may also change exposure rates to certain infectious and communicable diseases, altering population disease patterns in this age group.

An additional problem that has implications for disease rates is institutionalization. About 5 percent of Americans over age 65 years live in long-term care institutions, as do over 20 percent of those 85 years and above. This likely increases the transmission of nosocomial agents, particularly since those residing in institutional long-term care settings are likely to be frail and perhaps more susceptible than those in the ambulatory population.

Within both the family and institutional setting, however, there is another category of problem that sets the elderly apart from middle-aged adults: abuse and neglect by family members, acquaintances, and caregivers (Homer and Gilleard, 1990; Rounds, 1992). These are often difficult for health professionals to recognize and are frequently unreported by older adults because they may be very dependent on those responsible for the problem. The manifestations are varied and often nonspecific. Thus, this issue is particularly challenging to detect and particularly resistant to epidemiological surveillance. However, this should always be considered when patients or clients are not progressing as expected in a social or clinical program.

Lower Rates of Substance Abuse

While substance abuse remains a problem among older adults, the rates of abuse are clearly diminished compared to younger adults. This includes tobacco, alcohol, illicit drugs, and abuse of prescription medications. Age differences in the prevalence of substance abuse may be due in part to selective survival—in that fewer persons who abuse substances reach old age. Sometimes this decreased substance abuse may follow the onset of serious or chronic illness, but other times it is not easily explained. Whatever the causes, some of the conditions related to these substances might be expected to decrease in incidence with increasing age. However, the amount of health benefit associated with specific substance abuse interventions in older persons remains to be experimentally determined.

Changing Participation in Clinical Preventive Practices

It is established that older adults are currently less likely to partake of some clinical preventive practices such as mammography or cervical cytology screening. This problem is demonstrably more severe among minority older adults (Yee and Weaver, 1994). While the reasons for this are complex and include altered priorities and desires on the part of patients—as well as perhaps geographic and fiscal access to health professionals—the result must be that various conditions will present at a more advanced stage. Varying usage of some clinical preventive interventions such as immunization may lead to important differences in population incidence rates of target infections. A particularly important problem for preventive services in elders is the lack of research studies to provide a firm scientific footing for clinical guidelines and recommendations, although many programs have been promulgated and the issues thoroughly discussed (German and Fried, 1989).

Altered Clinical Practices Among Health Professionals

It is demonstrable that older persons with specific index conditions, such as certain cancers, are managed differently from middle-aged adults. The reasons for this are not always apparent, and may range from overt or tacit value judgments about the virtues of a given treatment, to patient refusals, to an increased prevalence of medical contraindications. This in itself may lead to altered disease patterns and outcomes. To the extent that there is reticence to employ aggressive diagnostic or therapeutic procedures in older persons, there will be less antemortem identification of some important conditions, and that will alter the estimates of community disease rates and patterns.

Varying Manifestations of Disease and the Impact on Disability

Both the physiological changes with age and various medical conditions and their treatments lead to varied levels of dysfunction and disability within individuals and populations. But just as these age-related changes and conditions are diverse and individual, so are the consequent disability and dysfunction levels. The methods for comprehensively assessing disability in population surveys or clinical programs are challenging, as is attributing the disabilities to various causes (Verbrugge and Patrick, 1995). For example, someone reporting difficulty with walking across a room may have one or more of the following: plantar fasciitis, an above-the-knee amputation, paralytic poliomyelitis from childhood, blindness, dyspnea from advanced pulmonary disease, excessive use of sedatives or alcohol, peripheral neuritis, a prior stroke with residual weakness, or many other conditions. Aside from the difficulty in measuring severity of dysfunction, population levels of disability can be expected to vary merely because of the varied physiological patterns and disease rates and distributions.

However, in addition to varied comorbidity and treatment patterns, individual and population variation in disability rates has other causes as well. Disability may be manifest only in terms of incompatibility of function with a particular environment. For example, someone may not appreciate that a disability is present if there are sufficient handrails or other devices to allow coping with an increasingly unsteady gait. Modest cognitive dysfunction may not be appreciated if it is never suitably challenged. What is extremely difficult to assess in individuals as well as in populations is individual ability and resourcefulness in coping and adapting to decreasing function, even though it certainly occurs. Thus, the environmental setting and adjustment to it could be extremely important in understanding and explaining population differences in disability rates and their consequences.

Population variability in disability rates may also be due to a more practical reason: Some communities are more hospitable to disabled persons than others; communities with more clinical care resources, long-term care, and rehabilitation facilities or physical and social adaptation programs may provide more effective services as well as attract more disabled residents. Either of these situations will alter population disability rates. In fact, elder mobility and relocation are important explanatory factors for interpopulation variation in disability rates.

Despite the possible explanations for interpopulation variation in disability, there are subgroups of older populations that have clear differences in age- and sex-specific disability prevalence rates. Most of these have been minority racial or ethnic populations or impoverished socioeconomic subgroups, as identified in geographically based surveys (Manton, Patrick, and Johnson, 1987). In general, in the United States racial and ethnic minorities and economically disadvantaged populations tend to have higher disability-prevalence rates. Of interest, after controlling for economic status and ethnicity distribution, only small urban-rural differences in disability prevalence have been found.

Progression of Illness and Degradation of Diagnoses

One important feature of disease and disability among older persons is that in the latter stages there may be progression of multiple conditions and secondary phenomena that make the clinical situation even more complex. For example, there may be a series of secondary events that obscure or challenge therapy for the original underlying conditions. Important examples are falls, delirium, malnutrition, and secondary infections that may be a consequence of serious illness. This may make it difficult for health professionals to prioritize and sort out the extant management problems in a patient. In effect, complex, multisystem illnesses, with their secondary but sometimes severe health sequelae, lead to a degradation of diagnostic information (Fairweather and Campbell, 1991) and loss of specificity for programmatic or clinical management purposes.

While the disease patterns of individuals vary dramatically, prospective, population-based studies suggest a pattern of increasing morbidity and disability in the two-to-three year period before death (Guralnik et al., 1991). Because of high mortality rates in the oldest old, preterminal phenomena can be an important part of population morbidity and dysfunction rates, and thus have important implications for epidemiology and public health. Clinically, preterminal patients are more likely to have higher levels of physical, social, and cognitive dysfunction, to consume more health care and family and institutional resources and, if living at home, to place enormous stresses on family and friends. From a public health perspective, distinguishing preterminal populations from others is most important for planning health services and resource allocation, assessing community-based programs, and applying different types of preventive interventions. While it is not always possible to define preterminal patients in advance, some attention to this phenomenon will help clarify interpopulation differences in disease and disability rates and intervention outcomes.

Diseases and Dysfunction: Implications for Programs, Public Health, and Society

Given what appears to be sustained and high levels of defined medical conditions, physiological changes, and physical, social, and mental dysfunctions that dominate older populations, several clear implications for public health and program fostering and management are present. Most, if not all, have been previously recognized, but some have been inadequately regarded, and their consideration has been sporadic.

To begin, the public health community and those in charge of specific programs must change the way they acquire information on older and disabled populations. Among older adults, the problem of disease recognition is complicated by multiple conditions and treatments, altered clinical manifestations, a background of physiological abnormalities, and a decreased propensity for intensive diagnostic activities. Even for major identified conditions, there will need to be more modern and efficient ways to capture disease occurrence from automated clinical databases. Additionally, the taxonomy and nomenclature of public health surveillance systems will need to be expanded beyond selected diseases and hygienic behaviors to incorporate multiple interactive conditions (comorbidity) as well as the presence and severity of dysfunctions and physiological abnormalities. It is not too difficult to imagine a time when public health surveillance will include population levels of bone density, aspirin prophylaxis consumption, immune competence, DNA repair capacity, frictional resistance of prosthetic knees, the need for assistance in toileting, and the ability to shop at home using a computer system. It will also be important to follow populations *longitudinally*, from the onset of disability, in order to be certain that community disability outcomes are subject to appropriate surveillance and intervention.

For older populations, there will need to be a whole new set of tertiary prevention programs that address the needs of the increasing number of older persons who have chronic illness and disability. There must be increased emphasis on preventing the progression of established chronic conditions, the deleterious interactions with other conditions, and the disabilities these interacting conditions engender. Examples include whether impediments to ambulation have been removed, whether the temperature of the hot water in the household of a patient with diabetes has been moderated, and whether heart attack patients are receiving appropriate medications to prevent recurrences. Very few public health programs target this area of prevention. Also, there should be a special effort to understand the provision of primary and secondary prevention in older persons with existing, even severe, disease and disabilities, from both an efficacy as well as a cost-benefit perspective. For example, what should the policy be on cervical pap smear or mammography application in women with active coronary disease or rheumatoid arthritis?

From a clinical perspective, there will need to be improved geriatric clinical diagnosis and problem management, because the multiple, interactive biological and social processes are not necessarily efficiently or optimally manageable with only the linear "problem list" of many clinical records. Rather, computer-assisted databases may become an essential tool in treating the complex patient. Even the logic of clinical activities will need refinement and change because of the challenges of diagnosis and treatment in the oldest old.

Most important, from an organizational perspective, there need not always be special public health or community agencies to attend to elders with these special problems—because they all occur in younger populations, only to a lesser extent. All ages and communities have a substantial occurrence of disability and multiple illnesses, sometimes leading to institutionalization. The challenge is to develop effective surveillance and assessment tools to identify individuals of all ages who either have these sets of health conditions or are at high risk of them, in order to deliver comprehensive and effective programs with appropriate evaluation techniques.

Conclusions

There is great heterogeneity in the health and functional status of older populations, due to great variation among populations and within individuals in the presence and rates of age-related physiological changes and specific medical conditions, with their incumbent dysfunction and disability. Because of the complexity of this situation and the altered manifestations and reporting of health problems by older persons, it is difficult and challenging to conduct effective population surveillance and case-finding for programatic purposes. The clinical problems are often so diverse that almost all programs will require multidisciplinary, team-management approaches. Because the majority of older persons have had a disease or disability experience, a major preventive and public health challenge is to provide tertiary preventive services that retard the progression of established disability and disease as well as prevent the emergence of new conditions. As better measurement devices emerge to assess and evaluate this complex situation, it will become easier to describe and explain the burden of illness in older populations, perhaps leading to increased managerial responsiveness and greater persuasiveness in dedicating resources to these problems.

References

Chrischilles, E. A., Segar, E., and Wallace, R. B. 1992. Self-reported adverse drug reactions and related resource use. *Annals of Internal Medicine* 117:634–40.

Fairweather, D. S., and Campbell, A. J. 1991. Diagnostic accuracy: The effects of multiple etiology and the degradation of information in old age. *Journal of the Royal College of Physicians* (London) 25:105–9.

German, P. G., and Fried, L. P. 1989. Prevention and the elderly. *Annual Review of Public Health* 10:319–32.

Guralnik, J. M., LaCroix, A. Z., Branch, L. G., Kasl, S. V., and Wallace, R. B. 1991. Morbidity and disability in older persons in the years prior to death. *American Journal of Public Health* 81:443–47.

Homer, A. C., and Gilleard, C. 1990. Abuse of elderly people by their carers. *BMJ* 301:1359–1362.

LaCroix, A. Z., Wienpahl, J., White, L. R., Wallace, R. B., Scherr, P. A., George, L. K., Cornoni-Huntley, J., and Ostfeld, A. M. 1990. Thiazide diuretics and the incidence of hip fracture. *New England Journal of Medicine* 322:286–90.

Manton, K. G., Patrick, C. H., and Johnson, K. W. 1987. Health differentials between blacks and whites: Recent trends in morbidity and mortality. *Milbank Quarterly* 65(Supplement 1):129–99.

Minaker, K. L., and Rowe, J. 1985. Health and disease among the oldest old: A clinical perspective. *MMFQ/Health and Society* 62:324–49.

Rounds, L. 1992. Elder abuse and neglect: A relationship to health characteristics. *Journal of American Academic Nurse Practitioners* 4:47–52.

Verbrugge, L. M., and Patrick, D. L. 1995. Seven chronic conditions: Their impact on U.S. adults' activity levels and use of medical services. *American Journal of Public Health* 85:173–82.

Weindruch, R., Walford, R. L., Fligiel, S., and Guthrie, D. 1986. The retardation of aging in mice by dietary restriction: Longevity, cancer, immunity and lifetime energy intake. *American Journal of Nutrition* 116:641–54.

Yee, B. W. K., and Weaver, G. D. 1994. Ethnic minorities and health promotion: Developing a "culturally competent" agenda. *Generations* 18:39–44.

Chapter

6

Disability Outcomes of Chronic Disease and Their Implications for Public Health

Marcel E. Salive, M.D., M.P.H., and
Jack M. Guralnik, M.D., Ph.D.

Public health professionals have long been active in dealing with the problems of disability. For example, the disability and death caused by poliomyelitis motivated the development of a vaccine that subsequently eliminated polio from the Western world. Now that much work has been done to mitigate the effects of infectious diseases, public health is facing a new challenge—the disability among older adults caused by a multitude of modifiable factors and chronic diseases. In its health objectives for the year 2000, the U.S. Department of Health and Human Services (1991) listed the prevention of disability along with the prevention of disease and premature mortality among its top three goals. This chapter will focus on four major issues: the definition and measurement of disability, the diseases that cause disability, the outcomes of disability as they affect both the individual and society, and the role of public health in preventing the functional consequences of disease.

What Is Disability?

Disability is commonly defined as incapacity, or "a lack of the ability to function normally, physically or mentally" (Dorland, 1981). The World Health

Organization defines disability similarly but places it in a sequence arising from disease, which then may cause an impairment that leads to disability and which may result in a handicap (a disadvantage that prevents an individual from fulfilling a normal role) (World Health Organization, 1980). The potential impact of disability on quality of life, the ability to remain independent in the community, and the need for long-term care is of great importance to older individuals, their families, and the health care system. Informal care, provided by family and friends, and formal care, provided by paid providers in the community and in nursing homes for those unable to remain in the community, represent a substantial and growing human and financial cost for the older disabled population. The size of the disabled older population and the personal and societal toll of disability at older ages are a major public health concern.

Disability may be measured using a number of functional scales that have been developed and validated since the early 1960s. These include the activities of daily living (ADLs) needed for self-care, the instrumental activities of daily living (IADLs) needed to maintain independent living in the community, mobility measures and measures assessing more vigorous activities such as ability to climb stairs or walk a certain distance, and objective measures of physical performance of specific tasks. Six basic ADLs frequently assessed include walking across a small room, bathing, dressing, eating, transferring from bed to chair, and using the toilet; any activity is considered limited if a person reports either an inability to perform the task or requires help from another person (Katz et al., 1963; Branch, Katz, Kniepmann, and Papsidero, 1984). The IADLs assess tasks such as the ability to shop for groceries or clothes, prepare meals, perform light housework, use the telephone, take medications, and manage money or pay bills (Lawton and Brody, 1969). A wide variety of other measures have been developed and are reviewed elsewhere (Kane and Kane, 1981; Branch and Meyers, 1987; Applegate, Blass, and Williams, 1990). Physical performance tests are standardized assessments of tasks such as walking four meters, putting on a blouse, and rising from a chair and sitting back down (Guralnik, Branch et al., 1989).

The Prevalence of Disability in the Older Population

A standard or universally accepted method of assessing disability in the population is lacking, therefore estimates of disability prevalence in the older population vary across surveys. The ADLs are the most frequently assessed disability measure. A core set of these items is generally included in disability research; they are the measures most often used to express disability prevalence in older populations. Wiener, Hanley, Clark, and Van Nostrand (1990) reviewed the prevalence rates for receiving ADL help from several national surveys conducted between 1982 and 1987 with the same items (bathing, dressing, eating, transferring, and toileting), and reported a range from 5.0 percent to 8.1 percent among noninstitutionalized adults aged 65 years and older.

Figures 6.1 and 6.2 present ADL and IADL prevalence rates according to age, race, and sex using recent national data from the Assets and Health Dynamics of the Oldest-Old (AHEAD) study sponsored by the National Institute on Aging (NIA). In general, disability prevalence rises with increasing age, and is higher for white women than white men in the age group 85 years and older. Most striking, however, are the rates among African Americans, who have considerably higher rates of ADL disability than whites in each age group for both sexes, with the exception of women aged 85 years and older, who have similar rates. Racial differences in disability level may be explained in part by differences in educational attainment, a measure of socioeconomic status (Guralnik, Land et al., 1993).

While these data indicate that disability prevalence is substantial, it is important to realize that they are based only on older adults living in the community. To understand the full picture of disability in the total older population, persons living in nursing homes must be added in. National estimates of this kind have been developed by supplementing the data from the National Health Interview Survey with data from the National Nursing Home Survey (National Center for Health Statistics, 1989; Hing and Bloom, 1990; Schneider and Guralnik, 1990). Figure 6.3 presents estimates of the percentages of the population living in a nursing home, living in the community but needing assistance from another person for selected ADLs and IADLs, and living independently in the community.

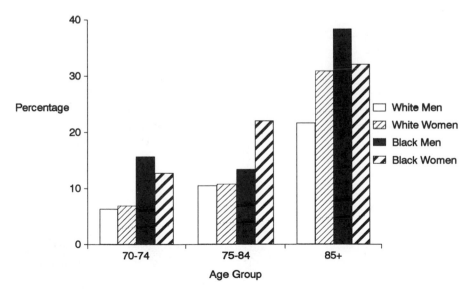

FIGURE 6.1 Dependency in one or more activities of daily living among community-dwelling adults age 70 years and older, by age, race, and sex, United States, 1994. Dependency is defined as receiving help in one or more of the following activities: bathing, dressing, using the toilet, getting into and out of bed, and eating.

Source: Assets and Health Dynamics of the Oldest-Old (AHEAD), unpublished data analysis by M. Salive.

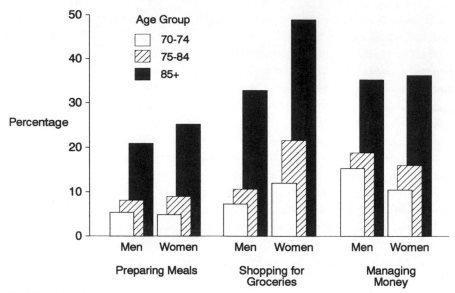

FIGURE 6.2 Dependency in three instrumental activities of daily living among community-dwelling adults age 70 years and older, by age and sex, United States, 1994. Dependency is defined as having difficulty with or being unable to perform a specific activity oneself because of a health problem.
Source: Assets and Health Dynamics of the Oldest-Old (AHEAD), unpublished data analysis by M. Salive.

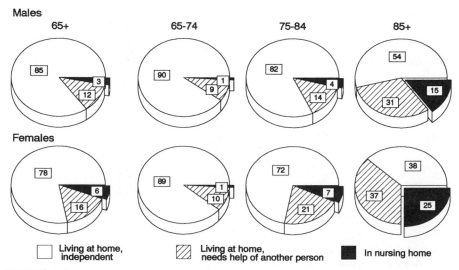

FIGURE 6.3 Percentage of the older population who live at home independently, live at home but require the help of another person, or live in a nursing home.
Source: Schneider and Guralnik, 1990.

Overall, 3 percent of men and 6 percent of women aged 65 and older reside in nursing homes, while 15 percent and 22 percent, respectively, either need help to live in the community or are institutionalized. In the younger age group, the proportion disabled is not significantly different for men and women. The proportion disabled rises with age, more steeply for women than for men, with nearly two-thirds of women and nearly half of the men aged 85 years and older either requiring help at home or living in a nursing home. The proportion institutionalized rises dramatically with increasing age, from 1 percent in the lowest age group to 15 percent and 25 percent for men and women, respectively, in the oldest age group. Understanding the extent of disability in persons 85 years and older requires recognition of those persons who are in the community as well as those in institutions, although the needs of both groups— from a public health system perspective—might be quite different.

The percentage of men and women at age 50 years who can expect to live to age 90 years has risen from about 2 to 3 percent in 1900 to 12 percent and 29 percent, respectively, in 1990, based on life table analysis. These changes in longevity have implications for the level of disability in the population. Since disability levels rise with age (Figures 6.1 and 6.2), an increase in longevity could, if these age-specific prevalence rates do not change, result in a population of older adults burdened with higher levels of disability. Many other factors relate to the incidence of disability, however, making the need for disability surveillance a high priority along with research on its etiology.

The EPESE Populations

Many of the data presented in subsequent sections are derived from the four Established Populations for Epidemiologic Studies of the Elderly (EPESE), which comprise a collaborative multiyear longitudinal study of men and women in the community aged 65 years and older (Cornoni-Huntley et al., 1993). Between 1981 and 1983, over 10,000 noninstitutionalized participants aged 65 years and older were enrolled in three EPESE communities: East Boston, Mass.; Iowa and Washington counties, Iowa; and New Haven, Conn. A fourth community was enrolled in five counties in northcentral North Carolina during 1986 and 1987, where African Americans were oversampled.

The Relation of Chronic Conditions with Disability

Physical disability is an important consequence of acute illness, chronic conditions, and injuries in older adults. While the natural history and pathophysiology of illness have received considerable attention, less work has been done in examining the functional consequences of the illnesses associated with aging. This relationship can be acute and quite obvious, such as the motor and cognitive deficits that can occur after a stroke and the functional consequences of a hip fracture. Alternatively, for chronic conditions such as arthritis and diabetes, functional decline may occur over many years, and it may be difficult to differentiate the functional consequences of illness from those of other processes of aging, or from other comorbid conditions.

Table 6.1 summarizes six prospective studies published in the last decade that examined the association of disease with disability. A variety of self-reported disabilities and diseases have been examined. Only the Framingham study (Pinsky et al., 1985) used clinical examination for the ascertainment of disease. Four of the five studies that examined arthritis found that it was associated with development of disability. Each of the three studies of stroke found such a relationship. The findings with respect to diabetes, hypertension, and heart disease were mixed. Only the study by Guralnik, LaCroix et al. (1993) was able to use information from several interviews that allowed differentiation between prevalent disease and incident disease, which developed after a baseline assessment. In this manner, prevalent diabetes and incident cancer predicted onset of mobility disability, whereas prevalent cancer and incident diabetes were not associated with the development of disability. The table also demonstrates that few studies have been able to study comprehensively the full range of diseases that become prevalent at older ages.

A report from the Cardiovascular Health Study of 5,201 community-dwelling older adults describes the disabilities present in the population and the diseases that participants stated were the causes of specific disabilities. Among those persons with difficulty in performing any one of 17 tasks, the largest proportion reported that the underlying cause of their difficulty was arthritis (49 percent of participants), followed by heart disease (14 percent), injury (12 percent), old age (12 percent), lung disease (6 percent), and stroke (3 percent) (Ettinger, Fried et al., 1994). Arthritis was associated with the whole panoply of tasks in a nonspecific manner. Conversely, heart disease was associated with difficulty in activities requiring endurance, and stroke was associated with upper extremity and self-care tasks. While it may be argued that individuals may not know the cause of their disability, these data suggest where to focus our initial efforts in understanding the disease-disability relationship. The next sections review the relationships of specific diseases with disability, first focusing on diseases that may be fatal and then on chronic, generally nonfatal diseases that can cause disability. This is followed by a consideration of comorbidity, or the co-occurrence of multiple diseases, and its effect upon disability.

Potentially Fatal Diseases That Cause Disability

Among persons aged 65 years and older, coronary heart disease (CHD) is the leading cause of both death and hospitalization in the United States, but it is not the

TABLE 6.1. Diseases and Conditions Associated with Disability: Selected Longitudinal Studies

Study Author	Study Population	Disability Outcome	Disease Ascertainment	Significant*	Not Significant
					Diseases and Conditions Studied
Pinsky et al., 1985	n = 2021 Framingham free of CHD	ADL, Rosow-Breslau, Nagi	Examination	Hypertension	Diabetes (men) Diabetes (women)
Mor et al., 1989	n = 852 LSOA age 70–74 years, intact ADL/IADL, 2 years followup	ADL, Rosow-Breslau, Nagi	Self-report	Diabetes Stroke Visual impairment Arthritis Falls	Cataracts Osteoporosis Hypertension Any heart disease Confusion
Harris et al., 1989	n = 1791 LSOA age ≥80 years, intact 2 years followup	ADL, Rosow-Breslau, Nagi	Self-report	Cardiovascular disease Arthritis	Vision problems Hearing problems
Guralnik and Kaplan, 1989	n = 841 Alameda County, 19 years followup	ADL/IADL	Self-report	Hypertension Arthritis Back pain	Heart disease Chest pain Shortness of breath Joint pain/stiffness
Guralnik, La Croix et al., 1993	n = 6981 EPESE age ≥65, intact 4 years followup	Mobility	Self-report	Heart attack Stroke Hip fracture Cancer (incident) Diabetes (prevalent) Exertional leg pain Dyspnea	Cancer (prevalent) Angina Arthritis Diabetes (incident)
Boult et al., 1994	n = 2605 LSOA age ≥70 years, intact 4 years followup	ADL, Rosow-Breslau	Self-report	Stroke Arthritis	Coronary artery disease Hypertension, cancer diabetes, osteoporosis

*Associated with disability at p < 0.05 level.

leading cause of disability. Nevertheless, coronary artery disease is the second or third leading cause of disability, through its manifestations of angina and myocardial infarction as well as through its complications, such as congestive heart failure. A cross-sectional analysis of data from the Framingham study (Guccione et al., 1994) mapped the manifestations of CHD to disabilities in specific sets of tasks. The presence of angina or history of myocardial infarction was significantly associated with difficulty walking a mile, performing heavy and light housework, and grocery shopping. Congestive heart failure was significantly associated with difficulty climbing stairs, performing heavy and light housework, and carrying bundles.

Another study of the Framingham cohort identified the onset of angina pectoris as a critical point in the development of Rosow-Breslau disability—that is, inability to walk a half-mile, climb stairs, or perform heavy housework without help (Pinsky et al., 1990). Moreover, angina pectoris was a better predictor of disability than either myocardial infarction or coronary insufficiency (chest pain lasting at least one hour with electrocardiographic changes). Since angina is diagnosed by physicians in persons who have recurring chest pain, on exertion, that is relieved by resting or nitroglycerin treatment, it is perhaps not surprising that it is so closely related to the onset of disability. In spite of these associations, comprehensive assessments of a clinical series of male cardiac patients compared objective functional ability on a treadmill to self-reported limitations of activity and failed to find an impressive relation (Neill et al., 1985). In fact, many persons with mild or severe angina were still able to perform basic self care and household tasks and, in some cases, discretionary activities such as sports, although they had reported difficulty or limitations in these activities.

Although cancer is the second leading cause of death for older men and women, its relation to poor physical functioning is not well understood. Although cancer patients can clearly have ADL disability (Goodwin, Hunt, and Samet, 1991), reported prevalence rates do not appear to be much higher than those from the general population. In cancer patients, functional status appears to be more related to patient age and stage of cancer, but not to the type of cancer (Mor, 1987). In a case-control study of newly diagnosed breast cancer patients, only small decrements in functioning could be detected in the patients, and these were limited to upper-body tasks such as lifting (Satariano et al., 1990). These findings may relate to the types of treatments given for this disease. Nevertheless, functional status frequently declines in cancer patients as their health deteriorates and they near death.

Stroke remains the third leading cause of death among men and women aged 65 years and older, despite declining rates of stroke mortality in the United States during the 1970s and 1980s. The effect of a stroke on a person's ability to perform usual tasks depends upon the severity, location, and type of the stroke, as well as the natural history of recovery from it, the selective effect of mortality, and other factors. In a large community-based study of stroke patients, 12 percent of survivors were completely nondisabled (using the Barthel index, which includes ADLs and mobility) within 7 days after the stroke; this rose to 31 percent after three weeks and 47 percent by six months (Wade and Hewer, 1987). The prognosis for independence at six months was better in those with absence of urinary incontinence, lower age, better sitting balance, and better initial function level. In a study of postrehabilitation stroke patients, Ferrucci et al. (1993) demonstrated that recovery continued after discharge from an inpatient rehabilitation program. Furthermore, older patients were found to be more likely than younger patients to use compensatory strategies that help to overcome their functional deficits after a stroke.

Within the New Haven EPESE cohort, stroke survivors were studied six weeks after the event (Colantonio et al., 1993). Controlling for key confounders, persons with a larger social network were more likely to improve in physical function after the stroke and less likely to be institutionalized. This illustrates the need to study the interaction of medical and psychosocial factors in relation to the occurrence of and recovery from disability.

Nonfatal Diseases That Cause Disability

Nearly half of all adults aged 65 years and older report that they have arthritis, and about one-quarter of these persons state that arthritis limits them in some everyday activities (CDC, 1994). The high prevalence of arthritis, combined with its association with moderate disability, makes it the leading condition causing disability (Verbrugge, Lepkowski, and Imanaka, 1989).

Verbrugge reported that in a large national cohort of noninstitutionalized adults aged 55 years and older, arthritis was associated with disability in all of the tasks and activities examined, including mobility, strength, IADLs, and ADLs (Verbrugge, Lepkowski, and Konkol, 1991). The most disability was seen for physical functions such as walking, reaching, and stooping, which are affected by the joint pain of arthritis. Guccione et al. (1990) cautioned that studying the association of arthritis in general with a measure of disability that aggregates specific tasks into an overall disability scale can obscure the relationship of arthritis of specific joints with distinct disabilities. They found that knee osteoarthritis was, as expected, associated with lower extremity disability, as well as with difficulties with housekeeping and carrying bundles, but not with other IADLs. Also, disability may worsen when arthritis co-occurs with certain other health conditions discussed below.

In the total population, blindness in both eyes has been identified as the third leading cause of disability associated with need for help in eating, bathing, or getting around the house, while severe partial blindness (affecting one eye more than the other) ranked thirteenth (LaPlante, 1989). Observational cohort studies have demonstrated that self-reported visual impairment is related to decline in physical function over one to two years among physically intact or only mildly disabled elders (Mor et al., 1989; LaForge, Spector, and Sternberg, 1992). Visual decline has been associated with decreased mobility and unmet needs in grocery shopping, food preparation, housekeeping, and paying bills (Branch, Horowitz, and Carr, 1989). In a longitudinal study of individuals initially free of limitations in ADLs in the original three EPESE communities, we examined the relation of visual acuity with the incidence of ADL limitations (Salive et al., 1994). Six percent of the group with visual acuity of 20/40 or better developed ADL limitations, compared with 12 percent and 25 percent in the moderately and severely visually impaired, respectively (Figure 6.4). Severe visual impairment (visual acuity worse than 20/200) was associated with approximately threefold higher odds of incident ADL limitations after adjusting for demographic characteristics and disease history. Improvement of mobility limitations was also less likely to occur among those with visual impairment. Visual acuity is an important factor in maintaining physical function, particularly mobility.

Two intervention studies provide additional information about changes in vision and its influence on physical function. In a study using a crossover design, patients who had problems with both distant and near vision were able to optimize visual acuity and task performance when they used distant contact lenses and reading glasses together (Harris, Sheedy, and Gan, 1992). Cataract surgery has been associated with improved visual acuity as well as with improvement in objective measures of physical function that persisted from four months to one year after surgery (Applegate et al., 1987).

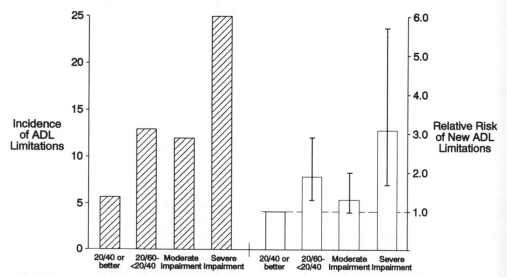

FIGURE 6.4 Incidence of dependency in one or more activities of daily living, by distant visual acuity, Iowa and New Haven Established Populations for Epidemiologic Studies of the Elderly, 1988–1990. *Relative risk is adjusted for age, sex, race, community, income, and history of diabetes and stroke. *Source:* Data from Salive et al., 1994.

Many of the diseases considered up to this point have physical effects that may result in disability. It is important to realize that cognitive impairment, whether mild or severe, can also cause difficulty in performing one's usual activities. Alzheimer disease is the leading cause of dementia in the United States. The prevalence of Alzheimer disease rises exponentially with age, beginning at age 65 years and doubling about every five years.

In a cross-sectional study of the East Boston EPESE population, persons with ADL limitations had significantly poorer scores on four tests of cognitive function (Scherr et al., 1988). However, the time course of this relation has not been extensively studied. A paper from the New Haven EPESE cohort reported on the three-year incidence of ADL limitations according to baseline cognitive functioning (Moritz, Kasl, and Berkman, 1995). Persons at baseline who were free of ADL limitations and who made four or more errors on a ten-item scale of cognitive function were two to three times more likely to develop ADL limitations compared with persons who made zero or one errors. The results were adjusted for age and several prevalent and incident health conditions. As with the chronic medical conditions, not all study subjects developed ADL disabilities, suggesting that a more detailed study of cognitive impairment and its course might suggest ways that disability may be ameliorated in this group.

Other mental health conditions, such as depressive symptoms and clinical depression, may be related to the occurrence of disability in older adults. A cross-sectional analysis of the New Haven EPESE population found that physical disability was associated with nearly all of the twenty depressive symptoms found on a commonly used questionnaire (Berkman et al., 1986). The North Carolina EPESE demonstrated that the prevalence of depressive symptoms increases with age because of the complex interrelationship of age, chronic diseases, functional and cognitive impairment, and socioeconomic status (Blazer et al., 1991). In a higher-functioning subgroup of men and women from three EPESE communities (known as the MacArthur Study of Successful Aging), high depressive symptoms were associated with an increased risk for the onset of ADL disability at a 30-month followup (Bruce et al., 1994). Taken together, this evidence suggests that both depressive symptoms and physical disability can combine to trigger a spiraling decline in physical and mental health. More research is necessary to understand the relationship of chronic conditions, reactive depression, and the incidence of ADL and other disabilities. This also highlights the necessity for considering comorbidities in all studies of disability.

The Relation of Comorbidity to Disability

The increasing prevalence of many diseases with aging leads to the coexistence of multiple chronic conditions, commonly referred to as comorbidity. A 1984 national survey found that considering the nine most common chronic conditions, nearly half of all adults aged 60 years and older had two or more conditions, with the most common examples being high blood pressure and arthritis (24 percent); cataract and arthritis (12 percent); and cataract and high blood pressure (10 percent) (Guralnik, LaCroix et al., 1989). Given the varying effects of single diseases on physical function and disability previously outlined, it is important to examine the effects of comorbidity on disability, to test the hypothesis that comorbidity may result in more severe levels of disability.

A prospective study of symptomatic knee osteoarthritis (OA) and disability illustrates the relation of comorbidity to functional outcomes. Persons with symptomatic knee OA were four times more likely to develop difficulty with both walking and transferring activities compared to persons without arthritis. However, persons with knee OA and either heart disease, pulmonary disease, or obesity were from eight to 13 times more likely to develop disability in ambulation or transferring (Ettinger, Davis, Neuhaus, and Mallon, 1994). Thus, while knee OA is clearly related to subsequent long-term disability in both men and women, those persons with certain comorbid conditions may have a substantially higher likelihood of subsequent disability and may be candidates for targeted interventions to reduce disability.

Population-attributable risk of disability. Although understanding the relationship of single and multiple diseases with overall disability is important, another key issue for public health is the percentage of disability attributable to individual diseases and comorbidity. The population-attributable risk is related to both the strength of the association between disease and disability and the prevalence of the specific disease. In a cross-sectional study of the Framingham cohort, Guccione et al. (1994) examined the relation of physician-diagnosed medical conditions and seven specific functional activities from the IADL and mobility domains. The investigators examined the relation of the conditions to the task disabilities, adjusting for age, sex, and comorbidity. Stroke was associated with disability in all seven tasks, hip fracture and depression were associated with disability in five tasks, while other diseases (knee OA, heart disease, congestive heart failure, and chronic obstructive pulmonary disease) were associated with four tasks each. Other conditions that were examined included diabetes, claudication, and cognitive impairment. The population-attributable risk (adjusted for age, sex, and comorbidity) for difficulty walking a mile was divided as follows: knee OA, 15 percent; depressive symptoms, 10 percent; stroke, 9 percent; heart disease, 9 percent; claudication, 7 percent; hip fracture, 5 percent; chronic obstructive pulmonary disease, 5 percent; diabetes, 4 percent; and congestive heart failure, 2 percent.

Modifiable risk factors for incident disability. Behavioral risk factors such as smoking, alcohol consumption, and obesity have been demonstrated to maintain their importance for disease, disability, and death into old age. Chapter 3, by Kaplan, has an overview of these risk factors, and a few examples—mainly derived from the EPESE studies of development of mobility disability (LaCroix et al., 1993)—will be presented here. For example, even after adjusting for age and several chronic diseases, current smokers have a significantly elevated risk of losing mobility, among both men and women. Among men, the risk of mobility loss was no higher among former smokers than among nonsmokers, suggesting that the benefits of smoking cessation may go beyond disease prevention to the prevention of functional outcomes such as mobility loss. After adjustment for age and other health behaviors, a higher risk of losing mobility was found for those who did not consume alcohol compared with those who consumed small-to-moderate amounts of alcohol. These are compatible with previous findings that low-to-moderate alcohol consumption is associated with greater longevity and decreased risk of coronary heart disease. The risk of losing mobility was also significantly associated with low levels of exercise in both men and women.

A longitudinal study of NHANES I participants found that middle-aged and older women who were overweight had a twofold higher incidence of mobility disability than women in the lowest tertile of weight (Launer et al., 1994). However, weight loss in older, heavy women was also associated with increased mobility problems, suggesting that more complex relationships with disease may also be important. Together, these studies suggest that public health interventions aimed at smoking cessation, moderate alcohol consumption, physical exercise, and preventing obesity, may prevent or decrease disability.

Outcomes and Consequences of Disability

Disability is one of the strongest predictors of adverse outcomes in the older population. It tends to progress in a downhill course and result in further disability. This spiraling course leads to the use of health care services such as home health care, to nursing home and hospital admission, and eventually to mortality. However, most longitudinal studies of aging populations reveal that persons may exhibit either decline, stability, or improvement in function over time.

Nursing home care is primarily sought by older adults with severe physical disabilities or cognitive impairment, with the need for care compounded by the lack of financial or social resources necessary to obtain community-based care, or the lack of access to informal care. In a prospective study of the North Carolina EPESE population, predictors with the highest risk for nursing home admission included disability in multiple ADLs and cognitive impairment for whites, and prior nursing home admissions for African Americans (Salive et al., 1993). Disability in IADLs were also a significant predictor of nursing home admissions among African

Americans. Other characteristics that predicted nursing home admission included age, white race, Medicaid eligibility, urban residence, living alone, being unmarried, and having either low perceived availability of support or fewer children. Thus, while disability places individuals at increased risk, many other factors play a role in determining whether an individual becomes institutionalized.

In many analyses of aging populations, after age, disability is consistently the strongest predictor of mortality. Mortality occurs much more frequently among those with ADL disabilities, compared to nondisabled persons.

In the three original EPESE communities, four-year all-cause mortality rates were four to six times higher among ADL disabled persons compared with nondisabled persons above age 70 years, while rates for persons with mobility disability were two and a half times higher (Corti et al., 1994). After adjusting for age, race, education, smoking, comorbidity, overweight, and serum albumin, persons with mobility disability were 70 to 90 percent more likely to die than the nondisabled, while the ADL disabled were 150 to 160 percent more likely to die. Figure 6.5 demonstrates the risk of death according to serum albumin and disability levels. In general, lower levels of serum albumin and greater ADL disability was associated with greater relative risk of mortality in women. This demonstrates, among women, the striking increase observed in the risk of dying as albumin levels became lower and

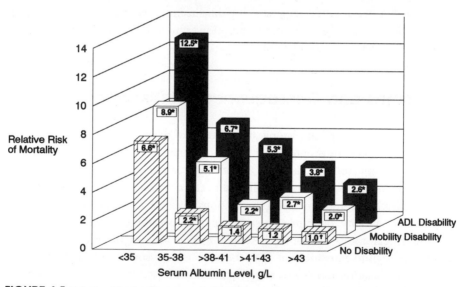

FIGURE 6.5 Relative risks for all-cause mortality in women, by serum albumin level and disability status, Established Populations for Epidemiologic Studies of the Elderly, 1988–1992. Risks were adjusted for age and are compared with the reference group (indicated by the dagger) of nondisabled women with serum albumin greater than 43 g/L.
*Significance at $p < 0.05$.
Source: Corti et al., 1994.

disability became greater. In general, at each level of disability there was an increased risk of death as albumin decreased, and at each albumin level, there was an increasing risk of death as disability increased. Women who had both ADL disability and hypoalbuminemia (albumin <35 g/L) had a risk of death twelve times that of the reference group. Similar results were obtained for men. Using low serum albumin and disability as two dimensions of "frailty" captures a vulnerable subset who are at high risk of mortality, and might be a useful tool for targeting public health interventions among older adults.

Informal and Formal Care Burden Resulting from Disability

Disabled persons receive care from sources that appear to relate to their level of disability. Figure 6.6 displays the type of care received according to disability level. These estimates were made in the same manner as Figure 6.3, using data from two national surveys (Hing and Bloom, 1990). The majority of persons with IADL difficulties receive informal care only, and few reside in a nursing home. The proportion living in nursing homes rises with the severity of disability, reaching 59 percent of persons with five to seven ADLs. Significantly, over half a million older adults with this high level of disability live at home and receive a combination of formal and informal care.

Disabled persons who can remain in the community need a considerable amount of informal care to meet their daily needs. Although the less severely disabled, those with IADLs only, can meet their needs with formal care alone, few persons with one or two ADLs and almost no one with three or more ADLs lives in the community with formal care only. Living arrangements of disabled community-dwelling older adults can have a profound effect on their need for formal care services. The most likely source of informal care is first the spouse (if living and able), followed by children, and others. The tremendous reliance of older disabled people on informal care illustrated in Figure 6.6 will be of major public health importance as the older population expands and the young and middle-aged populations contract.

Public Health Interventions on the Functional Consequences of Disease

The identification of interventions with the potential for prevention of disability is a prominent public health concern. These can occur at all three levels of prevention: primary, secondary, and tertiary. The traditional primary prevention of incident disease is of utmost importance but is less relevant when considering the older

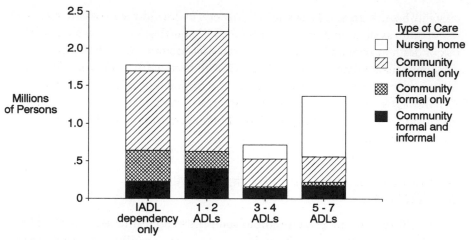

FIGURE 6.6 Number of persons who receive nursing home care and informal and formal care in the community, by level of disability. Community-dwelling persons represented in the figure actually receive help for one or more activities of daily living or instrumental activities of daily living. ADLs include bathing, dressing, transferring, walking, eating, using the toilet, and continence. IADLs include preparing meals, shopping, managing money, doing light and heavy housework, and getting outside.
Source: Guralnik and Simonsick, 1993. Copyright © The Gerontological Society of America.

population, who generally have prevalent disease. Secondary and tertiary preventions (e.g., after disease is present and preventing the impact of disease) may be more relevant for prevention of disability. Potential interventions can target medical care, technological interventions in the home, behavioral changes, and social factors that relate to provision of informal care in the home. However, current knowledge is quite limited, though provocative. Two examples can be cited. We have evidence that an exercise intervention can lead to improved performance such as faster walking time (Fiatarone et al., 1994), and that better performance is ultimately associated with lower rates of disability (Guralnik et al., 1995). Studies have documented that ophthalmology intervention (surgery or refraction) leads to improved vision, and that better vision is associated with lower incident rates of disability (Salive et al., 1994). Studies must be conducted to demonstrate the full effect of these interventions in the general or "at-risk" population: Does an intervention both improve physical performance and prevent disability? Does an intervention improve vision and prevent disability? For the former, these studies are just starting to be conducted. For the latter, although cataract surgery appears to have adequate data from a single trial (Applegate et al., 1987), other vision interventions should be tested. Further evidence should be gathered from research that includes health service utilization outcomes such as nursing home admission, the critical final common pathway of disability. Additional research and demonstration projects are needed that address the practical issues—such as compliance—that will be necessary prior to full-scale clinical trials.

Priorities for Future Research

Further study of gender differences in disability in older populations is a priority. Factors that underlie the observation that older men are more likely to die while older women live and develop disability are just beginning to be understood. Gender differences in survival in older populations is well documented, while Figures 6.1 and 6.2 demonstrate gender differences in the prevalence of disability in the aged. As life expectancy continues to rise and contributes to greater disability in men, what will be the consequences for society, particularly regarding the provision of formal and informal care? Which high-risk groups benefit from prevention interventions and why? One important group may be the moderately to severely disabled elderly still residing in their homes, with the goal of preventing further deterioration and perhaps initiating rehabilitation strategies that make it more likely for them to remain in the community.

Design and test interventions are required that can prevent or mitigate disability, especially in older women. Interventions could be public health interventions, and may be based in clinical practice or in other community settings. Once the research is completed, these interventions may need to be translated into public health programs for practicing physicians and lay audiences. Cost-effectiveness of the programs may be an important issue for gaining changes in public policy.

Developing specific interventions will require more in-depth understanding of the process by which disability develops and its relation to disease. More detailed studies, incorporating severity of illness and comorbidity, are needed of the relation of specific diseases with specific functional limitations and disability.

In conclusion, community-based longitudinal research has provided important information on the causes and consequences of disability in older populations. The association between disability and disease in older adults is complex and synergistic. Behavioral risk factors play a role in the development and cause of disability, and studies are urgently needed that further define the predictors of disability and interventions that can prevent disability.

References

Applegate, W. B., Blass, J. P., and Williams, T. F. 1990. Instruments for the functional assessment of older patients. *New England Journal of Medicine* 322:1207–14.

Applegate, W. B., Miller, S. T., Elam, J. T., Freeman, J. M., Wood, T. O., and Gettlefinger, T. C. 1987. Impact of cataract surgery with lens implantation on vision and physical function in elderly patients. *Journal of the American Medical Association* 257:1064–66.

Berkman, L. F., Berkman, C. S., Kasl, S., Freeman, D. H. Jr., Leo, L., Ostfeld, A. M., Cornoni-Huntley, J., and Brody, J. A. 1986. Depressive symptoms in relation to physical health and functioning in the elderly. *American Journal of Epidemiology* 124:372–88.

Blazer, D., Burchett, B., Service, C., and George, L. K. 1991. The association of age and depression among the elderly: An epidemiologic exploration. *Journal of Gerontology* 46:M210–15.

Boult, C., Kane, R. L., Louis, T. A., Boult, L., and McCaffrey, D. 1994. Chronic conditions that lead to functional limitation in the elderly. *Journal of Gerontology* 49:M28–36.

Branch, L. G., and Meyers, A. R. 1987. Assessing physical function in the elderly. *Clinical Geriatric Medicine* 3:29–51.

Branch, L. G., Horowitz, A., and Carr, C. 1989. The implications for everyday life of incident self-reported visual decline among people over age 65 living in the community. *Gerontologist* 29:359–65.

Branch, L. G., Katz, S., Kniepmann, K., and Papsidero, J. A. 1984. A prospective study of functional status among community elders. *American Journal of Public Health* 74:266–68.

Bruce, M. L., Seeman, T. E., Merrill, S. S., and Blazer, D. G. 1994. The impact of depressive symptomatology on physical disability: MacArthur studies of successful aging. *American Journal of Public Health* 84:1796–99.

Colantonio, A., Kasl, S. V., Ostfeld, A. M., and Berkman, L. F. 1993. Psychosocial predictors of stroke outcomes in an elderly population. *Journal of Gerontology* 48:S261–68.

Cornoni-Huntley, J., Ostfeld, A. M., Taylor, J. O., Wallace, R. B., Blazer, D., Berkman, L. F., Evans, D. A., Kohout, F. J., Lemke, J. H., Scherr, P. A., and Korper, S. P. 1993. Established populations for epidemiologic studies of the elderly: Study design and methodology. *Aging* 5:27–37.

Corti, M. C., Guralnik, J. M., Salive, M. E., and Sorkin, J. D. 1994. Serum albumin and physical disability as predictors of mortality in older persons. *Journal of the American Medical Association* 272:1036–42.

Dorland's Illustrated Medical Dictionary. 1981. (26th ed.). Philadelphia: W. B. Saunders Co.

Ettinger, W. H. Jr., Davis, M. A., Neuhaus, J. M., and Mallon, K. P. 1994. Long-term physical functioning in persons with knee osteoarthritis from NHANES I: Effects of comorbid medical conditions. *Journal of Clinical Epidemiology* 47:809–15.

Ettinger, W. H. Jr., Fried, L. P., Harris, T., Shemanski, L., and Schulz, R. J., for the CHS Collaborative Research Group. 1994. Self-reported causes of physical disability in older people. The Cardiovascular Health Study. *Journal of the American Geriatrics Society* 42:1035–44.

Ferruci, L. F., Badinelli, S., Guralnik, J. M., Lamponi, M., Bertini, C., Falchini, M., and Baroni, A. 1993. Recovery of functional status after stroke. A post-rehabilitation follow-up study. *Stroke* 24:200–205.

Fiatarone, M. A., O'Neill, E. F., Ryan, N. D., Clements, K. M., Solares, G. R., Nelson, M. E., Roberts, S. B., Kehayias, J. J., Lipsitz, L. A., and Evans, W. J. 1994. Exercise training and nutritional supplementation for physical frailty in very elderly people. *New England Journal of Medicine* 330:1769–75.

Goodwin, J. S., Hunt, W. C., and Samet, J. M. 1991. A population-based study of functional status and social support networks of elderly patients newly diagnosed with cancer. *Archives of Internal Medicine* 151:366–70.

Guccione, A. A., Felson, D. T., and Anderson, J. J. 1990. Defining arthritis and measuring functional status in elders: Methodological issues in the study of disease and physical disability. *American Journal of Public Health* 80:945–49.

Guccione, A. A., Felson, D. T., Anderson, J. J., Anthony, J. M., Zhang, Y., Wilson, P. W. F., Kelly-Hayes, M., Wolf, P. A., Kreger, B. E., and Kannel, W. B. 1994. The effects of specific medical conditions on the functional limitations of elders in the Framingham study. *American Journal of Public Health* 84:351–58.

Guralnik, J. M., and Kaplan, G. A. 1989. Predictors of healthy aging: Prospective evidence from the Alameda County Study. *American Journal of Public Health* 79:703–8.

Guralnik, J. M., and Simonsick, E. M. 1993. Physical disability in older Americans [Special issue]. *Journal of Gerontology* 48:3–10.

Guralnik, J. M., Branch, L. G., Cummings, S. R., and Curb, J. D. 1989. Physical performance measures in aging research. *Journal of Gerontology* 44:M141–46.

Guralnik, J. M., LaCroix, A. Z., Everett, D. F., and Kovar, M. G. 1989. Aging in the eighties: The prevalence of comorbidity and its association with disability. (Advance data from vital and health statistics, No. 170.) Hyattsville, MD: National Center for Health Statistics.

Guralnik, J. M., LaCroix, A. Z., Abbott, R. D., Berkman, L. F., Satterfield, S., Evans, D. A., and Wallace, R. B. 1993. Maintaining mobility in late life. I. Demographic characteristics and chronic conditions. *American Journal of Epidemiology* 137:845–57.

Guralnik, J. M., Land, K. C., Blazer, D., Fillenbaum, G. G., and Branch, L. G. 1993. Educational status and active life expectancy among older blacks and whites. *New England Journal of Medicine* 329:110–16.

Guralnik, J. M., Ferruci, L., Simonsick, E. M., Salive, M. E., and Wallace, R. B. 1995. Lower extremity function in persons over the age of 70 years as a predictor of subsequent disablity. *New England Journal of Medicine* 332:556–61.

Harris, M. G., Sheedy, J. E., and Gan, C. M. 1992. Vision and task performance with mono-vision and diffractive bifocal contact lenses. *Optometry and Vision Science* 69:609–14.

Harris, T., Kovar, M. G., Suzman, R., Kleinman, J. C., and Feldman, J. J. 1989. Longitudinal study of physical ability in the oldest-old. *American Journal of Public Health* 79:698–702.

Hing, E., and Bloom, B. 1990. Long-term care for the functionally dependent elderly. National Center for Health Statistics. *Vital Health Statistics* 13(104).

Kane, R. A., and Kane, R. L. 1981. *Assessing the Elderly: A Practical Guide to Measurement.* Lexington, MA: Lexington Books.

Katz, S., Ford, A. B., Moskovitz, A. W., Jackson, B. A., and Jaffe, M. W. 1963. Studies of illness in the aged. The Index of ADL: A standardized measure of biological and psychosocial function. *Journal of the American Medical Association* 185:914–19.

LaCroix, A. Z., Guralnik, J. M., Berkman, L. F., Wallace, R. B., and Satterfield, S. 1993. Maintaining mobility in late life. II. Smoking, alcohol consumption, physical activity and body mass index. *American Journal of Epidemiology* 137:858–69.

LaForge, R. G., Spector, W. D., and Sternberg, J. 1992. The relationship of vision and hearing impairment to one-year mortality and functional decline. *Journal of Aging Health* 4:126–48.

LaPlante, M. P. 1989. Disability risks of chronic illnesses and impairments. *Disability Statistics Report* 2:1–39.

Launer, L. J., Harris, T., Rumpel, C., and Madans, J. 1994. Body mass index, weight change, and risk of mobility disability in middle-aged and older women: The epidemiologic follow-up study of NHANES I. *Journal of the American Medical Association* 271:1093–98.

Lawton, M. P., and Brody, E. M. 1969. Assessment of older people: Self-maintaining and instrumental activities of daily living. *Gerontologist* 9:179–86.

Mor, V. 1987. Cancer patients' quality of life over the disease course: Lessons from the real world. *Journal of Chronic Disease* 40:535–44.

Mor, V., Murphy, J., Masterson-Allen, S., Willey, C., Razmpour, A., Jackson, M. E., Greer, D., and Katz, S. 1989. Risk of functional decline among well elders. *Journal of Clinical Epidemiology* 42:895–904.

Moritz, D. J., Kasl, S. V., and Berkman, L. F. 1995. Cognitive functioning and the incidence of limitations in activities of daily living in an elderly community sample. *American Journal of Epidemiology* 141:41–49.

National Center for Health Statistics, Hing, E., Sekcenski, E., and Strahan, G. 1989. The National Nursing Home Survey; 1985 summary for the United States. *Vital Health Statistics*, series 13, no. 97. DHHS pub. no. (PHS)89-1758. Washington, DC: U.S. Government Printing Office.

Neill, W. A., Branch, L. G., DeJong, G., Smith, N. E., Hogan, C. A., Corcoran, B. J., Jette, A. M., Balasco, E. M., and Osberg, S. 1985. Cardiac disability: The impact of coronary heart disease on patients' daily activities. *Archives of Internal Medicine* 145:1642–47.

Pinsky, J. L., Branch, L. G., Jette, A. M., Haynes, S. G., Feinleib, M., Cornoni-Huntley, J. C., and Bailey, K. R. 1985. Framingham disability study: Relationship of disability to cardiovascular risk factors among persons free of diagnosed cardiovascular disease. *American Journal of Epidemiology* 122:644–56.

Pinsky, J. L., Jette, A. M., Branch, L. G., Kannel, W. B., and Feinleib, M. 1990. The Framingham disability study: Relationship of various coronary heart disease manifestations to disability in older persons living in the community. *American Journal of Public Health* 80:1363–68.

Salive, M. E., Collins, K. S., Foley, D. J., and George, L. K. 1993. Predictors of nursing home admission in a biracial population. *American Journal of Public Health* 83:1765–67.

Salive, M. E., Guralnik, J. M., Glynn, R. J., Christen, W., Wallace, R. B., and Ostfeld, A. M. 1994. Association of visual impairment with mobility and physical function. *Journal of the American Geriatrics Society* 42:287–92.

Satariano, W. A., Ragheb, N. E., Branch, L. G., and Swanson, G. M. 1990. Difficulties in physical functioning reported by middle-aged and elderly women with breast cancer: A case-control comparison. *Journal of Gerontology* 45:M3–11.

Scherr, P. A., Albert, M. S., Funkenstein, H. H., Cook, N. R., Hennekens, C. H., Branch, L. G., White, L. R., Taylor, J. O., and Evans, D. A. 1988. Correlates of cognitive function in an elderly community population. *American Journal of Epidemiology* 128:1084–1101.

Schneider, E. L., and Guralnik, J. M. 1990. The aging of America: Impact on health care costs. *Journal of the American Medical Association* 263:2335–40.

U.S. Department of Health and Human Services. 1991. *Healthy People 2000.* National Health Promotion and Disease Prevention Objectives. DHHS Pub. No. (PHS) 91-50212. Washington, DC: U.S. Government Printing Office.

U.S. Department of Health and Human Services, Centers for Disease Control. 1994. Arthritis prevalence and activity limitations, United States, 1990. *Morbidity and Mortality Weekly Report* 43:443–48.

Verbrugge, L. M., Lepkowski, J. M., and Imanaka, Y. 1989. Comorbidity and its impact on disability. *Milbank Quarterly* 67:450–84.

Verbrugge, L. M., Lepkowski, J. M., and Konkol, L. L. 1991. Levels of disability among U.S. adults with arthritis. *Journal of Gerontology* 46:S71–83.

Wade, D. T., and Hewer, R. L. 1987. Functional abilities after stroke: Measurement, natural history and prognosis. *Journal of Neurology, Neurosurgery and Psychiatry* 50:177–82.

Wiener, J. M., Hanley, R. J., Clark, R., and Van Nostrand, J. R. 1990. Measuring the activities of daily living: Comparisons across national surveys. *Journal of Gerontology* 45:S229–37.

World Health Organization. 1980. *International Classification of Impairments, Disabilities and Handicaps.* Geneva: World Health Organization.

Chapter

7

Evidence of Modifiable Risk Factors in Older Adults as a Basis for Health Promotion and Disease Prevention Programs

Gilbert S. Omenn, M.D., Ph.D., Shirley A. A. Beresford, Ph.D.,
David M. Buchner, M.D., Ph.D., Andrea LaCroix, Ph.D., M.P.H.,
Mona Martin, M.P.A., B.S.N., Donald L. Patrick, Ph.D.,
Jeffrey I. Wallace, M.D., and Edward H. Wagner, M.D., M.P.H.

The Policy Framework

Health care in the United States is notorious for exerting all-out diagnostic and treatment efforts once serious illnesses and injuries have occurred, while neglecting any significant investment in prevention (Omenn, 1994a, 1994b). This paradox is particularly striking in our approach to caring for older men and women (Omenn, 1990). Until the 1980s, most research on the effectiveness of health promotion and disease prevention initiatives excluded people over age 60. For example, the Multiple Risk Factor Intervention Trial (MRFIT) to reduce heart disease was restricted to men aged 35 to 57. The Lipid Research Centers Coronary Primary Prevention Trial recruited only men aged 35 to 59. The same was true for studies organized in Finland, in Norway, and by the World Health Organization.

Belatedly, a positive message of health promotion and social value is taking hold, with attention to new concepts of "successful aging," "productive aging," "active life expectancy," "preventive gerontology," and "compression of morbidity."

Health promotion activities, enhanced social function, improved physical and mental expectations, greater autonomy, and successful postponement of chronic illnesses can provide much-needed balance against the pervasive gloomy images of older people facing risks of dementia and of inevitable admission to nursing homes, with attendant social and financial consequences.

The landmark U.S. health policy document, *Healthy People: The Surgeon General's Report on Health Promotion and Disease Prevention* (U.S. DHHS, 1979), established major goals by age group. For older adults, the primary goal was to improve the quality of life and functional independence—"adding life to years, rather than years to life." The measure chosen was a decrease in the number of days with limitations on activities of daily living. Available data indicated that nearly half of the people aged 65 and older limited their activities primarily because of preventable chronic health conditions, with an overall average of 31 to 38 days of limitations per year. The series of documents from the Office of Disease Prevention and Health Promotion in the Public Health Service establishing Health Objectives for the Nation has mobilized concerted state and local as well as private and voluntary efforts.

Elsewhere, we have reviewed the three major sets of recommendations for older adults' prevention activities: the Lifetime Health-Monitoring Program by Breslow and Somers, the Canadian Task Force's Periodic Health Examination, and the U.S. Preventive Services Task Force *Guide to Clinical Preventive Services* (Omenn, 1990). Community-wide health protection and health education programs complement the preventive services provided by various health professionals. In general, a successful prevention strategy requires the individual reinforcement of community-based public health programs, office-based clinical preventive services, and health-promoting social, regulatory, economic, and educational policies (U.S. DHHS, 1979; Omenn, 1994b).

The primary policy conclusions for older adults are these: It is never too late to begin health promotion activities. Current levels of preventive services are severely deficient for older adults in most settings. Well-targeted prevention programs, with appropriate follow-up, can meet a reasonable benefit/cost test. And a broadly coordinated effort is needed, bridging clinical practitioners, patients and families, the private sector (including insured retirees), and all levels of government (including the Veterans Affairs Department and military and civilian retirees) responsible for interrelated social, economic, and health policies (Omenn, 1990).

A Model of Frailty and Its Implications

Most elderly persons are not nearly as concerned about death as about living for a long period of years with what has come to be called "frail health" or "frailty." Katz et al. (1983) introduced the concept of active life expectancy—the number of years a person can expect to live without deficits in activities of daily living (ADL).

It is striking that most of the increased longevity of women, compared with men, is time spent with ADL deficits, so that the active life expectancy of men and women is fairly similar. Screening for indicators or predictors of frail health before ADL deficits appear may be important in increasing active life expectancy. Thus, the focus of geriatric care has shifted from treatment of specific conditions to assessment of functional status, prevention of disability, and protection of independence (Buchner and Wagner, 1992). Prevention of disability requires identification of modifiable risk factors and good methods for assessing the risk factors and related physical, mental, and social functioning (Guralnik and LaCroix, 1992; Wallace and Woolson, 1992).

The conceptual model of frailty and disability developed by our Center for Health Promotion in Older Adults is shown in Figure 7.1. The crucial biological characteristic associated with aging is a progressive reduction in the capacity of the organism/person to withstand stressors. Thus, stress tests such as insulin and glucose responses to glucose load show larger age-related reductions than do resting or basal measures (fasting glucose/fasting insulin levels). Like others (Verbrugge, 1991; Larson, 1991; Speechly and Tinetti, 1991; Young, 1986), we use the term *frailty* to define the state of reduced physiological reserve associated with increased susceptibility to disability. Frailty is thereby defined and measured independently of disability.

The model in Figure 7.1 describes a physiological state that is the result of combined effects of biological aging, chronic conditions, and disuse. The model predicts

Demonstration - Conceptual Model

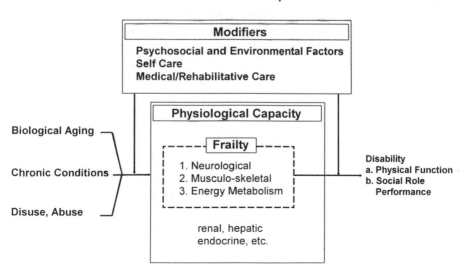

FIGURE 7.1 Conceptual model of frailty and disability.
Source: Buchner and Wagner, 1992, p. 3.

disability and can be modified for appropriate interventions. Deficits in three major physiological domains have the greatest impact on subsequent function: neurological control for complex tasks, including most activities of daily living and walking without falling; integrity of the musculoskeletal system of joints, bones, and muscles; and energy capacity, reflecting primarily the cardiovascular and pulmonary systems and conveniently measured by maximal aerobic capacity. Other organ systems contribute, of course.

It is clear that aging per se is not always associated with serious declines of function. Many octogenarians and even centenarians are quite active in their personal lives and communities; some famous individuals stand out, including Rubenstein and Casals in music; Picasso and Grandma Moses in painting; Verdi in opera; and Martha Graham in choreography. Thus, the MacArthur Foundation and various researchers have focused on the theme of "successful aging" to reflect the positive prospect when negative risk factors can be averted or overcome.

Chronic or acute inactivity can trigger loss of functional capacity. Measures of the rate of loss of aerobic capacity, for example, suggest that one day of bed rest may cause the same loss as one year of sedentary lifestyle (about 1 percent, or 0.3–0.5 mL/kg/min) (Convertino, 1986). Muscle strength may decline as much as 5 percent per day of bed rest. More active adults also show less decline in strength, bone mass, and cognitive function (Buchner and Wagner, 1992). Dementia is the most prevalent chronic condition in hip fracture patients (Buchner et al., 1994), and a major factor in falls.

Figure 7.2 depicts how risk factors cause frailty, emphasizing episodes of acute and subacute loss and the capacity for recovery upon resumption of normal activities (without any special exercise). Recovery is determined by the baseline level of capacity and by psychosocial and iatrogenic barriers, most importantly recommendations from health professionals and from well-intentioned caregivers for unnecessary rest. Medications, falls, stressful life events, and depression are other common and preventable inhibitors of resumption of normal activity.

It will be no surprise, then, that the following five elements can help prevent the development of frailty: monitoring physiological reserve, regular exercise, avoiding episodes of loss (as by immunization against influenza), increasing physiological reserve before elective hospitalizations ("prehab"), and removing obstacles to recovery noted above (Buchner and Wagner, 1992).

Modeling Preventable Causes of Restricted Activity Days

The number of restricted activity days experienced by an individual in the course of a year is an important and fairly robust measure of functional well-being, partic-

Demonstration - Results

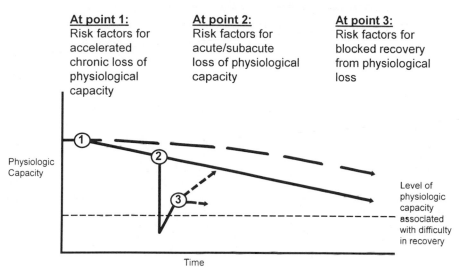

At point 1:
Risk factors for accelerated chronic loss of physiological capacity

At point 2:
Risk factors for acute/subacute loss of physiological capacity

At point 3:
Risk factors for blocked recovery from physiological loss

Physiologic Capacity

Level of physiologic capacity associated with difficulty in recovery

Time

FIGURE 7.2 Conceptual model of how risk factors cause frailty.
Source: Buchner and Wagner, 1992.

ularly for older adults (Scholes et al., 1991). A restricted activity day, as defined in the National Health Interview Survey (NHIS) (Fitti and Kovar, 1987), is a day in which an individual spends over half of the day in bed, home from work or school, or cutting down on usual activities because of illness or injury. Kosorok et al. (1992) used data from the 1984 Supplement on Aging of the NHIS to estimate the relationship between restricted activity days reported and age, gender, and the presence or absence of selected chronic conditions and falls for all noninstitutionalized individuals aged 65 years and older. The results were quite striking and are informative for planning health promotion/disease prevention programs.

Of an annual average of 31 restricted activity days, 6 days were associated with falls; 4 each with heart disease and arthritis/rheumatism; 2 each with high blood pressure, cerebrovascular disease, and visual impairment; and 1 day each with atherosclerosis, diabetes, major malignancies, and osteoporosis, totalling 24 of the 31 days. Multivariate analyses were performed on the association of health conditions with restricted activity days, with results shown in Table 7.1. When age by sex interaction and all interactions between each health condition and either age or sex were examined, none was statistically significant. When all 59 two-way interactions among the health conditions were examined stepwise in the final main effects model, only four interactions were significant at the .05 level (Table 7.1). The estimated baseline level in the final interaction model of 8.4 restricted activity days per year is

TABLE 7.1. Estimated Average Annual Days of Restricted Activity per Person Directly Associated with Various Conditions

| Condition | Prevalence per 1000 | Days Directly Associated with Condition | | | |
| | | Main Effects Model | | Interaction Model | |
		Number	Percent	Number	Percent
(Overall average)	N/A	31.4	100.0	31.4	100.0
Baseline level	1000.0	6.2	19.6	8.4	26.9
Visual impairment	112.8	1.8	5.9	1.9	6.0
Falls	203.7	5.6	17.8	5.7	18.1
Osteoporosis	33.1	0.9	2.9	0.9	2.8
Hip fracture	35.8	0.5	1.5	0.5	1.5
Atherosclerosis	105.5	1.4	4.6	1.5	4.7
High blood pressure	440.5	2.0	6.3	2.3	7.4
Ischemic heart disease	144.9	2.2	6.9	2.2	7.0
Other heart disease	89.1	2.2	7.2	2.3	7.2
Cerebrovascular disease	66.1	2.3	7.4	2.3	7.4
Diabetes	97.8	1.4	4.6	1.5	4.7
Major malignancy	52.2	1.1	3.6	1.1	3.6
Arthritis and rheumatism	495.2	3.7	11.7	4.1	13.0
Falls × arthritis and rheumatism	123.7	N/A	N/A	1.7	5.4
Atherosclerosis × diabetes	16.4	N/A	N/A	0.6	2.0
High blood pressure × other heart disease	50.4	N/A	N/A	0.9	2.9
Other heart disease × hearing impairment	30.5	N/A	N/A	(0)	(0)

Source: Kosorok et al., 1992, Table 3.

remarkably close to the 10.5 restricted activity days per year that was the actual average from the data for people with none of the 17 selected conditions.

Neither age, sex, nor any interaction with age or sex was significantly associated with restricted activity days after the effects of self-reported health conditions were accounted for in the model. This important finding supports the concepts of successful aging and of disease-triggered frailty described in the previous section of this chapter. Verbrugge, Lepkowski, and Imanaka (1989) obtained similar results from regression analyses. Falls were clearly the biggest risk factor for restricted activity days. Suppose we have an intervention against falls that can reduce by 50 percent the total number of people experiencing a fall in one year; from Table 7.1 we know that falls are associated with about 18 percent of all restricted activity days; we would, therefore, estimate that the proposed intervention could reduce the total number of restricted activity days by about 9 percent.

The effects of interventions with multiple benefits, such as smoking cessation (which was demonstrated by Hermanson et al., 1988, to be remarkably beneficial in older adults) and control of high blood pressure, could be estimated similarly by determining the interrelationships between the various risk factors and health conditions involved. Then one would multiply the resulting reductions in health condition prevalences by the direct effect estimates found in Table 7.1, subtracting for certain overlaps. For example, a 50 percent reduction in both falls and arthritis/rheumatism would result in an estimate of $(50\% \times 18.1\%) + (50\% \times 13.0\%) - (50\% \times 5.4\%) = 12.9$ percent reduction, where 5.4 percent is the overlap in percentage of days associated with the falls by A/R interaction.

A Randomized Demonstration of Health Promotion Interventions

Group Health Cooperative (GHC) of Puget Sound has a long standing policy commitment to health promotion and disease prevention. Beginning in 1986, Wagner and Beery and colleagues at Group Health developed and implemented a multiple-faceted senior health promotion program as part of the University of Washington/Group Health Cooperative Center for Health Promotion in Older Adults. The program emphasized increase in physical activity, reduction of excessive prescription drug use, reduction of excess alcohol use, identification and amelioration of hazards in the home, and detection and correction of visual and hearing deficits (Wagner et al., 1994). A separate demonstration called "A Healthy Future" (supported by the Health Care Financing Administration [HCFA]) addressed fifteen interventions in a package of preventive services that might be offered to all Medicare-eligible elderly (Patrick et al., 1994). Relevant features of the two demonstrations are summarized in Table 7.2.

The dependent variables for the Wagner and colleagues demonstration were restricted activity and other indicators of dysfunction; incidence of falls, motor vehicle accidents and other injuries; and health care utilization among these senior enrollees in the Group Health HMO. The linked data systems at GHC make these analyses feasible and allow comparisons with nonparticipating subscriber-members of GHC. After randomization, 600 eligible older adults received the experimental multifaceted health promotion program from trained nurse-educators; 300 received a routine GHC health assessment visit; 600 received usual care without a health assessment visit; and another 300 received usual care from a different GHC primary care clinic. That fourth group was added to assess whether physician or nurse behavior might be influenced by the involvement of some of their patients in the in-

TABLE 7.2. Multiple-Component Health Promotion Intervention Package: Rationale, Description, Source, and Previous Experience with Intervention Components

Intervention Target Area	Rationale	Recommended Intervention	Previous Approaches*	Lessons Learned from Previous Experience
Exercise	Cornerstone intervention	Walking, strength and balance training with partial or no supervision and at least monthly follow-up	Wide variety, from informational and motivational classes to intense supervised exercise	Most cost-effective approach is multicomponent intense program with minimal, although continuous, supervision
Depression	Depression impairs motivation to exercise, leading to deconditioning	For those too depressed to exercise, offer psycho-educational group program or written materials	Series of classes on life events, stress, and life satisfaction	Classes well received but expensive and not effective in reducing depressive symptoms
Alcohol	May block benefits of exercise on mood and sleep and increase risk of injury during exercise	CAGE screening for high-risk drinking behaviors with referral to M.D. or use of self-help booklet and telephone follow-up	Same as current	Increased awareness of the problem but no change in high-risk drinking behaviors
Smoking	Decreases exercise tolerance, strong correlate of sedentary life style	As desired, referral to classes in community or choice of two self-help programs	Motivational self-quit booklet with self-help programs	Low prevalence of smoking in HMO enrollees (9%) probably limited intervention effects; no change in rate of smoking

Psychotropic	May block benefits of exercise on mood and sleep and increase risk of injury during exercise	Self-help booklet on alternatives to medication for symptom management; encouragement to discuss discontinuation with private M.D.	Pharmacist's review of medication profile with recommendations for changes made to primary care M.D.	Expensive, labor-intensive approach that failed to result in changes in regime
Nutrition	Exercise and nutrition are linked in many respects	Tip sheets in four areas: fiber and carbohydrates, fats and cholesterol, calcium and sodium, calories and water; follow-up by nurse educator	Self-help materials and tip sheets, targeted to dietary fat	Approach successful at reducing intake of dietary fat in Healthy Future Project; tip sheets well received in NorthShore pilot, with majority reporting some behavioral change
Home safety	Home-based exercise programs require a safe environment	Self-administered hazard checklist with telephone follow-up by nurse educator	Hazard evaluation by a home visit or, if preferred, self-administered; telephone follow-up by nurse educator	Self-administration of hazard checklist much better received than home visit; intervention effective at reducing home hazards by self-report in HPOA demonstration

*Data from University of Washington experiences from Group Health Cooperative Demonstration of Center for Health Promotion in Older Adults; A Healthy Future Project (Health Care Financing Administration demonstration); MOVE-IT and FICSIT trials; and NorthShore Senior Center pilot project.

terventions. These study participants were representative of the 37,000 persons 65 years of age and older who comprised 11 percent of the GHC total enrollee population. Costs were quite modest: Expenditures in the experimental arm of the GHC demonstration are estimated to be $100 to $150 per participant. The up to 15 interventions in "A Healthy Future" were supported by HCFA at $180 per person per year (Patrick et al., 1994).

The group receiving the health promotion intervention had significantly fewer restricted activity and bed disability days during the first year of follow-up, compared with the usual care controls. They had significantly less functional decline, as 730 measured by the MOS physical function scale. In addition, significantly fewer persons fell during the first year of follow-up than among the usual care controls (Wagner et al., 1994). Figure 7.3 shows the percent of GHC seniors by intervention arm who had increases in disability measures or experienced new falls during the first year. After two years, with no additional intervention, the intervention group still was doing better, though the differences had diminished, as might be expected.

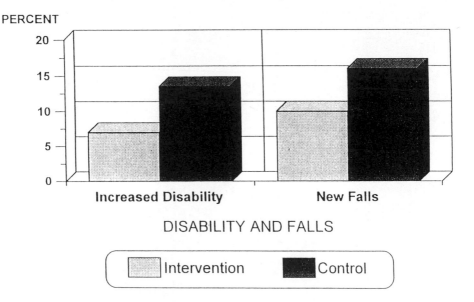

FIGURE 7.3 Results from the Group Health Cooperative Demonstration: percentage of seniors with increased disability or new falls, by treatment.
Source: Wagner et al., 1994.

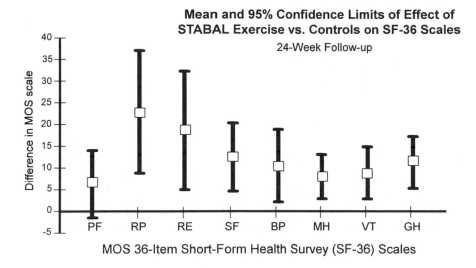

FIGURE 7.4 Results from the NorthShore Senior Center Intervention, emphasizing exercise regimen. *Source:* STABAL exercise, Buchner et al., unpublished.

Can Similar Results Be Obtained in Community Settings?

It is a truism of all kinds of prevention programs—and even treatment programs—that those individuals with the greatest risk factors are often the least likely to come for care or to join health promotion/disease prevention activities, especially at health care facilities (Carter et al., 1991). Our Center for Health Promotion in Older Adults conducted a pilot study at a local senior center, the NorthShore Senior Center in Bothell, Washington. The main objectives were to evaluate the feasibility of recruitment, interventions, data collection, and follow-up in such settings, utilizing components from the Group Health Demonstration previously described.

A total of 100 senior center participants were randomized to receive, or not receive, the redesigned multiple-component health promotion intervention by trained nurse-educators. The intervention emphasized physical activity, including organized exercise classes for group walks and for use of weights in certain maneuvers. The results were dramatic, as shown in Figure 7.4, using the MOS 36-item short form (SF-36) scales at 24 weeks of follow-up (Buchner et al., unpublished). The participants were so enthusiastic about the program that it was sustained by the Senior Center staff themselves, and a similar intervention was then offered for the 50 control participants. With the senior centers, our strategy is to partner with these community-based organizations serving older adults and to build stepwise with incremental improvements until all sites will have appropriate and cost-effective offerings.

Can Health Promotion Be Stimulated in Low-Income Populations?

An even harder-to-reach older adult population can be found in low-income housing facilities. In cooperation with the Seattle Housing Authority (SHA) and the Seattle/King County Health Department, staff of the Center for Health Promotion in Older Adults first approached the manager and the residents of Barton Place, in the low-income, southeast section of Seattle. Residents were not interested; their prime concerns were physical security—both outside the building and crossing the street to a grocery store and inside the building, where policies to mix residents of different ages and physical and mental states had produced highly heterogeneous populations that frightened many older residents. The manager and the SHA officials were dubious about the whole concept.

Persistence and attention to the expressed needs of the residents paid off. Our staff person gained the confidence of the residents over several months of weekly visits for several hours at a time, and gradually the whole place came alive (King, 1993). We call this process "social activation," overcoming major barriers to interest and to participation. The general model is shown in Figure 7.5 and the specific application to our low-income housing sites is shown in Figure 7.6.

The approach integrates three areas of behavioral science research: (1) the Stage Model of Behavior Change (Prochaska and DiClemente, 1983) describing the readi-

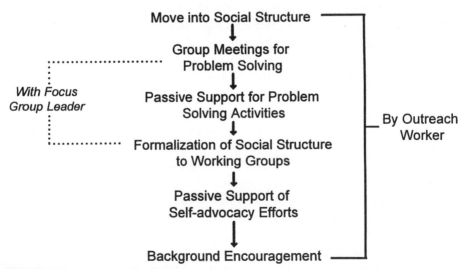

FIGURE 7.5 General model of social activation.
Source: Patrick, Beresford, Buchner, et al., unpublished.

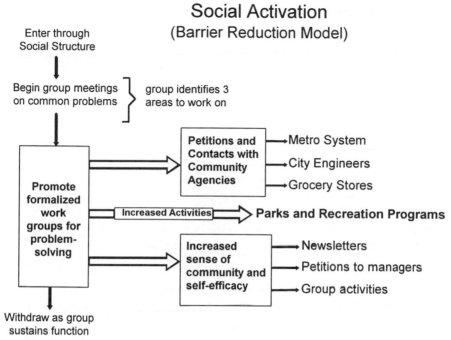

FIGURE 7.6 Model of social activation applied to low-income housing setting.
Source: Beresford, Buchner, Patrick, et al., unpublished.

ness of the individual for change through precontemplation, contemplation, preparation, action, and maintenance; (2) empowerment, comprising social support, change, and community organization theories to facilitate group process and foster indigenous leadership for group problem solving (Minkler, 1985; Alinsky, 1972); and (3) community-wide intervention programs with sustained, multiple-component approaches to enhance participation in health promotion/disease prevention activities (Freire, 1973; Abrams et al., 1986; Abrams, 1992).

Simply (actually, not so simply) increasing regular social activities, without an explicit focus on health behavior change, can be beneficial to older individuals. Increasing regular contact with other individuals can help identify health problems, such as cognitive and emotional illnesses. Social support and social networks have been shown consistently to enhance mental and physical health and quality of life (House, Landis, and Umberson, 1988).

The Seattle Housing Authority does not have computerized records with descriptive information about the SHA residents; therefore, we conducted a survey of a 7 to 10 percent sample of residents aged 60+ at 29 SHA facilities. The SHA population differs strikingly in every parameter from the community-based sample of participants in the Group Health Demonstration previously described, as shown in Table 7.3. The SHA residents were living alone, low-income, less well educated, more

TABLE 7.3. Comparison of Seattle Housing Authority Residents with a Community Sample

Characteristics	SHA Sample (n = 198) (%)	Community Sample (n = 2289) (%)
Male	25	39
Living alone	90	9
Income under $10,000	85	17
Currently married	8	56
Ethnic minority	25	12
Report health is "fair or poor"	42	18
Limited in kinds of work	90	9

Source: University of Washington Health Promotion in Older Adults, unpublished.

nonwhite, and less often male; they rated their health much worse; and almost all had difficulty with activities of daily living. In two facilities, all residents were surveyed about their major concerns. Neighborhood safety (35 percent), building safety (21 percent), transportation and social opportunities (10 percent), and personal health (7 percent) were cited most frequently. No one mentioned health promotion or any equivalent.

The pilot intervention increased physical activity and social integration, and reduced physical security fears and transportation barriers. The residents learned, for example, that if eight of them signed up and showed up they could have the services of a van and driver from the county agency to take them grocery shopping, for a walk in a park, to their doctor appointments, or even to a City Council budget hearing at which they successfully testified in favor of reinstating the Parks and Recreation staff person who leads their physical activity sessions! Social activation and increased physical activity were associated with slower decline in measures of physical, social, and emotional function, as shown in Figure 7.7.

Nutritional Interventions

We are introducing multiple-component interventions emphasizing exercise and nutrition in several SHA low-income housing facilities. Our combination of exercise and diet change interventions relates to at least 14 *Healthy People 2000* objectives: to reduce the proportion of people aged 65+ with difficulty in personal care activities (17.3); African Americans with activity limitations (17.2c); people with fall injuries (9.4a, 9.4b, 9.7); people with too little exercise and leisure time activity (1.3, 1.5a), par-

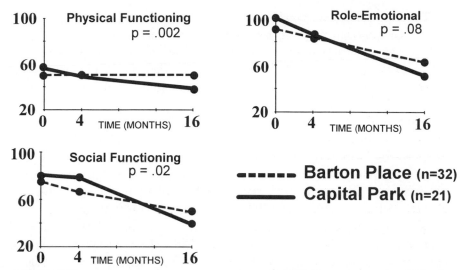

FIGURE 7.7 Effects of social activation intervention on MOS SF-36 scores among Seattle Housing Authority residents at Barton Place over 16 months and compared with Capital Park (preintervention). Higher scores indicate better health; the slope of the change is indicated for 4- and 16-month follow-up.
Source: Bucher et al., unpublished.

ticularly low-income adults (1.4a, 1.5c); people who don't do strengthening exercises (1.6); people who are overweight (2.3, 2.7); and people with inappropriate dietary intakes of fat (2.5), complex carbohydrates, and fiber (2.6) (U.S. Department of Health and Human Services, 1991). The self-help component of the low-intensity intervention to reduce dietary fat, increase fiber, and increase intake of green and yellow vegetables included in the low-income housing facility intervention has been shown (Beresford et al., 1992) to be effective in modifying both fat and fiber intake in the context of primary care, and bears the hallmarks of a strategy designed to be accessible to the general population, without regard to disease risk factors.

We also employ multilevel interventions, based on the conceptual model of behavior change described above. Studies by others find that at least 40 percent of adults are in the action and maintenance stages of changing dietary fat, and another 5 to 10 percent are preparing to change their diets (Bowen, Meischke, and Tomoyasu, 1994; Henderson et al., 1990). A "high-intensity" intervention is appropriate for many such receptive adults; a modification of the high-intensity group sessions used effectively in the Women's Health Trial (Insull et al., 1990) has been incorporated into our low-income housing intervention. The other adults, however, are in the precontemplation and contemplation stages of change; a low-intensity intervention that seeks to advance them to preparation and action stages is more appropriate. Combined high- and low-intensity interventions have proved effective in reducing dietary fat (Bowen et al., 1995).

The acceptability of dietary behavior change programs to older adults is largely untested. Low-intensity tip sheets have been used in a trial of persons over the age of 65 years with modest benefit at two years followup (Beresford, unpublished). As efforts to devise acceptable and effective components for population-wide dietary intervention come to fruition, we expect to see more studies with multilevel interventions, as illustrated here.

While the health hazards of obesity are well established, recent NIH sponsored reviews of the potential risks and benefits associated with weight loss indicate limited knowledge in this area (Kuller and Wing, 1993; Pamuk et al., 1993; Andres, Muller, and Sorkin, 1993). Studies in older adults suggest that weight loss in the elderly is common and is associated with increased morbidity and mortality (Manson and Shea, 1991; Dwyer and Campbell, 1991; Morley et al., 1988). Further, in the few studies that have made the distinction, similar increases in mortality have been observed regardless of whether weight loss was volitional or not (Williamson and Pamuk, 1993; Wallace et al., 1995). The extent to which weight loss is a marker of underlying potentially reversible psychosocial and medical conditions, or is itself a causal factor leading to increased frailty, remains to be determined. Community-based health promotion studies can help clarify these issues by prospectively evaluating the association between nutrition, weight change, and health status in the elderly.

Partnerships for Health Promotion Interventions

These examples of effective interventions and of necessary social activation illustrate, also, the importance of relevant partnerships in community settings. Schools of public health have a major role to play in training of prevention researchers and public health practitioners. The Northwest Center for Health Promotion in Older Adults developed and conducted needs assessment surveys in local communities and statewide assessement of training needs of public health and other agency staff. The Northwest Center for Public Health Practice at the University of Washington School of Public Health and Community Medicine developed a health promotion curriculum for older adults as an offering in its annual Summer Institute for Public Health Practice. Together with CDC and other prevention research centers, we are engaged in active sharing and testing of instruments for measuring health status and change in health status, physical activity, depression, and other variables. We are working with the Harlem Columbia Prevention Center on a lifespan approach to social activation and health promotion. The goal, it must be emphasized, is improved health of the people in the community; the community agencies and citizens can join with the research institution to conduct sustainable community-based studies. The elements of a successful partnership are shown in Figure 7.8. New linkages are needed

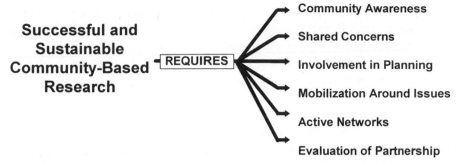

FIGURE 7.8 Elements of a successful partnership for community-based interventions.

to tie together the quite separate and separately funded public health and aging networks, both for services and for research. Community-based research can facilitate the development of such linkages.

Recommendations for Future Research

The combination of epidemiological analyses of the prevalence and significance of risk factors for frailty and disability with well-controlled studies of the modifiability of those risk factors and preventability of frailty and disability is a powerful and much-needed area of research for older adults.

Older adults should be included in important risk-reduction trials. Until just a few years ago, older adults were routinely neglected in major prevention trials. Inclusion of older adults in the Coronary Artery Surgery Study (N = 24,959, of whom 10 percent were 65+ at enrollment) permitted later analyses of the effects on survival, adjusted for numerous other factors, of smoking status and of smoking cessation in older adults, compared with middle-aged and younger participants in the same trial (Hermanson et al., 1988; Principal Investigators of CASS, 1981). Older adults are also a significant proportion of participants in the Beta-Carotene and Retinol Efficacy Trial (CARET) to try to prevent lung cancer (and coronary heart disease and cataracts) in high-risk populations—heavy smokers, former heavy smokers, and asbestos-exposed workers who are/were smokers (Omenn et al., 1994).

Intermediate endpoints and biomarkers of behavior change and early disease states are becoming more commonplace elements of epidemiological studies and prevention trials, so that mechanistic underpinnings for clinical and public health decisions and planning will improve. The generalizability of results is always suspect when only rather small percentages of target populations participate in studies or are reached with services. Therefore, it is essential to conduct well-monitored and well-controlled studies in community settings, and to reach out to hard-to-reach individuals and subgroups. Until very recently there was considerable skepticism that such research could be performed rigorously and could produce significant results; therefore, funding from NIH was quite unfavorable (Omenn, 1994c). We have presented here early evidence of strikingly favorable results from health promotion interventions in community and especially low-income settings and with low-income older adults populations. Much more such research and then appropriate dissemination of services will be necessary in order to achieve the quality-of-life goals and the many specific relevant objectives of *Healthy People 2000*.

Finally, partnerships across the public health and aging networks and between academia and community organizations and agencies are essential for effective community-based interventions to improve the health of older people. We hope this conference and its proceedings will galvanize formation of such bridges between the public health and aging networks everywhere; we are committed to doing so in Seattle.

References

Abrams, D. B. 1992. Conceptual models to integrate individual and public health interventions: The example of the work place. In Henderson, M. M., Chair. *Conference Proceedings. Promoting Dietary Change in Communities: Applying Existing Models of Dietary Change to Population-Based Interventions* (pp 173–94). Seattle: Fred Hutchinson Cancer Research Center.

Abrams, D. B., Elder, J. P., Carleton, R. A. 1986. Social learning principles for organizational health promotion: An integrated approach. In Cataldo, M. F., and Coates, T. J., eds., *Health and Industry: A Behavioral Medicine Perspective* (pp. 28–51). New York: Wiley Interscience Publications.

Alinsky, S. 1972. *Rules for Radicals.* New York: Random House.

Andres, R., Muller, D. C., and Sorkin, J. D. 1993. Long-term effects of change in body weight on all-cause mortality: A review. *Annals of Internal Medicine* 119(7pt2):737–43.

Beresford, S. A. A., Farmer, E. M. Z., Feingold, L., Graves, K. L., Sumner, S. K., and Baker, R. M. 1992. Evaluation of a self-help dietary intervention in a primary care setting. *American Journal of Public Health* 82:79–84.

Bowen, D. J., Meischke, H., and Tomoyasu, N. 1994. Preliminary evaluation of the processes of changing to a low-fat diet. *Health Education Research* 9:85–94.

Bowen, D. J., Henderson, M. H., Inversion, D., Burrows, D., Henry, H., and Forety, J. 1995. Reducing dietary fat: The Women's Health Trial. *Cancer Prevention International* 1:21–30.

Buchner, D. M., and Wagner, E. H. 1992. Preventing frail health. In Omenn, G. S., Larson, E. B., Wagner, E. H., and Abrass, I., eds. *Health Promotion and Disease Prevention in the Elderly.* Clinics in Geriatric Medicine 8:1–17.

Buchner, D. M., Koepsell, T. D., Abrass, I. B., and Karlen, P. 1994. Chronic illness as a risk factor for hip fracture: Results of a case-control study and review of the literature. In Apple, D. F., and Hayes, W. C., eds., *Prevention of Falls and Hip Fracture in the Elderly* (pp. 9–18). Rosemont, IL: American Academy of Orthopedic Surgeons.

Carter, W. B., Elward, K., Malmgren, J. A., Martin, M. L., and Larson, E. 1991. Participation of older adults in health programs and research: A critical review of the literature. *Gerontologist* 31:584–92.

Convertino, V. A. 1986. Exercise responses after inactivity. In Sandler, H., and Vernikos, J., eds., *Inactivity: Physiological Effects* (p. 149). Orlando: Academic Press.

Diehr, P., Patrick, D. L., Grembowski, D., and Picciano, J. 1993. Accounting for deaths when measuring health status over time. In *Proceedings of the 1993 Public Health Conference on Records and Statistics: Toward the Year 2000; Refining the Measures* (pp. 34–37). Washington, DC: U.S. Department of Health and Human Services, Public Health Service, Centers for Disease Control and Prevention.

Dwyer, J. T., and Campbell, D., eds. 1991. *Screening older Americans' nutritional health: Current practices and future possibilities.* Washington, DC: Nutrition Screening Initiative.

Fitti, J. E., and Kovar, M. G. 1987. The Supplement on Aging to the 1984 National Health Interview Survey. DHHS publication PHS 87-1323. Hyattsville, MD: National Center for Health Statistics.

Freire, P. 1973. *Education for Critical Consciousness.* New York: Seabury Press.

Guralnik, J. M., and LaCroix, A. Z. 1992. Assessing physical function in older populations. In Wallace, R. B., and Woolson, R. F., eds. *The Epidemiologic Study of the Elderly* (pp. 159–81). New York: Oxford University Press.

Henderson, M., Kushi, L., Thompson, D., Gorback, S., Clifford, C., and Insull, W. 1990. Feasibility of a randomized trial of a low-fat diet for the prevention of breast cancer: Dietary compliance in the Women's Health Trial Vanguard Study. *Preventive Medicine* 19:115–30.

Hermanson, B., Omenn, G. S., Kronmal, R. A., and Gersh, B. J. 1988. Beneficial six-year outcomes of smoking cessation in older men and women with coronary artery disease: Results from the CASS registry. *New England Journal of Medicine* 319:1365–69.

House, J. S., Landis, K. R., and Umberson, D. 1988. Social relationships and health. *Science* 241:540–45.

Insull, W., Henderson, M. M., Prentice, R. L., Thompson, D. J., Clifford, C., Goldman, S., Gorbach, S., Moskowitz, M., Thompson, R., and Woods, M. 1990. Results of a randomized feasibility study of a low-fat diet. *Archives of Internal Medicine* 150:421–27.

Katz, S., Branch, L. G., Branson, M. H., Papsidero, J. A., Beck, J. C., and Greer, D. S. 1983. Active life expectancy. *New England Journal of Medicine* 309:1218–24.

King, M. 1993, 13 June. Back to Life: Now There's Plenty to Do at Barton Place. Seattle *Times*, pp. L1-2.

Kosorok, M. R., Omenn, G. S., Diehr, P., Koepsell, T. D., and Patrick, D. L. 1992. Conditions associated with restricted activity days among older adults. *American Journal of Public Health* 82:1263–67.

Kuller, L., and Wing, R. 1993. Weight loss and mortality. *Annals of Internal Medicine* 119:630–32.

Larson, E. B. 1991. Exercise, functional decline, and frailty. *Journal of the American Geriatrics Society* 39:635–36.

Manson, A., and Shea, S. 1991. Malnutrition in elderly ambulatory medical patients. *American Journal of Public Health* 81:1195–97.

Minkler, M. 1985. Building supportive ties and sense of community among the inner-city elderly; The Tenderloin Senior Outreach Project. *Health Education Quarterly* 12:303–14.

Morley, J. E., Mooradian, A. D., Silver, A. J., Herber, D., and Alfin-Slater, R. B. 1988. Nutrition in the elderly (clinical conference). *Annals of Internal Medicine* 109:890–904.

Omenn, G. S. 1990. Prevention and the elderly: What are appropriate policies? *Health Affairs* 9:80–93.

Omenn, G. S. 1994a, August 2. Don't forget community public health services in the debate on health. Washington *Post*, p. C5.

Omenn, G. S. 1994b. Prevention: What Does it Save? What Does it Cost? Prevention: Benefits, Costs and Savings, (pp. 1–8). A report prepared for Partnership for Prevention. Washington, DC: Partnership for Prevention.

Omenn, G. S. 1994c. Prevention policy: Perspectives on the critical interaction between research and policy. Presented at NIH Conference on Disease Prevention Research at NIH: An Agenda for All, October 6, 1993. *Preventive Medicine* 23:612–17.

Omenn, G. S., Goodman, G., Thornquist, M., Grizzle, J., Rosenstock, L., Barnhart, S., Balmes, J., Cherniack, M., Cullen, M., Glass, A., Keogh, J., Meyskens, F., Valanis, B., and Williams, J. 1994. The β-carotene and retinol efficacy trial (CARET) for chemoprevention of lung cancer in high-risk populations: Smokers and asbestos-exposed workers. *Cancer Research* 54:2038s–43s.

Omenn, G. S., Goodman, G. E., Thornquist, M. D., Balmes, J., Cullen, M. R., Glass, A., Keogh, J. P., Meyskens, Jr. F. L., Valanis, B., Williams, Jr. J. H., Barnhart, S., and Hammar, S. 1996. Effects of a combination of beta-carotene and vitamin A on lung cancer incidence, total mortality, and cardiovascular mortality in smokers and asbestos-exposed workers. *New England Journal of Medicine* 334:1150–55.

Pamuk, E. R., Williamson, D. F., Serdula, M. K., Madans, J., and Byers, T. E. 1993. Weight loss and subsequent death in a cohort of U.S. adults. *Annals of Internal Medicine* 119(7pt2):744–48.

Patrick, D. L., Grembowski, D., Diehr, P., Durham, M., Beresford, S., Ehreth, J., Hecht, J. A., Picciano, J., Beery, W., and Odle, K. 1994. A Healthy Future: The Cost Utility of Medicare Reimbursement for Preventive Services in an HMO. Final report: Health Care Financing Administration, Cooperative Agreement #95-C-99161: July 31.

The Principal Investigators of CASS and Their Associates. 1981. The National Heart, Lung and Blood Coronary Artery Surgery Study (CASS). *Circulation* 63(Suppl I):I–I81.

Prochaska, J. O., and DiClemente, C. C. 1983. Stages and processes of self-change of smoking: Toward an integrative model of change. *Journal of Consulting and Clinical Psychology* 51:390–95.

Scholes, D., LaCroix, A. Z., Wagner, E. H., Grothaus, L. C., and Hecht, J. A. 1991. Tracking progress towards national health objectives in the elderly: What do restricted activity days signify? *American Journal of Public Health* 81:485–88.

Speechly, M., and Tinetti, M. 1991. Falls and injuries in frail and vigorous community elderly persons. *Journal of the American Geriatrics Society* 39:46.

U.S. Department of Health and Human Services. 1979. *Healthy People, The Surgeon General's Report on Health Promotion and Disease Prevention.* DHEW (PHS) Pub. No. 79-55071. Washington, DC: U.S. Government Printing Office.

U.S. Department of Health and Human Services. 1991. *Healthy People 2000.* DHHS (PHS) Pub. No. 91-50212. Washington, DC: U.S. Government Printing Office.

Verbrugge, L. M. 1991. Survival curves, prevalence rates and dark matters therein. *Journal of Aging and Health* 3:217.

Verbrugge, L. M., Lepkowski, J. M., and Imanaka, Y. 1989. Comorbidity and its impact on disability. *Milbank Quarterly* 67:450–84.

Wagner, E. H., LaCroix, A. Z., Grothaus, M. S., Leveille, S. G., Hecht, J. A., Artz, K., Odle, K., and Buchner, D. M. 1994. Preventing disability and falls in older adults:

A population-based randomized trial. *American Journal of Public Health* 84:1800–1806.

Wallace, J. I., Schwartz, R. S., LaCroix, A. Z., Uhlmann, R. F., and Pearlman, R. A. In press. Involuntary weight loss in elderly outpatients: Incidence and clinical significance. *Journal of the American Geriatrics Society* 43:329–37

Wallace, R. B., and Woolson, R. F., eds. 1992. *The Epidemiologic Study of the Elderly.* New York: Oxford University Press, 387 pp.

Williamson, D. F., and Pamuk, E. R. 1993. The association between weight loss and increased longevity: A review of the evidence. *Annals of Internal Medicine* 119(7pt2):731–36.

Young, A. 1986. Exercise physiology in geriatric practice. *Acta Medica Scandinavica* 711(Suppl):227.

Part

III

Program Planning and
Development for Older
Populations

Chapter

8

Integrating Research into Program Planning and Development

Terrie Wetle, Ph.D.

Substantial resources, energy, and effort are devoted to research on topics of direct relevance to public health policy and programs. The findings of this research hold the potential to enhance our understanding of health and disease in old age, enrich programs for older persons, and improve the quality of life for the elderly. Similarly, program personnel and policy makers have important knowledge and information and can provide access to data and people essential for research investigations. Moreover, they have the capacity to implement practical strategies for applying research findings to improve the lives of older persons. Unfortunately, these worlds of research, policy, and practice infrequently interact effectively around topics of mutual interest and even more rarely work together for mutual benefit. This chapter describes opportunities for improved integration of research into everyday planning and practice of public health programs and services, using two case examples of community-based, public health projects focused on common problems among older persons.

The chapter first describes an ideal dynamic relationship between research and program development and then uses a model planning process to illustrate the utility of research at each step of the process of implementing the program. Other less ideal, but nonetheless pragmatic, uses of research are also described in this section. Two case examples are then described: (1) the Hartford Puerto Rican Alzheimer's

Education Project, in Hartford, Connecticut, and (2) the Educational Demonstration of Urinary Continence Assessment and Treatment for the Elderly (EDUCATE) project, in Massachusetts. The specific benefits of integrating research into planning are described, as are problems, constraints, and special considerations. The chapter ends with suggested strategies for research-based program planning and development.

The Dynamic Relationship between Research and Program Development

The relationship between research and program development is—or at least should be—dynamic. Ideally, policy development and program planning and implementation are based on data, and each step of the implementation process is defined, structured, informed, evaluated, and driven by high-quality, objective, and timely research.

However, the reality of policy formation and program planning today can be quite different and considerably more chaotic. Relevant research may not be readily available to policy makers and practitioners, and available research findings may not be in a format easily applied to public health programs. Most scientists write for their peers, such as reviewers for, and readers of, professional and specialty journals, and not for potential users of research findings. Researchers tend to speak a separate language, have a different focus, and operate on a timeline removed from the current issues and needs of policy and program decision makers. Moreover, in an approach that invariably frustrates program professionals on the front lines, research often raises more questions than it answers. Practitioners and policy makers wince at what they so often hear from the ivory tower: "More research is needed."

The notion that policy and programs flow from a knowledge base developed by research is often stymied by the real-world considerations of public finance and politics. Studies are widely used to justify policy decisions after the fact or to sell programs to those who might provide financial support. Findings that lend credence to a program or help to prove its value take on enormous significance as programs compete for scarce resources. It is not uncommon for research to be conducted not as a part of planning a program, but rather to market it.

As we look at ways to include research more systematically in the planning process, the very definition of "research" becomes important. Our thinking about what constitutes research often has been too narrowly focused and limited, for example, to epidemiology or evaluation. A broader definition is in order, one that recognizes the multifaceted nature of research and involves the collection of information and development of data from an extensive array of sources, using a wide continuum of procedures and analytic strategies. In addition to the collection of primary data through interviews and surveys, research may encompass review of existing reports, secondary analysis of available data, or the collection of new data in innovative and sometimes unobtrusive ways.

A Model Planning Process

With this wider view, a model can be developed for incorporating research as a relevant part of each step of the planning process. Identifying the individual steps in this process can help planners ascertain what kinds of research might be useful and efficient methods for gaining needed information. Table 8.1 outlines a model planning process. Though twelve steps are described, the process may be conceptualized in fewer steps. On the other hand, it is likely that the process will go through several iterations as program development progresses.

Applying the model in the real world also involves corollary activities for the success of a program's development and implementation. These include, among others: identifying and "grooming" constituencies and support groups for the project, responding to funding opportunities, handling budget reductions, facilitating community organization and political action, and developing collaborations and interest groups.

Case Studies Integrating Research and Program Development

Two case studies are useful to illustrate these concepts for integrating research into planning and practice: the Hartford Puerto Rican Alzheimer's Education Project and the Educational Demonstration of Urinary Continence Assessment and Treatment for the Elderly (EDUCATE). Each project illustrates a collaboration be-

TABLE 8.1. A Model Process for Developing a Program

1. Identify the problem(s)
2. Select/develop a theoretical base/model
3. Develop goals
4. Assess needs
5. Identify resources
6. Set program objectives and identify deliverables
7. Identify alternative strategies
8. Calculate likely costs and outcomes of each alternative
9. Make choices and design program
10. Implement the program
11. Evaluate the process and outcomes of the program
12. Refine the program (Return to step 1)

tween university-based research and community-based services to improve the lives of older persons through public health interventions.

Hartford Puerto Rican Alzheimer's Education Project

Community leaders and service providers in the Greater Hartford area noted that Puerto Rican elders were not fully using health services in the community, particularly services relevant to the assessment and treatment of the memory loss and behavioral changes associated with Alzheimer disease. A partnership of community agencies, service providers, and university-based researchers was formed to address this problem. The first member of this partnership was the Institute for Community Research, a nonprofit, freestanding research and service agency in Hartford, Connecticut. The Institute for Community Research, which had developed out of the Hispanic Health Council, had a long history of innovative community program development and research. The second partner was the Braceland Center for Mental Health and Aging, a research and education unit of the Institute of Living, a large psychiatric hospital and mental health system. The third partner was the Travelers Center on Aging at the University of Connecticut Health Center. The University of Connecticut Alzheimer's Assessment Coalition had worked for several years in the Greater Hartford area to improve Alzheimer assessment protocols and services for patients and families. The coalition had the cooperation and participation of six hospital-based assessment sites.

The Hartford Puerto Rican Alzheimer's Education Project developed a series of interrelated research and service activities to improve understanding of the issues and to implement public health responses to this problem. Over a three-year period, projects were supported with funding from the Administration on Aging, the Howard and Bush Foundation, and the State of Connecticut. Interventions involved community education programs for consumers and service providers, design of improved and new services, and identification of community resources to increase access to care. Research was an integral part of the process of planning and implementing the program. Table 8.2 shows how research methods and findings were used at each implementation stage of the project.

Problem identification first occurred as an expressed concern by clinicians in the Alzheimer assessment clinics, but data from a doctoral dissertation and from interviews with service providers and minority community service personnel clarified issues. The problem was defined as inappropriate response to symptoms of Alzheimer disease within the Puerto Rican community and underuse of available assessment and treatment services. Contributing factors included lack of understanding of memory loss, misinterpretation of symptoms by Puerto Rican elders and their families, lack of culturally appropriate information, a service system that was not user-friendly for older Puerto Ricans—particularly those with limited English—and

TABLE 8.2. Planning and Research Interaction: Case Studies

Planning Stage	Peurto Rican Alzheimer's Education Project	EDUCATE Project
Identify the problem(s)	Survey of community leaders; previous research: community-based survey of elder Peurto Ricans (doctoral dissertation); previous demonstration project	Clinicians; focus group with experts, health advocates; previous research (EPESE East Boston Community Survey)
Select a theoretical model	Literature search	Literature search; key informant interviews
Develop goals	Focus group: project advisory board, including community service providers, academics	Team process including academics, clinicians, public health professionals
Assess needs and resources	Focus groups of community leaders, focus groups of clinicians; interviews with community informants	Data analysis from prior survey; evaluation data from former Massachusetts Influenza Vaccination Project
Set program objectives	Literature review; team process; advisory group	Literature review; team process
Identify alternatives	Literature review; key informant interviews; qualitative study of elder project; data from UCONN Alzheimer's Alliance	Literature review; data from EPESE follow-up, Massachusetts Influenza Project; HRCA clinical studies; housing resident interviews
Calculate costs/ outcomes of each alternative	Data from prior ICR community studies; literature review	Data from Massachusetts Influenza Project; review of literature
Design the program	Symptom depiction cards from anthropological study; interviews and focus groups with senior center elders, clinical staff, service providers	Clinical and public health experts; granting agency input (CDC)
Implement the program	Staged implementation; process data, provider input	Collect process data; problem solving; targeted implementation
Evaluate the process/ outcomes	Process data; outcome exit; 6 month/- 1 year follow-up data	Process data; outcome exit data pre-, postsurvey; utilization data; comparisons between intervention and control counties
Refine the program	Implementation special services	Project advisory group, team to identify ongoing services

lack of personnel and materials for Spanish-speaking patients. The theoretical model was identified by literature review and was based in educational theory as well as help-seeking strategies. Symptom interpretation and help-seeking behaviors are determined by a variety of factors that have been organized into several theoretical models. One such model (Anderson and Newman, 1973) suggests three categories of factors—predisposing, enabling, and need factors, each of which may have ethnic and cultural influences. This model was used to identify variables and to design the interventions.

Goals were developed using two focus groups, one comprised of the advisory board supplemented by community service providers and the other comprised of academic geriatricians and other community clinicians. The primary goal was to develop a system of Alzheimer disease services and resources for the Greater Hartford area. The focus groups also assessed the needs and resources available in the community. Follow-up interviews with community informants provided additional detail and clarification. Identified needs included improved knowledge regarding symptom experience and interpretation and help-seeking strategies, improved information for service providers regarding memory loss and health behaviors of older Puerto Ricans, and enhanced resources for the service system. At this point, a formal application was submitted to the Administration on Aging to conduct research to better understand Alzheimer disease experience and knowledge among older Puerto Ricans and to develop educational materials for the community.

Program objectives were set using research methods including a literature review, small group process using the research team, and a meeting of the project advisory group. Program objectives were multifaceted and involved several iterations of the planning process. Alternative approaches to meeting these objectives were developed using literature review, key informant interviews, data from the qualitative study of elders and data from the UCONN Alzheimer's Alliance Assessment program. Costs and likely outcomes of each alternative were weighed and the project strategy was selected. Data for this process were derived from prior Institute for Community Research community studies, literature review, and other community-based service projects.

The project developed several important resources and service improvements in the community. An educational strategy was developed and published, including a study guide, "Alzheimer's Disease among Puerto Rican Elderly: Educational Materials and Innovative Dissemination Strategies" (Schensul et al., 1992), with accompanying script, slide set, and case studies. This was published in both English and Spanish after testing in a community demonstration process. The research team, working with a Puerto Rican artist, developed a set of "Symptom Depiction Cards" to be used with persons of limited literacy to discuss symptoms of memory loss and behavior change associated with Alzheimer disease, as well as other health conditions. Dr. Schensul, working with other anthropologists in developing countries, had used similar cards to successfully discuss childhood symptoms and diseases. A coloring book (Rivera, Wetle, and Oritz, 1992) was published in Spanish and English to help children better understand Alzheimer-related behavior changes in their grandparents and other older persons. Papers for scientific communities were also published (Schensul, Wetle, and Torres, 1993; Schensul and Wetle, 1992; Wetle et al., 1990).

Resources were developed in the service community as well. Public education for elders was conducted in concert with development of culturally appropriate assessment outreach and assessment strategies. Translators were trained in the Alzheimer assessment process and were made available for Alzheimer clinics. Hartford Hospital's geriatrics program developed a specialized clinic for minority elders with support from the Howard and Bush Foundation and worked with community-based services to identify persons appropriate for assessment. Connecticut Community Care, Inc., cooperated in bringing case management services to elders and their families, using Spanish-speaking case managers and staff. Spin-off projects, supported by the local Area Agency on Aging, included educational programs for Puerto Rican and other minority elders on topics of patient rights, living wills, and improved communication with physicians and other care providers.

Educational Demonstration of Urinary Continence Assessment and Treatment for the Elderly (EDUCATE)

Clinicians and epidemiologists have noted a high prevalence of unreported and, therefore, untreated urinary incontinence among older people living in the community. A countywide, multifaceted intervention project was designed to step up reporting of symptoms by elders to health professionals and to improve the response of clinicians to incontinence symptom reporting. The Centers for Disease Control and Prevention provided funding to the Massachusetts Department of Public Health to conduct and evaluate this collaboration. The project involved faculty from Harvard Medical School, Boston University, and the University of Connecticut, working with staff from state health departments and local senior centers.

The EDUCATE project was implemented in two matched counties in Massachusetts, an intervention county (Essex) and a comparison control county (Norfolk), using a multifaceted, multi-focused intervention strategy. A full-day educational seminar was targeted toward urologists and gynecologists in the intervention county, providing them with educational materials, slide kits, and presentation guides as well as encouragement to present educational grand rounds at local area hospitals. All hospitals and HMOs in the intervention county had some type of educational program during the study period. Urology practices were visited by a geriatrician with special expertise in urinary incontinence, and educational programs were presented to groups of nurses in various practice settings. The message to professionals was to seek information from patients regarding symptoms of urinary incontinence and to respond appropriately. Seniors were targeted with a media campaign and with educational programs at senior centers, congregate living facilities, and other sites where seniors gather. The message to seniors was that urinary incontinence is a common but treatable problem, and they were encouraged to report urinary incontinence symptoms to health professionals. The success of the project was measured via pre- and postintervention random telephone surveys of health professionals and similar surveys of seniors in the intervention and control counties.

Table 8.2 describes the interaction between planning and research during development and implementation of the projects. Problem identification involved clinical experience and findings from a major epidemiological study conducted in East Boston, Massachusetts, with support from the National Institute on Aging as part of the Established Populations for the Epidemiological Study of Elderly (EPESE). The EPESE identified a variety of health problems and conditions among older, community-dwelling persons (Cornoni-Huntley et al., 1986). The study documented urinary incontinence as both a common health condition among older persons and a problem that frequently was not reported to health professionals (Wetle et al., 1995). Moreover, respondents to the survey indicated that, even when the problem was reported to health providers, the most frequent recommendation was to use pads rather than more appropriate assessment and treatment. Staff of the Massachusetts Public Health Department were also aware of the problem from their work with elders in senior centers and other settings. Together they identified the problem as being one of lack of information on the part of both elders and their health providers.

The theoretical model was identified through literature review and discussion with public health education specialists and involved a public health education model. Interventions focused on the patient are based on the health belief model, which postulates that health behaviors are determined by the extent to which help-seeking actions are viewed as valuable (Becker, 1974). The most successful interventions are multimodal, including the use of media and direct contact with target groups, as well as with the community more generally (Kottke et al., 1988; Puska et al., 1985; Farquhar, Maccoby, and Solomon, 1984). Interventions focused on physicians and other health professionals are based on the observation that direct training increases not only skills in health promotion but also response to symptom reports (Ockene, 1987; Levine, 1987).

Goals were developed by a team using a small-group process and involving academic researchers, clinicians, and public health professionals. To improve the continence status of older persons, elders must be encouraged to report symptoms accurately to health providers, and health providers must respond appropriately to those reports. Needs and resources were assessed using data from a prior community education project, the Massachusetts Influenza Vaccination Project—a highly successful educational program to improve vaccination rates. This information was supplemented by literature review as well as clinical research and a survey of senior housing residents, which was a collaboration between Harvard and Boston University faculty.

Program objectives were developed using the MASS Influenza project as a model, the team process, and data from the surveys. Alternative strategies were identified via literature review, EPESE data, and the surveys, and the costs and potential outcomes of each of the strategies were analyzed using data from the influenza project. The program was designed using clinical and public health experts, with input from the Centers for Disease Control and Prevention, from whom project support had been requested.

Program implementation involved the collection of process data for tracking objectives and for solving problems as they arose. The implementation was targeted so that problems could be identified early and midcourse corrections made. Project evaluation was both formal and informal and occurred at planned periods during and after the implementation phase. The formal evaluation involved pre- and post-intervention surveys of elders and of physicians in the intervention and comparison counties. The evaluation strategy also included evaluations of presentations and educational programs, knowledge tests of program participants, documentation of intervention activities, and informal discussions with community informants and the project advisory committee. Based on these evaluation activities the program was refined to improve educational and media interventions and to implement additional interventions with providers and elders.

In addition to the educational programs and media campaign, the project has had several reports and publications for a variety of audiences. An educational film, "Enjoy Life Today: Don't Let Bladder Control Problems Spoil Your Good Times," was produced and distributed to cable television stations and senior centers.

Informational brochures were developed and published in several languages including English, Spanish, Italian, Portuguese, Cambodian, Vietnamese, and Russian. Findings were also incorporated into ongoing training programs for geriatric physicians, nurses, and other health professionals at Harvard University, Boston University, and the University of Connecticut Health Center.

The Benefits of Integrating Research and Planning

At each step of the way for each of these case studies, from identifying the problem to fine-tuning an up-and-running program, the benefits of a process that integrated research and program development were obvious. At the design stage, research helped planners steer clear of failed approaches, adopt strategies that had been proven successful, and more effectively target programs to identified needs. It enabled planners to fashion programs that were responsive to community needs and that built on community strengths. Ultimately, planning in this way meant more efficient use of the community's human and fiscal resources. By demonstrating the credibility of the approach and documenting successes and future needs, the incorporation of research into planning also encouraged community support and the buy-in of influential constituencies and financial supporters. In addition, by documenting the project's outcomes and by providing additional data to be disseminated to other communities, programs could more efficiently be developed elsewhere, broadening the impact of the original project.

Challenges, Problems, and Constraints

Despite these positive aspects, the marriage of research and planning is not without problems and constraints. Many programs are fragmented, and there is little coordination among states and communities facing similar issues. The programmatic and policy system is often characterized by weak or nonexistent relationships between and among several key players—most important, university-based researchers and community-based public health services. An important question arises as to just how productive collaborative relationships are forged between researchers and service providers or policy makers. At times, ad hoc partnerships are focused on a specific project. More productive, however, are longer-term relationships that span several projects and allow opportunities for the development of trust and deeper understanding of the constraints, concerns, resources, and limitations imposed by the environments of academe and by the service and policy worlds. Several avenues provide opportunities for matchmaking between researchers and program personnel. One strategy involves internships that place students in agencies and programs for practical experience. Well-run student programs involve close working relationships between supervisory faculty and agency mentors. A second strategy would bring health administrators and practitioners serving older populations into the classroom. This would provide students and research faculty a perspective on the challenges and priorities faced by the health care system for the aged population. A third strategy is the organization of local conferences and workshops focused on topics of mutual interest and planned by representatives from both research and practice. For example, in past years, The Gerontological Society of America has sponsored a nationwide program to match and place university-based researchers into agencies and programs to conduct applied gerontological research on short-term assignments (Hofland et al., 1987).

Practitioners in programs for elderly persons frequently face societal ageism and a geriatrics nihilism that takes an inappropriately negative view of older persons and their prospects for productive lives. Public health professionals and policy makers often focus on younger populations, while medical personnel and the health system focus on the treatment of illness rather than on prevention of disease and excess disability. More recently there has been increased interest in the concept of "successful" aging and in identifying strategies to improve health, function, and quality of life even in very advanced years.

Lack of conceptual models and information on successful program strategies makes program development of community-wide service systems difficult and inefficient. Dissemination of information about successful programs is limited, and information about unsuccessful programs and how to avoid their pitfalls is almost nonexistent. Researchers often fail to provide clear outcome data relevant to the aging network that can be meaningfully used in specific strategies. The academic goals of the scientists are often inconsistent with the needs of the planning and policy process, and they may hold very different views on appropriate time lines and dissemination strategies.

How can these difficulties be overcome? A strategy for research-based program planning and development is comprised of several components. There is a need for multifaceted and multidimensional approaches. Public health concerns are complex, particularly for older individuals, and successful programs coordinate multiple efforts to "get the message across" and to change health behaviors. For example, the EDU-CATE project used print and electronic media to raise awareness, talks and focus groups at senior centers to educate and encourage symptom reporting, and brochures and posters to publicize the project. At the same time, physicians were being educated and provided materials to improve their response to reported symptoms.

Developing knowledge of resources in academic and service networks is another component of the strategy. The most important resources are human, and knowledge not only about the expertise of individuals, but also about who can provide access to information as well as other resources, is key. Another resource is funding for projects, research, or services. Collaborative relationships increase the likelihood of funding, not only because proposals are better written and more relevant, but because researchers and practice personnel may have access to different sources of support. In-kind and educational resources are another asset. Access to target populations is also a highly valuable, but sometimes overlooked, resource.

Being sensitive to the constraints and valued "payoffs" of each world is important. Researchers may not be aware that state health departments have mandated programs, personnel caps, and service populations targeted by legislative language or regulation. Area Agencies on Aging may have mandated programs, but may also have grant resources and a long history of coalition building among community agencies. Academic programs may have a strong knowledge base, technical expertise, and perhaps clinical personnel or services, but also may be constrained by the academic calendar and may view academic publications as the most important "payoff." Clinicians also have time constraints, may be focused by necessity on reimbursable services, and may be constrained by the bureaucracies and inefficiencies of the environments in which they work. Elder populations are also a resource, for purposes of needs identification, program planning and implementation, advice, and access to other elders. Early and real involvement of consumers is a key aspect of effective program planning and of successful research involving older persons.

Configuring programs to be culturally appropriate for specific subgroups of the heterogeneous elder population is key. Certainly, individual ethnic groups hold health beliefs, engage in health behaviors, and interact with the health care system in ways unique to their culture and experience. "User friendly" services are designed with these differences in mind. Similarly, persons in separate age cohorts may also have different experiences, education, and expectations of the service system. Efficient and effective services are carefully targeted to the specific populations most likely to benefit from the service. This targeting may be along cultural lines, but also may be determined by risk factors, health status, or functional ability.

Conclusion

The benefits of strong working relationships between the worlds of research, policy, and practice are many. The scientific community, program planners, and policy makers can take steps toward each other to strengthen research-based planning efforts. Practitioners should be proactive in reaching out to universities for assistance in accessing existing and relevant research and should play a role where appropriate in developing new research projects and in implementation of selected studies. This chapter has provided successful examples of the process and benefits of such a strategy.

The benefits of a renewed effort to blend research and planning will cut both ways. The value of research in improving the lives of older people and their families will be enhanced, and the programs and policies developed will be based on proven interventions. In an era of tightening resources and an increasingly elderly population whose need for services is likely to escalate, the importance of an integrated approach cannot be overstated.

References

Anderson, R., and Newman, J. F. 1973. Societal and individual determinants of health services utilization in the United States. MilBANK Memorial Fund Quarterly/Health and Society 51:95–124. New York: MilBANK Memorial Fund Commission.

Becker, M. H., ed. 1974. *The Health Belief Model and Personal Behavior.* Thorofare, NJ: Slack, Inc.

Branch, L. G., Rosen, A. T., and Stoner, D. 1994. Post-intervention Survey of Physicians for an Evaluation of the Educational Demonstration of Urinary Continence Assessment and Treatment for the Elderly (EDUCATE). Report to the Massachusetts Department of Public Health. Cambridge, MA: Abt Associates.

Branch, L. G., Rosen, A. T., and Stoner, D. 1995. Post-intervention Survey of Community Dwelling People 65 Years and Older for an Evaluation of the Educational Demonstration of Urinary Continence Assessment and Treatment for the Elderly (EDUCATE). Report to the Massachusetts Department of Public Health. Cambridge, MA: Abt Associates.

Branch, L. G., Walker, L. A., and Stoner, D. 1993. Pre-intervention Survey of Physicians for an Evaluation of the Educational Demonstration of Urinary Continence Assessment and Treatment for the Elderly (EDUCATE). Report to the Massachusetts Department of Public Health. Cambridge, MA: Abt Associates.

Branch, L. G., Walker, L. A., Wetle, T. T., Resnick, N. M., and DuBeau, C. E. 1994. Urinary incontinence knowledge among community-dwelling people 65 years of age and older. *Journal of the American Geriatrics Society* 42(12):1229–1329.

Cornoni-Huntley, J., Brock, D. B., Ostfeld, A. M., Taylor, J. O., and Wallace, R. B. 1986. Established Populations for Epidemiologic Studies of the Elderly. NIH Publication No. 86-2443. Washington, DC: National Institute on Aging.

Farquhar, J. W., Maccoby, N., and Solomon, D. S. 1984. Community applications of behavioral medicine. In Gentry, W. D., ed., *Handbook of Behavioral Medicine*. New York: Guilford Press.

Hofland, B., Smyer, M., Wetle, T., and Walter, A. 1987. Linking research and practice: The fellowship program in applied gerontology. *Gerontologist* 27(1):39–45.

Kottke, T. E., Battista, R. N., DeFriese, G. H., and Brekke, M. L. 1988. Attributes of successful smoking cessation interventions in medical practice: A meta-analysis of 39 controlled trials. *Journal of the American Medical Association* 259:2882–89.

Levine, D. M. 1987. The physician's role in health-promotion and disease prevention. *Bulletin of the New York Academy of Medicine* 63:950–56.

Ockene, J. D. 1987. Physician delivered interventions for smoking cessation: Strategies for increasing effectiveness. *Preventive Medicine* 16:723–37.

Puska, P., Nissinen, A., Tucmilehto, J. 1985. The community-based strategy to prevent coronary heart disease: Conclusions from the ten years of the North Karelia project. In Breslow, L., Fielding, J. E., and Lave, L. B., eds., *Annual Review of Public Health*. Palo Alto, CA: Annual Reviews 6:147–61.

Rivera, Z., Wetle, T., and Ortiz, J. 1992. *Learning about Alzheimer's Disease Coloring Book*. Hartford, CT: Institute for Community Research.

Schensul, J., and Wetle, T. 1992. *A New Technique for Obtaining Data on Symptoms of Dementia from Puerto Rican Elders*. Hartford, CT: Institute for Community Research.

Schensul, J. J., Wetle, T., and Torres, M. 1993. The Health of Puerto Rican Elders. In: Sotomayor, M., and Garcia, A., eds., *Elderly Latinos: Issues and Solutions for the Twenty-first Century* (pp 59–77). Washington, DC: National Hispanic Council on Aging.

Schensul, J., Wetle, T., Torres, M., Rivera, Z., and Rivera, M. 1992. *Alzheimer's Disease among Puerto Rican Elderly: Educational Materials and Innovative Dissemination Strategies*. Hartford, CT: Institute for Community Research.

Siegal, D., and Wetle, T. 1993. Film. Enjoy Life Today: Don't Let Bladder Control Problems Spoil Your Good Times. Massachusetts Department of Public Health: Fast Forward Productions.

Wetle, T., Schensul, J., Torres, M., and Mayen, M. 1990. Alzheimer's disease symptom interpretation and help seeking among Puerto Rican Elderly. *Geriatric Education Center Newsletter* (University of Connecticut) 4(2):1–3.

Wetle, T., Scherr, P., Branch, L. G., Resnick, N. M., Harris, T., Evans, D., and Taylor, J. O. 1995. Difficulty with holding urine among older persons in a geographically defined community: Prevalence and correlates. *Journal of the American Geriatrics Society* 43(4):1–7.

Chapter

9

Surveillance, Needs Assessment, and Evaluation

Susan L. Hughes, D.S.W.

The selection and evaluation of preventive interventions should be based on reliable and valid information about the health status, needs, and preferences of the specific population of interest. Recent advances in data collection have great potential to increase the relevance and impact of preventive interventions with older people in the United States. This chapter reviews the kinds of data that are routinely collected by public health and aging network data collection systems, reviews the strengths and weaknesses of the data, describes recent advances in data collection, and provides examples of how available data can be used to plan and evaluate the success of interventions. It also reviews the designs and methods that agencies can use to evaluate the impact of interventions and concludes with suggestions about how data can be improved in the future.

At present, state departments of public health and aging are funded by different sources at the federal level and serve different but overlapping constituencies. The two agencies also use different terminology and methods to monitor and collect data. Table 9.1 lists the types of data that are monitored by state systems and by national or regional surveys. As this table demonstrates, public health departments have traditionally tracked diseases and their risk factors using "surveillance systems." In contrast, state units and area agencies on aging use "needs assessments" to track unmet needs for a wide array of services that older people with all levels of ability-disability need in a given community. In many cases, needs assessments conducted by the Aging Network also include inventories of available services and providers.

TABLE 9.1. Different Types of Surveillance Systems

Public Health	Aging Network	Other National Data

Numerator
• Mortality
• Morbidity
  • Hospital discharge data
  • Trauma registry
  • Cancer registry
• Behavioral Risk Factor
  Surveillance Survey
• Community needs assessments
  and health plans
Denominator
• Census data
• HCFA beneficiaries
	• Regional (multistate needs
	  assessments)
	• State client demographic,
	  functional status, use data
	• State and local needs
	  assessments
	• National Aging Program
	  Information System
		• National Health and Nutrition
		  Examination Survey
		• National Health Interview Survey
		  Supplement on Aging
		  Longitudinal Study on Aging
		• National Nursing Home Survey
		• Minimum Data Set

Experience over the last twenty to thirty years has taught us that both kinds of information are vital for the design of preventive interventions with older people. Knowledge about impairment or disability informs us about services that are needed by older people. However, these data do not tell us which diseases cause the lion's share of disability and therefore should be high priorities for preventive interventions. Similarly, knowledge about the prevalence of a disease, absent information about its functional impact, does not enable us to prioritize disease-prevention interventions in terms of their impact on the quality of life or health care expenditures. Thus, disease-specific functional impairment/disability data are needed if we are to select and/or justify funding for interventions in a rational way and evaluate their impact.

Public Health Surveillance Systems

Historically, public health departments have used surveillance systems to track disease-specific mortality and the incidence and prevalence of communicable and sexually transmitted diseases. Public health surveillance is defined as "the ongoing, systematic collection, analysis, and interpretation of data on specific health events for use in the planning, implementation, and evaluation of public health programs" (Thacker and Berkelman, 1988).

Behavioral Risk Factor Surveillance System

In 1984 the scope of surveillance systems was expanded to include behavioral risk factors that give rise to disease. Originally, the Centers for Disease Control (CDC)

Behavioral Risk Factor Surveillance System (BRFSS) was limited to fifteen participating states. It has recently been expanded to include all states. The BRFSS is an ongoing series of monthly telephone surveys of adults that uses a standardized questionnaire regarding self-reported health behaviors (U.S. Department of Health and Human Services, 1995). It is conducted as a joint effort of state departments of public health and CDC. The state department of public health conducts the surveys and CDC provides financial assistance, the questionnaire methodology, and training. The questionnaire has three parts: core questions used by all states, standard modules on selected topics that each state may choose to add, and questions added by states on topics of special interest.

The sampling frame for the survey is based on random-digit dialing, with respondents chosen by chance from persons residing in the household who are 18 years of age and older. Thus, the BRFSS sample excludes persons without telephones. The survey asks adults about health behaviors and knowledge related to chronic diseases, injury, and HIV infection. Other topic areas covered include access to health care, self-awareness of conditions such as hypertension and diabetes, use of tobacco and alcohol, diet, participation in physical activity, weight and height, and women's health issues. Demographic data (sex, race, age, ethnicity, marital status, educational attainment, employment, household income) are also obtained. The BRFSS can be used by states to answer questions of particular interest, such as attitudes toward mammography among women over age 50 with different educational backgrounds, races, and geographic locations. These data can be used to tailor prevention strategies to particular market segments. In addition, the data from the core questions can be compared across states and between any state and all states combined. Thus, a state can rate its comparative progress in having an impact on important health-related behaviors.

Nationally, data from the BRFSS have been used to investigate the relationship between leisure-time physical activity and dietary fat in adults (Simoes et al., 1995). In 1990, twenty-four states collected data on participation in any of fifty-six specific physical activities and consumption of 13 foods known to account for more than 65 percent of intake of dietary fat in U.S. adults. Findings demonstrated that the two risk behaviors were strongly and inversely associated, independent of nine other demographic and behavioral risk factors. This relationship indicates that public health education interventions targeting one of these behaviors should also address the other.

Data from the BRFSS can also be used at the state level to assess progress in meeting targeted national public health goals. Current findings from the BRFSS in Illinois (Table 9.2) indicate, for example, that the proportion of the adult population that is currently overweight will have to be reduced by 14 percent, the proportion that smokes needs to be reduced by 36 percent, and the proportion currently not participating in leisure-time physical activity will have to be reduced by 19 percent in order to meet the goals of *Healthy People 2000*.

TABLE 9.2. Sample Findings from the Illinois Behavioral Risk Factor
Surveillance Survey

Risk Behavior	Population Currently at Risk %	Population at Risk Targeted by Year 2000 %	Reduction in Behavior Needed %
Overweight	23.3	20.0	14.0
Smoke	23.6	15.0	36.0
No participation in leisure-time physical activities	61.5	50.0	19.0

Source: Data from Illinois Department of Public Health, 1993.

Efforts at the State Level

In addition to national goals such as *Healthy People 2000,* states set their own internal public health goals. Illinois state goals regarding chronic disease, for example, are (1) to continue to reduce heart disease mortality, cerebrovascular disease, and cirrhosis; (2) to improve detection and treatment of colorectal cancer to meet Year 2000 objectives; (3) to increase screening for female breast and cervical cancer with the goal of improving the stage at which disease is detected in order to improve mortality; (4) to reduce alcohol and drug abuse; (5) to reduce smoking; and (6) to modify dietary, alcohol, and physical activity behaviors.

These state goals are being met through I-Plan, an attempt to mobilize and involve local health departments in meeting the goals of *Healthy People 2000.* In collaboration with a team of university-based health educators, the Illinois Department of Public Health works with local health departments to use focus groups and health indicators to identify needs and establish priorities and strategic plans for preventive interventions. I-Plan has replaced ten local health department program standards, known as basic health services, with public health practice standards and accompanying performance indicators that measure the core functions of public health. The new standards require local health departments to perform a community needs assessment every five years and to develop and implement a community health plan that addresses at least three priority health problems. The state also provides an important incentive for compliance with the standards. Specifically, fulfillment of the standards qualifies a local health department for certification, thereby entitling it to Local Health Protection Grants and preference for state grants for community direct service.

It is important to note that surveillance data constitute the numerators that are used by public health departments to compute rates. The denominators for specific age subgroups are generally obtained from the decennial census. However, more timely information is available for 95 percent of older persons using Health Care Financing Administration annual data on total number of Medicare beneficiaries by state. The availability of these data should enable states to monitor the need for and progress in meeting prevention needs of elderly persons both rapidly and reasonably accurately.

In addition to monitoring age-specific causes of death for persons over age 65, states collect a wealth of other indicators of the health of their populations. In Illinois, for example, the Department of Public Health uses Illinois Hospital Cost Control Commission data tapes to monitor age- and sex-specific hospital discharges by International Classification of Disease codes that can be matched with mortality data. All Level 1 trauma centers also submit data on an ongoing basis to the state's trauma registry. These data can be useful for the design of prevention interventions. For example, the number of admissions for hip fractures can be tracked at the county and even the individual hospital level. These data have been used by the state as a resource in putting together a recent application to CDC for funding to conduct an osteoporosis education/nutrition intervention. The advisory board for this intervention includes staff members from the Department on Aging whose role on the proposed project is to disseminate information about the intervention, mobilize the Aging Network, and facilitate access to groups of high-risk women.

National Health and Nutrition Examination Surveys

To summarize, in general, good data exist regarding causes of mortality and hospital use by older persons, and behavioral risk factors at the county, state, and national levels. However, data on chronic conditions associated with disability and functional limitations are considerably more sparse. Three ongoing national surveys provide some of these data. The National Center for Health Statistics (NCHS) conducts the National Health and Nutrition Examination Survey (NHANES), the National Health Interview Survey (NHIS), and the National Nursing Home Survey (NNHS). The NHANES I obtained detailed information based on physical exams, laboratory tests, and interviews about a limited set of chronic conditions and nutritional status in a national probability-based sample of noninstitutionalized persons aged 1 to 74 (NCHS, 1994a). For example, NHANES I reported both radiologic and physical examination findings for osteoarthritis of the hip, knee, and sacroiliac joints. However, the dataset is limited insofar as the timing of repeat surveys is variable, the set of conditions addressed in the survey is limited, the prevalence of disease is based on a physical exam—thereby excluding persons who are unable to come to an office for an examination—and the survey was limited to persons under age 75. Thus, elderly persons who are most functionally impaired were not included in measurement.

The sample that participated in NHANES I has been followed in a longitudinal study (the NHANES I Epidemiologic Followup Study or NHEFS) that to date has encompassed three waves of data collection in 1982–84, 1986, and 1987. The NHEFS has succeeded in identifying approximately 90 percent of survivors of the original survey and obtained substantial data on demographic characteristics (including household composition), medical history, overnight hospital and nursing home stays, ADLs, cigarette smoking, use of alcoholic beverages, weight, vision and hearing, female medical history, use of community programs for elderly persons, activity level, urinary incontinence, changes in memory, and location of death. These data can be used to identify physical and dietary risk factors at baseline for a number of outcomes, and can be generalized to the same age cohorts in the U.S. population. Thus, the data can be used to understand the natural history of the progression of specific chronic diseases and disability and the relationship between disease, disability, and use of health services.

The NHANES I was conducted between 1971 and 1974 and was followed by NHANES II in 1976–80. NHANES II followed the same format and design but focused on additional conditions. Specifically, NHANES II includes data on demographics, medical histories, diet, medications and vitamin use, and behavior associated with coronary heart disease. For persons included in the physical exam, data include X rays of the cervical and lumbar spine, chest X rays, spirometry, EKGs, body measurements, audiometry, speech, allergy tests, urine tests, and blood tests (McDowell et al., 1981). Finally, NHANES III was conducted during 1988–91 and 1991–94, with oversampling for children, older persons, African Americans, and Mexican Americans to allow for more precise estimates for these population subgroups. Some of the topics covered include high blood pressure, high blood cholesterol, obesity, passive smoking, lung disease, osteoporosis, HIV, hepatitis, helicobacter pylori, immunization status, diabetes, allergies, growth and development, blood lead, anemia, food sufficiency, dietary intake including fats, antioxidants, and nutritional blood measures (NCHS, 1994a). In addition a Hispanic Health and Nutrition Examination Survey was conducted (1982–84) to provide one-time data on three major Hispanic subgroups: Mexican Americans, Cubans, and Puerto Ricans (NCHS, 1994b).

National Health Interview Survey

In contrast to the NHANES, which is conducted at somewhat unpredictable time intervals, the NHIS is an annual survey that has been completed continuously since 1957 on a proportional household sample of adults (NCHS, 1986). It provides estimates of specific acute conditions, episodes of persons injured, restriction in activity, prevalence of chronic conditions, limitation of activity due to chronic conditions, respondent-assessed health status, and use of medical services—including physician contacts and short-stay hospitalization. All data are based on self-reports, and adults with all levels of disability are included; however, persons in institutions are excluded. A Supplement on Aging (SoA) was added to the NHIS in 1984 to track functional impairment associated with major chronic diseases (Fitti and Kovar, 1987). The cohort identified in this supplement was then tracked longitudinally for approximately ten years by the Longitudinal Study on Aging (LSoA). The LSoA yielded previously unavailable estimates concerning prevalence of disability in elderly persons. The LSoA may be repeated, but funding has not yet been obtained for this purpose. LSoA datatapes are available for public use and can be used to develop estimates of rates of ADL and IADL impairment per 1,000 elderly persons.

Data on disease-specific functional status represent a new and very significant enhancement of the NHIS for persons who are planning and designing preventive interventions for elderly persons. During the 1980s, NHIS obtained data on the number of bed days and days lost from work but did not track disease-specific limitations with respect to IADLs or ADLs. Thus, although it was possible to use NHIS data to estimate the prevalence of chronic limitations in older people, it was not possible to determine their functional significance. For example, we have known for a long time that the prevalence of arthritis increases dramatically with age and that it is by far the most prevalent chronic condition among persons over age 65. However, until recently we have not had good information about its functional significance. Recently the NHIS questionnaire was revised to ask whether anyone in the household needs personal assistance with ADLs and IADLs, what condition causes the limitations, what other conditions cause it, and *which* condition is the *main cause of limitation.*

Recently, the staff at CDC used the NHIS data tapes to assess the linkage between arthritis and functional impairment in a national sample of older persons. Findings showed that 2.8 percent of the total U.S. population experienced some or total limitation in activity because of arthritis. This estimate increased to 7.1 percent for persons aged 55 to 64, 9.9 percent for persons 65 to 74, 13.1 percent for persons 75 to 84, and 18.5 percent for persons over age 84, indicating a strong relationship between age and arthritis-specific disability. The age-adjusted prevalence of activity limitation due to arthritis was higher for women (3.4 percent) than for men (2.0 percent), higher for blacks (4.0 percent) than for whites (2.6 percent), and higher for persons with eight or fewer years of education, persons earning $10,000 per year or less, persons in the Midwest and South, and persons in rural areas. When these data were applied to 1990 census data and projected forward to the elderly portion of the population in the year 2020, the estimated number of persons with arthritis was projected to increase by 57 percent and activity limitation associated with arthritis by 66 percent, largely as a function of the high prevalence of arthritis among older persons and the increasing age of the U.S. population (U.S. Department of Health and Human Services, 1994).

National Nursing Home Survey

Although the NHIS now provides detailed data on chronic disease prevalence and disease-specific functional status annually on noninstitutionalized elderly persons, it does not include older persons receiving care in nursing homes. Persons receiving care in nursing homes are tracked by the NNHS, which does not use the same nomenclature or units of measure used in the NHIS or the NHANES and bases prevalence of chronic conditions on chart review (NCHS, 1989). The NNHS provides substantial amounts of data on residents and facility characteristics but the timing of its administration varies, depending on the availability of funding. The National Nursing Home Survey Followup (NNHSF) is a longitudinal study that is following the cohort of current residents and discharged residents sampled from the 1985 NNHS. It encompasses three follow-up waves conducted in 1987, 1988, and 1989. The NNHSF Mortality Public Use Data tape contains multiple cause-of-death information for 6,506 subjects from the NNHSF found to be decreased after linking and matching files with the National Death Index. Information on the tape includes the date of death, underlying cause of death, multiple conditions, site of death, region of occurrence, and residence. All NNHSF tapes include a patient identification number that is common across files to enable linkage between them. These types of data can be used to examine a number of different issues related to the mortality of elderly nursing home residents over time. For example, the use of a similar dataset showed that the place of death shifted after the implementation of the Medicare Prospective Payment System (PPS) for acute hospital care in 1984–86. Previous research showed that mortality rates decreased in hospitals after PPS was implemented but increased in nursing homes. This shift indicated that hospitals could be responding to fixed payment per admission by discharging patients to nursing homes who previously would have remained in the hospital until death.

Minimum Data Set

Although data from the NNHS are somewhat sporadic with respect to periodicity, a new source of very reliable data on nursing home residents is expected to be published in the near future. In 1987, in response to recommendations of the Institute of Medicine's Committee on Nursing Regulation, the Omnibus Reconciliation Act mandated the development and implementation of a uniform, standardized, comprehensive assessment instrument for all residents, regardless of payer. In 1990 the Department of Health and Human Services specified that the Minimum Data Set (MDS) be used to assess all nursing home residents residing in facilities participating in the Medicare and Medicaid programs (Morris et al., 1990). The MDS encompasses the Resident Assessment Instrument (RAI), which is conducted with each resident on admission, upon "significant change" in the resident's status, and at least annually thereafter. The RAI also encompasses Resident Assessment Protocols (RAPs), which are guidelines for more in-depth assessment of eighteen conditions that affect the functional well-being of nursing home residents (e.g., falls, urinary incontinence, cognition, use of physical restraints). In addition, residents are assessed quarterly on a subset of MDS items.

The reliability of the MDS has been tested in 13 nursing homes in five states. Findings indicate that items in the key areas of cognition, ADLs, continence, and diagnoses had an intraclass correlation of 0.7 or higher, indicating that the data are sufficiently reliable to be used for research purposes (Hawes et al., 1995). In 1995, HCFA issued a rule requiring facilities to computerize MDS data and submit them to state and federal agencies. Although the Congress attempted to reverse this ruling and to rescind the mandate for use of the MDS as part of its 1996 budget, public concern for continued regulation of nursing home care has forced the abandonment of this effort. Thus, it appears that very good data on nursing home residents will be available in the near future at the state and federal levels.

Reporting Methods, Controls, and the Future

It is important to note that reporting methods used in these national surveys vary from physical exam to self-report to chart abstract. This inconsistency in reporting method makes it difficult to compare rates across population subgroups. Our previous work indicates that the reporting method can affect prevalence estimates substantially. NHIS self-report data indicate that prevalence of arthritis is 631/1,000 in women and 481/1,000 in men over age 75. We recently studied the prevalence of arthritis based on self-report versus physical exam in a sample of 761 persons over age 60. Using the physical exam finding as the gold standard, we found that the self-report underestimated the prevalence by 16 percent (Hughes et al., 1993). Almost all respondents reported symptomatic or painful arthritis, but advanced age significantly reduced the probability of a valid self-report.

At present, except for the NHIS, surveys are conducted at sporadic intervals and use different classifications of disease and impairment. It also appears that secondary prevention or containment of morbidity associated with the presence of chronic conditions may not be as aggressively pursued as it could be at present. In Illinois, for example, state public health efforts have been devoted to closing a growing gap between white and African American mortality rates, reducing infant mortality, improving immunization rates for two-year-olds, and reducing the rate of unintentional injuries. Of ten health status priorities selected for concentrated efforts with respect to the Year 2000 national health objectives, only three—unintentional injuries, breast and cervical cancer, and chronic disease risk factors—relate to conditions that have high prevalence in persons over age 65 (Illinois Department of

Public Health, 1993). Furthermore, priority conditions appear to be selected on the basis of their relationship to mortality or communicable disease, rather than on the basis of their relationship to morbidity.

The types of items tracked in surveillance systems to date make sense, given the historic mission of public health to maximize life expectancy through the prevention of premature (e.g., preventable) deaths. However, we have reached a point as a mature industrialized society where the gains associated with a marginal increase in life expectancy at advanced ages may not be consistent with improved quality of life. Recent work by Olshansky and colleagues indicated that if we wish to avoid a pandemic of chronic disease and concomitant disability that is likely to be associated with increased survival at very old ages, we simply have no choice but to invest heavily in the prevention and/or management now of diseases that cause disability (Olshansky, Carnes, and Cassel, 1990; Olshansky et al., 1991).

The linking of disease prevalence and disability that is currently possible using NHIS data holds great promise for enabling us to identify diseases that are associated with high rates of morbidity. Using these data, public health departments can develop a set of target conditions for which secondary and tertiary preventive interventions are badly needed. To take the case of osteoarthritis again, little information is currently available about risk factors for its incidence. Persons with osteoarthritis have been shown to have decreased aerobic capacity, decreased ability to perform ADLs, and reduced mobility (Semble, Loeser, and Wise, 1990). However, a growing body of literature indicates that older people with osteoarthritis can participate safely in fitness walking and muscle-strengthening exercises (Kovar et al., 1992; Fisher et al., 1991). Trials to date have shown significant short-term reductions in arthritis pain and increases in physical activity (Kovar et al., 1992; Minor et al., 1989). However, the longer-term impact of these interventions is unknown and constitutes an important topic for future research.

Aging Network Needs Assessments

In contrast to reasonably systematic data that are currently available through public health surveillance systems, data currently collected by the Aging Network are considerably more variable and sparse. The Aging Network is headed by the Administration on Aging (AoA), which funds state Units on Aging (SUAs) in each state as well as Area Agencies on Aging (AAAs) at the local level within each state. The SUAs have voluntarily participated in periodic regional needs assessments, but these efforts are sporadic in nature. The AAAs conduct their own needs assessments on geographic catchment areas that may or may not coincide with catchment areas served by local public health departments. Generally, AAAs base these needs assessments on public hearings and publicly available data.

Recently, the types of data collected by the Network were significantly upgraded. Specifically, AoA mandated that AAAs collect systematic data on all clients who receive any of nine core services, including home-delivered meals, personal care, homemaker/chore services, adult day health care, and adult day care. The National Aging Program Information System (NAPIS) is expected to become operational by 1997, at which time it will include an identifier, Instrumental Activities of Daily Living (IADL) and basic Activities of Daily Living (ADLs), as well as demographic, service use, and cost data for each older person served by the Aging Network. At present, AAAs must use a unique identifier for each client but are not required to use a client's Social Security number for this purpose. The data are collected by the AAA and sent to the SUA. The SUA then aggregates the data and forwards the data in aggregate form to AoA. The NAPIS data provide for the first time a consistent numerator for the number of older people receiving Home and Community-Based Services (HCBS) at the federal, state, and local level. If these data are combined with functional impairment prevalence rates (denominators), they can be used to assess the extent to which the Aging Network is meeting HCBS service needs among the population at risk.

The extent to which AAAs collaborate with county health departments in the development of health plans and the extent to which AAAs have similar catchment areas is unclear. In general, the Aging Network tends to conduct screenings and multimedia health education campaigns. The Network appears to collaborate with health departments in an ad hoc way to promote interventions and facilitate access to high-risk participants.

Current Data Gaps

As the above review indicates, departments of public health generally collect data on disease-specific mortality, hospital utilization, and behavioral risk factors, but do not systematically monitor disability among older people. NCHS collects very good data on disability, but the periodicity of data collection across national surveys is uneven and the surveys use different reporting methods and measures, limiting the comparability of the data. The Aging Network is beginning to collect systematic disability data on users but does not monitor the relationship of disability to specific diseases. This chapter argues that both types of data are needed to plan preventive interventions for older people. Specifically, a critical need exists for valid and reliable information concerning the impact of specific chronic conditions and clusters of conditions in causing disproportionate levels of disability over time in older people.

Sepulveda and colleagues (1992) presented a set of criteria that should be used to gauge whether a health condition is a priority area for ongoing surveillance: (a) its relevance—is the problem a legitimate public health concern? (b) its vulnerability, the degree to which the problem is amenable to available interventions; and (c) the capacity of the health system to implement a control program. The application of these criteria to two different conditions illustrates how they can inform strategic decisions. Alzheimer disease is a highly prevalent chronic disease that is a major cause of severe disability and death in older persons. However, despite very promising biomedical research that is currently ongoing, no efficacious treatment is available at present. Therefore, Alzheimer disease may be a good candidate for surveillance, but may not be a good candidate for screening. In contrast, musculoskeletal disease is highly prevalent among older persons, and can cause differing levels of disability, but recent data indicate that the progression of arthritis-specific disability may be moderated by education and exercise. Thus, musculoskeletal disease would be a better candidate for inclusion in screening.

How can we use available data to prioritize the development and testing of public health interventions? We can determine from the NHIS which conditions have high prevalence and are major causes of disability among elderly persons, and from the literature ascertain which are amenable to secondary prevention aimed at the containment of disability and the maintenance of function. This list could include, for example, arthritis, arteriosclerosis, cardiovascular disease, vision impairment, hearing impairment, chronic obstructive pulmonary disease, diabetes, and cancer (Verbrugge, Lepkowski, and Imanaka, 1989; Yelin and Katz, 1990; Hughes et al., 1993; Patrick and Verbrugge, 1992). Thus, NHIS data can be used to select/prioritize a prevention strategic agenda.

In this regard a good example of a screening agenda was developed by Albert (1987). Based on a review of the literature, she compiled a list of sixteen screening interventions that providers could implement for clients. The list starts with immunization and ends with pharmacological iatrogenesis. Importantly, the second- and third-ranked interventions are exercise and diet, with more traditional topics like hypertension and cancer listed ninth and tenth, respectively.

Evaluation of Preventive Interventions

Once available data on prevalence and/or needs assessment have been examined and a decision made about the need to implement a specific intervention, planning for the evaluation of the intervention should occur as soon as possible. Evaluation research is essentially the application of social sciences to determine whether programs are implemented as intended and achieve their desired effects. Evaluations are very hands-on, applied, and practical. Many different types and levels of complexity of evaluation designs are possible. We begin first with a description of a more simple approach to evaluation known as formative evaluation and conclude with a review of summative or outcome evaluation.

Formative Evaluation

Formative evaluations assess the feasibility of implementing an effective intervention while the intervention is being developed and fine-tuned. They are appropriate in two situations. First, they are very appropriate to use when the intervention is new and in a developmental phase. At this stage, formative evaluations can include focus groups with key segments of the target population (for example, different ethnic groups or groups of male versus female seniors). The systematic use of focus groups with key stakeholders will enable intervention planners to assess consumers' views with respect to the importance, timing, and location of the intervention. This information will be critical to the successful marketing and promotion of the intervention. In some cases this marketing step can be bypassed by examining very specific data or market segments in BRFSS data.

The next step in a formative evaluation entails the specification of the target population, including its size, age, sex, and ethnic and geographic composition. This step should be relatively simple to accomplish because this information will already be available from the surveillance/needs-assessment data described earlier. At the outset of the intervention it also will be important to collect reliable and valid baseline information from intervention enrollees about the symptoms or functional domains that the intervention is expected to impact as well as their demographic, geographic, and other characteristics that would enable meaningful comparisons of enrollees versus nonenrollees. These comparisons can be used to fine-tune subsequent iterations of the intervention to improve its appeal to other segments of the target population.

Once the intervention is under way, it is important to monitor uptake among enrollees as well as adherence to the intervention. Certain hours of the day, days of the week, or seasons of the year, for example, may facilitate increased attendance. While the monitoring of attendance is straightforward, the measurement of adherence to an intervention is considerably more complex, especially with respect to behavior-modification interventions like exercise or dietary interventions that are implemented in enrollees' homes. Adherence in these cases is usually assessed on the basis of enrollees' self-reports, which have unknown validity. However, it is possible to bolster the accuracy of the self-report with preprinted diaries that participants can maintain at home and bring to group meetings at regular intervals. Although adherence to the intervention can be complicated to assess, it is important to measure, especially in cases where an intervention is in a developmental phase. Poor adherence is basically implementation failure, which can lead to the premature abandonment of an intervention that is theoretically sound but needs refinement to increase its acceptance by the target population.

Assuming the collection at baseline of good measures of the outcome of interest, and the measurement of outcomes at the close of the intervention, it will be possible to compare baseline/post-test differences in the outcome of interest to make some limited inferences about the effectiveness of the intervention. Although the absence of a control or comparison group limits the ability to infer effectiveness, good pre/post-test results in a formative evaluation can help agencies make persuasive arguments for further funding to test the intervention in more controlled circumstances in the future.

Assuming that some evidence of impact on the outcome of interest is observed, a next step in the evaluation would assess the duration of the impact over time once the intervention ends. This type of information is critical if we are to learn whether reinforcements are necessary to sustain change in behavior or lifestyle. It is also important to test the extent to which the intervention can be replicated and/or sustained using trained laypersons or by other equally inexpensive means. Finally, a debriefing with enrollees and/or a poll concerning their satisfaction with the intervention can be very helpful in further fine-tuning the intervention during its formative stage of development.

The preceding discussion illustrates the application of formative evaluation techniques to interventions that are themselves in a developmental stage. The other type of intervention for which a formative evaluation is appropriate is an intervention of demonstrated efficacy. If sufficient information is available from well-documented controlled trials of an intervention, there is no need to continue to test its effectiveness. However, it is important to monitor the intervention's uptake and its adherence among the target population. These data can enable interventions of known efficacy to be successfully replicated across ethnically and geographically diverse target populations (Mittelmark et al., 1993).

A description of the formative evaluation of an exercise intervention for older persons with musculoskeletal disease in Chicago may help illustrate the utility of a formative evaluation. Connell and Perlman and colleagues developed an Educize intervention in 1984 to test the feasibility of a multiple-component preventive intervention with middle-aged women with rheumatoid arthritis. The intervention combined low-impact aerobics with problem-solving discussions designed to promote self-care. Preliminary findings from a single-group pre/post-test evaluation showed significant improvements in physical and psychological functioning. Since the initial intervention was led by professional staff members, the next step involved training laypersons to conduct it. As part of this process, a videotape and manual were produced and eight lay leaders were trained. The success of the lay leader approach was tested with seniors with osteoarthritis in a series of sessions held at a senior center in suburban Cook County. The results were again encouraging, and funds are now being sought for a controlled outcome trial (Perlman et al., 1990; Connell, Gecht, and Conlon, 1993).

Summative/Outcome Evaluation

Summative evaluations are most appropriate when the intervention has been fine-tuned and has proved promising in previous single-group trials. Several different designs are possible, including interrupted time series, matched comparison group, and the randomized controlled trial. The interrupted time series design is by far the most economical choice, since it involves the pre/post comparison of existing trend data. However, in many cases valid historical trend data are not available on functional status or disability outcomes of interest. This design also is vulnerable to threats to validity, especially history. For example, if the intervention targets physical activity and the general population modifies its physical activity level as a result of widespread discussion of the advantages associated with this behavior change in the media, an intervention may show no effect.

Matched comparison group designs also are problematic because it is often difficult to accurately specify, a priori, the precise characteristics on which study groups should be matched (Cook and Campbell, 1959). Additionally, it is possible that two groups can be selected and matched on some measure that is unusually high at baseline, but later regresses to its mean value over time. Thus, the randomized trial offers substantial advantages vis-à-vis others discussed with respect to the ability to make clear and unambiguous inferences about the efficacy of an intervention. If this design also includes careful documentation of the costs of the intervention, comparative cost-effectiveness also can be computed, an issue that invariably must be addressed in assessing replicability. In addition to these advantages, a rigorous design can help attract funding for the evaluation and will also interest local academics who will be happy to collaborate in this type of effort. Collaboration with a local university school of public health, medical school, or center for health services research also can help the project access expert technical assistance for other aspects of the intervention, such as marketing and promotions.

One of the Multicenter Trials of Frailty and Injuries—Cooperative Studies of Intervention Techniques (FICSIT)—conducted in Boston provides a good example of an outcome evaluation. The FICSIT studies are a series of eight biomedical, behavioral, and environmental interventions to reduce the risks of frailty and injury among elderly persons. Seven of the eight interventions are being evaluated with randomized trials. The Boston site tested the comparative impact of strength training and nutritional supplements for ambulatory nursing home residents 80 to 99 years old who had history of, or were at risk of, falls at baseline. A multifactorial design compared progressive resistance exercise training, multinutrient supplementation, both interventions, and neither in 100 frail nursing home residents over a 10-week period. The mean age of enrollees was 87.1, with an impressive 94 percent completing the study. Findings included significant increases in muscle strength, gait velocity, stair-climbing power, and spontaneous physical activity in both of the exerciser groups. These findings enabled investigators to conclude that high-intensity resistance exercise training is a feasible and effective means of counteracting muscle weakness and physical frailty in very elderly people (Fiatarone et al., 1994).

Why Bother?

We cannot afford to conduct business as usual with respect to monitoring the health and functional status of older people. The likely alternative to doing nothing is a pandemic of disability that will accompany increased life expectancy. At present, 3 percent of health expenditures are devoted to prevention. If we are to increase funding for prevention, we need to have unequivocal evidence concerning interventions that work, can be replicated at low cost, and can be rapidly diffused. If we are to use existing dollars wisely, we need to target interventions at those conditions that have promise to yield the greatest payoff with respect to the reduction of disability. The new databases (NHIS, BRFFS, MDS, NAPIS) that are currently coming on line hold great potential to provide reliable, valid, and timely information regarding both chronic conditions in older people that cause disability, as well as the proportion of persons with disability who are enrolled in formal service systems. These data can be used to develop and test secondary preventive interventions aimed at minimizing disability among older people. During the 1960s and 1970s, targeted preventive interventions significantly reduced the mortality from heart disease and stroke. We now need to devote a similar type of effort to the containment of disability associated with chronic disease. Increased collaboration between state departments of public health and the Aging Network holds great promise to help systematic, effective, and widespread health-promotion interventions for older persons become a reality. The Aging Network can become involved in numerous ways, including assisting with public health needs assessments at the community level, helping specify conditions that should be tracked in existing surveillance systems, disseminating health education information, helping access target populations, and housing interventions in user-friendly environments. Collaborative efforts of this type have great potential to target scarce resources in order to maximize their payoff for society and for our future selves.

References

Adams, P. F., and Benson, V. 1992. Current estimates from the National Health Interview Survey, 1991. *Vital and Health Statistics*, (1992 Series 10, No. 184 DHHS Publication No. PHS 93–1512). Hyattsville, MD: National Center for Health Statistics.

Albert, M. 1987. Health screening to promote health for the elderly. *Nurse Practitioner* 12(5):42–58.

Cook, T. D., and Campbell, D. T. 1959. *Quasi-Experiments: Design and Analysis Issues for Field Settings.* Chicago: Rand McNally.

Cohen, B. B., Barbano, H. E., Cox, C. S., et al. 1987. Plan and operation of NHANES I Epidemiologic Follow-up Study, 1982-84. NCHS *Vital and Health Statistics* 1(22). Washington DC: Government Printing Office.

Connell, K. J., Gecht, M. R., and Conlon, P. 1993. Multi-media dissemination of EDUCIZE for arthritis. *Arthritis Care and Research* 6:622.

Fiatarone, M. A., O'Neill, E. F., Ryan, N. D., Clements, K. M., Solares, G. R., Nelson, M. E., Roberts, S. B., Kehayias, J. J., Lipsitz, L. L., and Evans, W. J. 1994. Exercise training and nutritional supplementation for physical frailty in very elderly people. *New England Journal of Medicine* 330:1769–75.

Fisher, N. M., Pendergast, D. R., Gresham, G. E., and Calkins, E. 1991. Muscle rehabilitation: Its effect on muscle and functional performance of patients with knee osteoarthritis. *Archives of Physical Medicine Rehabilitation* 72:367–74.

Fitti, J. E., and Kovar, M. G. 1987. Supplement on Aging to 1984 National Health Interview Survey. *Vital and Health Statistics* 1(21) DHHS No. PHS 87-1323. Washington DC: Government Printing Office.

Hawes, C., Morris, J. N., Phillips, C. D., Mor, V., Fries, B. E., and Nonemaker, S. 1995. Reliability estimates for the Minimum Data Set for nursing home resident assessment and care screening (MDS). *Gerontologist* 35(2):172–78.

Hughes, S. L., Edelman, P. L., Singer, R. H., and Chang, R. W. 1993. Joint impairment and self-reported disability in elderly persons. *Journal of Gerontology: Social Sciences* 48(2):S84–92.

Hughes, S. L., Edelman, P. E., Chang, R. W., Singer, R. H., and Schuette, P. 1991. The GERI-AIMS: Reliability and validity of the arthritis impact measurement scales adapted for elderly respondents. *Arthritis and Rheumatism* 34(7):856–65.

Illinois Department of Public Health. 1993. *Statewide Health Needs Assessment: Towards a Healthy Illinois 2000.* Springfield, Ill.: Dept. of Public Health.

Kovar, P. A., Allegrante, J. P., MacKenzie, C. R., Peterson, M. G. E., Gutin, B., and Charlson, M. E. 1992. Supervised fitness walking in patients with osteoarthritis of the knee: A randomized, controlled trial. *Annals of Internal Medicine* 116(7):529–43.

Kutner, N. G., Ory, M. G., Baker, D. I., Schechtman, K. B., Hornbrook, M. C., and Mulrow, C. D. 1992. Measuring the quality of life of the elderly in health promotion intervention clinical trials. *Public Health Reports* 107(5):530–39.

McDowell, A., Engel, A., Massey, J. T., and Maurer, K. 1981. Plan and operation of the second National Health and Nutrition Examination Survey, 1976–80. *Vital and Health Statistics* (Series I, No. 153, DHHS Pub. No. 81–1317). Hyattsville, MD: National Center for Health Statistics.

Minor, M. A., Hewett, J. E., Webel, R. R., Anderson, S. K., and Kay, D. R. 1989. Efficacy of physical conditioning exercise in patients with rheumatoid arthritis and osteoarthritis. *Arthritis and Rheumatism* 32(11):1396–1405.

Mittelmark, M. B., Hunt, M. K., Heath, G. W., and Schmid, T. L. 1993, winter. Realistic outcomes: Lessons from community-based research and demonstration programs for the prevention of cardiovascular diseases. *Journal of Public Health Policy*, pp. 437–62.

Morris, J. N., Hawes, C., Fries, B. E., Phillips, C. D., Mor, V., Katz, S., Murphy, K., Drugovich, M. L., and Friedlob, A. S. 1990. Designing the national Resident Assessment Instrument for nursing homes. *Gerontologist* 30:293–307.

National Center for Health Statistics. 1978. Plan and operation of the Health and Nutrition Examination Survey United States, 1971–1973. *Vital and Health Statistics* (Series 1, No. 10a, DHEW Publication No. PHS 79-1310). Washington, DC: U.S. Government Printing Office.

National Center for Health Statistics. 1979. Basic data on arthritis: Knee, hip and sacroiliac joints in adults ages 25–74, 1971–1975. *Vital and Health Statistics* (Series 11, No. 213, DHHS Publications No. PHS 79–1661). Washington, DC: U.S. Government Printing Office.

National Center for Health Statistics. 1986. Aging in the eighties, age 65 and over: Use of community services; Preliminary data from the Supplement on Aging to the National Health Interview Survey: United States, January–June, 1984. *Advance Data from Vital and Health Statistics* (No. 124, DHHS Publication No. PHS 86–1250). Hyattsville, MD: Public Health Service.

National Center for Health Statistics. 1989. The National Nursing Home Survey: 1985 summary for the United States. *Vital and Health Statistics* (Series 13, No. 97). Washington, DC: Government Printing Office.

National Center for Health Statistics. 1994a. Plan and operation of the third National Health and Nutrition Examination Survey, 1988–94. *Vital and Health Statistics* (Series 1, No. 32, PHS No. 94–1308). Washington, DC: Government Printing Office.

National Center for Health Statistics. 1994b. Investigation of nonresponse bias: Hispanic Health and Nutrition Survey. *Vital and Health Statistics* (Series 2, No. 119, PHS No. 94–1393). Washington, DC: Government Printing Office.

Olshansky, S. J., Carnes B. A., and Cassel C. 1990. In search of Methuselah: Estimating the upper limits to human longevity. *Science* 250:634–40.

Olshansky, S. J., Rudberg, M. A., Carnes, B. A., Cassel, C. K., and Brody, J. B. 1991. Trading off longer life for worsening health: The expansion of morbidity hypothesis. *Journal of Aging and Health* 3:194–216.

Patrick, D. L., and Verbrugge, L. M. 1992. Impact of and service needs for seven chronic conditions. Presentation at the American Public Health Association.

Perlman, S. G., Connell, K. J., Clark, A., Robinson, M. S., Conlon, P., Gecht, M., Caldron, P., and Sinacore, J. 1990. Dance-based aerobic exercise for rheumatoid arthritis. *Arthritis Care and Research* 3:20–35.

Semble, E. L., Loeser, R. F., and Wise, C. M. 1990. Therapeutic exercise for rheumatoid arthritis and osteoarthritis. *Seminars in Arthritis and Rheumatism* 20(1):32–40.

Sepulveda, J., Lopez-Cervantes, M., Frenk, J., Gomez de Leon, J., Lezana-Fernandez, M. A., and Santos-Burgoa, C. 1992. Key issues in public health surveillance for the 1990s. *Morbidity and Mortality Weekly Reports* 41(supplement):61–76.

Simoes, E. J., Byers, T., Coates, R. J., Serdula, M. K., Mokdad, A. H., and Heath, G. W. 1995. The association between leisure-time physical activity and dietary fat in American adults. *American Journal of Public Health* 85:240–48.

Thacker, S. B., and Berkelman, R. L. 1988. Public health surveillance in the United States. *Epidemiology Review* 10:164–90.

Thacker, S. B., Koplan, J. P., Taylor, W. R., Hinman, A. R., Katz, M. F., and Roper, W. L. 1994. Assessing prevention effectiveness using data to drive program decisions. *Public Health Reports* 109:187–94.

U.S. Department of Health and Human Services. 1994. Arthritis prevalence and activity limitations, United States, 1990. *Morbidity and Mortality Weekly Report* 43:433–38.

U.S. Department of Health and Human Services. 1995. *Chronic Disease Notes and Reports* 8:8–11.

Verbrugge, L. M., Lepkowski, J. M., and Imanaka, Y. 1989. Comorbidity and its impact on disability. *Milbank Quarterly* 67:450–84.

Yelin, E. H., and Katz, P. P. 1990. Transitions in health status among community-dwelling elderly people with arthritis. *Arthritis and Rheumatism* 33:376–80.

Chapter

10

Conceptual, Measurement, and Analytical Issues in Assessing Health Status in Older Populations

Anita L. Stewart, Ph.D., and Ron D. Hays, Ph.D.

From a public health perspective, health status needs to be defined in terms of aspects of health that can be addressed by the public health system and that are relevant to those who are the primary targets of public health interventions—namely, the more disadvantaged segments of the older population such as those of lower socioeconomic status and ethnic minorities (Markides and Mindel, 1987; Miles and Bernard, 1992). Issues in defining health are basically similar for older and younger populations, with the exception of issues pertaining to the increased diversity in health in older populations (Rowe and Kahn, 1987).

Defining Health

Among the many definitions of health status, the World Health Organization (WHO) definition is the broadest and most widely cited. The WHO defines health in terms of the physical, mental, and social well-being of individuals (World Health Organization, 1948). Most approaches to operationalizing this broad view reflect physical and mental health, but are less clear in terms of social well-being. For example, the Medical Outcomes Study defined health in terms of two underlying dimensions—physical and mental health—each with a number of indicators, although social health was recognized theoretically as a third dimension (Stewart, 1992; Hays and Stewart, 1990). Indicators of physical and mental health can be clinical (e.g., diagnosed disease, pathology) or they can reflect the perspective of individuals in terms of how they feel and function in their daily lives. Clinical status refers to diagnosed physical or mental conditions (chronic and acute) and physiological signs that reflect the perspective of clinicians and typically require clinical judgment. However, it is not the disease entities per se that are critical to individuals' daily lives, but rather how the conditions are manifested in terms of physical comfort, ability to function, and well-being. Further, many treatments can also adversely impact their lives. Assessment of generic rather than disease-specific concepts of health describe the "final common pathway" of various conditions and treatments. Generic functioning and well-being concepts also provide a way to characterize variations in health among those with no chronic or acute conditions.

There are numerous domains or components of health, such as physical and cognitive functioning, limitations in the performance of work and other daily activities, psychological distress and well-being, symptoms, energy and fatigue, and sleep problems. Although there is broad agreement on the various domains, there are nevertheless differences in how they are organized into an overall conceptual framework (Patrick and Bergner, 1990; Starfield, 1974; Stewart, 1992). Once domains are specified, each must be operationalized in terms of the content area or components and the response dimensions. Differences in content area and response dimensions account for substantial variation in definitions.

The content area pertains to how domains are defined. For example, physical functioning is nearly always defined in terms of walking, climbing stairs, and carrying loads. Some investigators distinguish various distances walked (across a room, one block, several blocks) or amounts of stairs climbed (one flight, several flights). Some definitions of physical functioning include complex tasks such as doing errands and laundry, and others include only basic physical functions such as walking and getting out of a chair. Some include discretionary activities such as walking long distances and participating in sports. There is also wide variation in the content areas of measures of functioning in daily activities, sometimes referred to as role functioning. Early definitions focused on major role activities such as work, housework, and school. However, as people age, these major roles may diminish in importance and/or may be replaced by other activities or roles such as hobbies, community activities, volunteering, and caregiving. Self-care (e.g., bathing, dressing) and self-maintenance (e.g., shopping, cooking) activities assume greater importance in older adult populations, as problems in these areas can affect people's ability to live independently.

From a public health perspective, which considers the entire population, the content areas of each domain should include the possibility of positive functioning and well-being in addition to limitations and difficulties. For example, when physical functioning is defined in terms of ability to walk long distances and/or participate in sports, it taps aspects of functioning that may be relevant to the more healthy segment of the population. Similarly, assessments of psychological domains tend to focus on negative feelings such as depression, anxiety, and loneliness. Underrepresented are positive aspects of well-being such as happiness, self-mastery, optimism, and overall satisfaction. Fatigue is a commonly assessed symptom, but assessment of levels of energy enables description of more positive aspects of well-being. One could argue that it is not within the purview of the health care system (or public health system) to improve these more positive aspects of health, but for descriptive studies, such definitions and measures enable characterization of the limits of good health.

Once the content area of each domain is determined, the next step is to clarify what it is about each content area that is of interest. Several types of response dimensions are possible. Because the various types of response dimensions yield different information, defining the response dimension is an important part of the conceptualization process. The majority of response dimensions for health measures focus on defining some level or state of a behavior, symptom, or feeling (e.g., how often a symptom has occurred, whether help is needed with self-maintenance activities, amount of time felt depressed, extent of difficulty walking). In addition, there is growing interest in determining the values or preferences of the respondents for the various health states in order to facilitate interpreting scores. One way to obtain such information is to ask respondents to *evaluate* their level of functioning or well-being in a particular domain (e.g., rate their satisfaction with their level of functioning or report how much they are bothered by a symptom). If people report being satisfied with an "objectively" poor level, it could reflect either a relatively low value placed on that domain or an adaptation or adjustment to poor health. Alternatively, there are a number of methodologies (e.g., standard gamble, time trade-off, category rating) that are designed to assess values or utilities associated with different combinations of health states (described below).

Table 10.1 presents a framework of potential domains, content areas, and response dimensions that could be useful in defining health status in aging studies. It includes physical, mental, and social aspects of health and, thus, is relevant for many types of public health studies. For each domain, various content areas are suggested as well as possible response dimensions, distinguished as either state/level or evaluative. The framework is intended to provide a menu of possibilities of measurement for any one concept.

The trajectory of health (e.g., prognosis, expected future health) is an important part of the conceptualization, although difficult to operationalize. Knowing the trajectory has implications for policy and planning as well as for the individual in terms of the meaning of the health state. If a person is improving or expecting to improve (e.g., recovering from surgery, responding to an intervention), a poor level

TABLE 10.1. Conceptual Framework of Health Status for Older Adults

Domain	Potential Content Areas	Potential Response Dimensions	
		State/Level	Evaluative
Physical functioning	Lower body (e.g., walking, climbing stairs, getting out of a chair)	Amount of difficulty (perceived or observed)	Satisfaction with level of functioning
	Upper body (e.g., reaching, carrying)	Need for help	Extent to which bothered by limitation
	Dexterity	Presence of problem	
	Basic movements (e.g., standing walking short distances, climbing a few stairs)	Extent of limitation	
		Able to perform	
	Discretionary movements (e.g., running, walking long distances)		
	Mobility, ability to go places		
Self-maintenance, self-care	Self-care (e.g., bathing, dressing, toileting, transferring, grooming)	Need for help	Satisfaction with abilities
		Amount of difficulty (perceived or observed)	
	Instrumental activities (e.g., shopping, errands, cooking, finances)	Extent of limitation	
		Able to perform	
Usual activities	Work, employment	Unable to do because of health	Satisfaction with ability to perform activity
	Child care	Any limitation because of health	Satisfaction with amount of activities
	Caregiving (of family, friends)		
	Volunteer, community work	Extent of limitation due to health in general or to physical health or to emotional problems	Quality of leisure time
	Hobbies, recreational activities		
	Work around the house	Extent of limitation due to specific health problem	
		Restricted activity days (e.g., number of days unable to perform activity, limited in activity)	
Social functioning	With friends	Amount of social contact	Satisfaction with amount of contact
	With groups	Extent of limitations in activities due to health in general, due to physical health, or due to emotional problems	Quality of social relationships
	With neighbors		
	Family		Extent to which bothered by limitations
	Spouse/partner	Extent of limitations due to specific health problems	

(continued)

TABLE 10.1. *Continued*

Domain	Potential Content Areas	Potential Response Dimensions	
		State/Level	Evaluative
Sexual functioning, intimacy		Frequency of sexual problems Presence of sexual problems	Satisfaction with sex life Extent bothered by sexual problems Satisfaction with level of intimacy
Psychological well-being and distress (subjective well-being)	Depression Anxiety Anger, irritability Loneliness Positive affect (e.g., interest in life, happiness, hopefulness/optimism, morale, enjoyment) Perceived stress Distress about health	Amount of time experienced various psychological states Presence of various psychological states Frequency of various psychological states	Satisfaction with psychological states
Cognitive functioning	Memory Confusion Attention Concentration Orientation Judgment Alertness	Frequency of cognitive problems Presence of cognitive problems	Worry about cognitive function Extent to which bothered by cognitive problems
Pain and discomfort	Pain in general Specific pains (e.g., back pain, angina)	Severity/intensity (on average, at its worst) Extent pain interferes with activities Duration of pain Frequency of pain	Extent to which bothered by pain Ability to tolerate pain Ability to manage pain Distress due to pain
Energy/ fatigue	Energy, pep Fatigue, tiredness	Frequency of states of fatigue Amount of time experienced states of energy, fatigue	Extent to which bothered by fatigue Satisfaction with level of energy "Enough energy to do everything"
Sleep	Sleep disturbance Daytime sleepiness	Frequency of sleep problems Amount of sleep	Perceived adequacy of sleep
Self-esteem	General esteem Physical self-esteem (e.g., physical appearance, competence)	Agreement with statements about self	Satisfaction with self

(continued)

TABLE 10.1. *Continued*

Domain	Potential Content Areas	Potential Response Dimensions	
		State/Level	Evaluative
	Social self-esteem Intellectual self-esteem		
Sense of mastery, control	General control Control over health	Agreement with statements about control	Satisfaction with level of control
Perceived health	Current health Future health, health outlook Past health Resistance to illness	Ratings of health Agreement with statements about health	Satisfaction with level of health
Life satisfaction	Current life in general Past life in general Components of life* (e.g., social life, life situation)		Satisfaction with life Extent to which needs met Contentment with life

Source: Stewart and King, 1994 (pp. 32–34). Reprinted with permission.

*Satisfaction with various components of life, such as social life, is sometimes defined by the evaluative response dimension in that category (e.g., satisfaction with social life is the evaluative dimension for social functioning).

may not be as distressing as if the person is getting worse. There are several approaches to assessing trajectories without actually collecting longitudinal data. Perhaps the simplest is to directly query if the person's health is better or worse than at some previous time point (Bindman, Keane, and Lurie, 1990; Ware and Sherbourne, 1992). Another approach is to assess perceptions about future health (Davies and Ware, 1981).

In considering concepts of health status as potential outcomes of interventions, we are assuming that such concepts are changeable or mutable. There is a growing literature suggesting that physical and mental health both deteriorate and improve in older populations (Chirikos and Neste, 1985; Schaie and Willis, 1986), even in those with substantial limitations (Manton, 1988).

Diversity in Health in Older Adult Populations

Whereas a younger population is fairly healthy on average on most health indicators, older populations are noted for their great diversity. Understanding more precisely the nature of this diversity can improve our ability to define and measure health in older populations. Increasingly it is noted that whereas in younger age groups the variation around good health is relatively small, older populations include a large proportion who remain extremely healthy as well as many who are doing very poorly on many of the domains of health (Rowe and Kahn, 1987). For example, Jette and Branch (1981) found that a great majority of older adults in the Framingham Disability Study were able to perform a variety of physical functions without help and without difficulty, even in the age category 75 to 84 years. This principle is illustrated graphically using national population data in which the average physical functioning scores declined with age but the variability increased (see Figure 10.1A) (McHorney, Kosinski, and Ware, 1994; Ware et al., 1993).

However, the extent to which the general pattern of decreasing average scores and increasing variation is observed may vary by domain of health. Schaie (1994) observed that there is no uniform pattern of age-related changes in adulthood across all intellectual abilities. Using longitudinal data, Schaie found that average scores of most components of intellectual functioning peak in the middle-aged groups (ages 40–60) and decline thereafter. When examining age group differences in pain or health perceptions, although there is some decline in average scores across the age groups, the variability remains relatively stable (Ware et al., 1993).

Some of the more subjective components of health may be more stable with aging, although results are somewhat inconsistent across studies. In a general population study (McHorney et al., 1994; Ware et al., 1993), average scores on psychological well-being remained approximately the same across age groups, as did the variability (see Figure 10.1B). In a longitudinal study of patients with chronic conditions, psychological well-being improved with age (Cassileth et al., 1984). McNeil, Stones, and Kozma (1986) summarized several studies indicating no association of age and subjective well-being; they also review studies suggesting that subjective well-being is stable in older populations. They concluded that subjective well-being may be a trait reflecting a tendency to interpret stimuli in certain ways; thus, it may be difficult to change. In the Medical Outcome Study (MOS), mental health scores were highest in the two older age groups (65–74, 75 and older), lowest in the youngest age group (18–44), and intermediate in the middle age group (45–64) (Hays, Sherbourne, and Mazel, 1995). Although research indicates that older persons may have relatively good mental health, the position of middle-aged persons is less well understood (Nelson et al., 1989). There is some indication that the extent of depressive symptoms such as depressed mood may be lowest among the middle-aged, but that rates of clinical depression (diagnosed according to clinical criteria) may be highest (Kessler et al., 1992; Mirowsky and Ross, 1992). Depressive symptoms are more prevalent among older adults (Kessler et al., 1992), but depressive disorder is less prevalent (Feinson, 1989; Weissman et al., 1988).

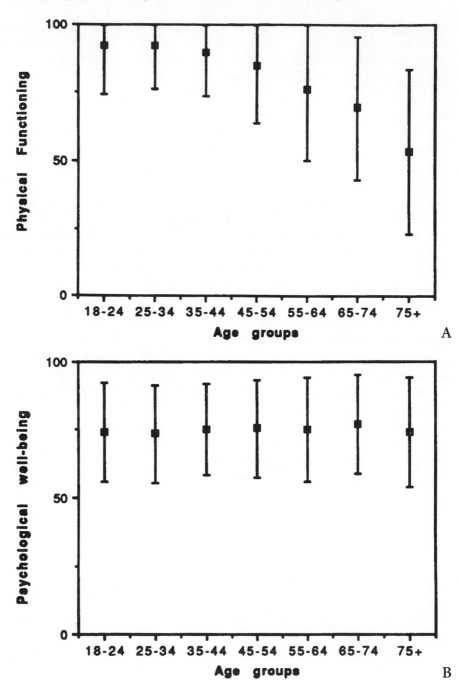

FIGURE 10.1 A: Physical functioning by age group. B: Psychological well-being by age group. *Source:* Data from Ware et al., 1993.

Measurement Issues

Data quality is of more concern in aging studies, primarily because of potential problems of subjects with memory, comprehension, vision, hearing, and dexterity. Data quality problems that can affect the reliability and validity of the health measures include not answering certain questions (omission), responding by not answering questions that are confusing or ambiguous (commission), tending to agree with questions regardless of content (acquiescent responding), and responding in socially desirable ways (Colsher and Wallace, 1989; Sherbourne and Meredith, 1992).

In any study, measures should meet standard psychometric criteria of variability, reliability, validity, and sensitivity to change. Because information on basic psychometric principles is widely available (Hays, Anderson, and Revicki, 1995; Nunnally, 1978; Stewart, Hays, and Ware, 1992a, 1992b), we discuss these issues only briefly and focus instead on some special issues concerning studies of older adults, which are not as widely discussed elsewhere.

Investigators often rely on prior evidence of the psychometric adequacy of measures in selecting appropriate measures. However, it is important to evaluate these psychometric features of measures in the group of individuals being studied to assure their adequacy for that particular population. This is especially important in studies of older adults because of potential problems with data quality.

Variability

Adequate variability means that the scores obtained reflect a full range of the concept being studied and that the distribution of the scores is approximately normal. Of major concern in assessing health in diverse populations is the potential for floor and ceiling effects. For example, if a substantial proportion of the sample score is close to or at the lowest possible score (a floor effect), very little information is obtained and change in the negative direction is less likely to be detected. Bindman and colleagues (Bindman, Keane, and Lurie, 1990) applied five standard Medical Outcomes Study (MOS) measures to a sample of patients who were recently discharged from a public hospital. Patients were followed for six months, and very small, nonsignificant changes were observed on the MOS measures. However, on parallel perceived change measures, substantially more patients reported getting worse than reported getting better. For example, on the physical function scale, 37 percent reported getting worse and 15 percent reported getting better. On closer evaluation, Bindman et al. determined that from 1 to 12 percent of the sample scored at the floor across the five measures. They concluded that the lack of measurable change was in part due to the floor effects that occurred by applying health measures designed for more typical patient populations to a severely ill population. The extent to which floor and ceiling effects occur depends on the measure being used.

Pretesting of potential measures can help determine the distribution of scores in the target population.

Reliability

Reliability is the extent to which scores are free of random error—that is, are reproducible, repeatable, and consistent. Because most health measures currently in use are based on Likert scaling principles (multiple-item summated ratings scales), internal consistency (also known as Cronbach's alpha) is the most commonly reported reliability coefficient (Cronbach, 1951). Cronbach's alpha indicates consistency of scores across parallel items administered at one time point. In contrast, test-retest reliability estimates repeatability of scores across two or more time points; thus, test-retest coefficients can supplement the internal consistency of multiple-item scales as well as provide reliability estimates of single-item measures. Although test-retest data collection is impractical in many studies, the importance of understanding repeatability warrants its assessment in at least a small subset (e.g., about 30–50 individuals). Reliability may diminish in older age groups, although it may still be acceptable (McHorney et al., 1994). For example, Sherbourne and Meredith (1992) found few differences in internal consistency for a variety of MOS measures across several age groups; when an older group had poorer reliability, it was still above 0.70. However, it should be noted that the MOS panel was selected, in part, based on the completeness of the data up to that point; thus, these reliability results may be somewhat inflated relative to a general patient sample.

Validity

Validity refers to the extent to which a measure or instrument actually assesses what it is intended to assess. Establishing the validity of a measure is an ongoing process, one that involves the acquisition of evidence about the meaning and interpretation of the measures from a variety of studies, settings, and samples. One validity issue that may be especially relevant in health assessment of older persons is that of socially desirable responding or "rosy" response bias (Carp, 1989). These reflect the tendency of respondents to provide responses either to appear favorably (e.g., active, functional, nondepressed) or well satisfied, even if they are not. Rosy response bias is more likely to occur when questions are asked in general rather than specific ways (e.g., overall life satisfaction as opposed to satisfaction with family life).

Sensitivity to Change

For purposes of describing populations or comparing subgroups of a population, validity in terms of an instrument's ability to discriminate among groups is sufficient (Guyatt et al., 1989). However, for studies attempting to examine changes in health over time, the measure must be able to detect small, but meaningful, changes over time. Thus, an additional validity indicator that is important when evaluating change over time is responsiveness (sometimes referred to as sensitivity to change) (Guyatt et al., 1989). Responsiveness refers to the ability of a measure to reflect true underlying change (Hays and Hadorn, 1992). The sensitivity of measures to change may be more important in studies of older populations than in other groups because of the importance of learning the extent to which dysfunction and diminished well-being can be reversed in older adults. In addition, because aging studies often attempt to use short-form or single-item measures to reduce respondent burden, and because as measures become shorter or more coarse they are less able to detect change over time, the evaluation of responsiveness is critical to the usefulness of such measures.

Although there is much written on methodological issues of sensitivity to change (Deyo and Centor, 1986; Guralnik and LaCroix, 1992), and appropriate methods for evaluating it are available (Deyo, Diehr, and Patrick, 1991; Tugwell et al., 1991), there is relatively little systematic knowledge regarding the sensitivity of particular measures or instruments. Changes in functioning and well-being can be compared to changes in clinical status, intervening health events, interventions of known or expected efficacy, and direct reports of change by patients or providers (Chambers et al., 1987; Wagner, LaCroix, Grothaus, and Hecht, 1993).

Some investigators are beginning to examine responsiveness (Bombardier and Raboud, 1991; Siu et al., 1993). For example, Wagner and colleagues (1993) found that restricted activity days measures were more responsive to change than were measures of physical functioning, self-rated health, or positive affect in a sample of older enrollees in a health maintenance organization.

Missing Data

Missing data are strongly correlated with age and frailty and occur more frequently among those minorities who are older, those who are in poor health, and those who are socioeconomically disadvantaged (McHorney et al., 1994; Wagner et al., 1993). The extent of missing data varies across health measures (Scholes et al., 1991; Sherbourne and Meredith, 1992), suggesting that some missing data may not be random and may be due to difficult characteristics of the question—including its difficulty and invasiveness. Because of these biases in the nature of missing data, the most important issue is how to handle it in analyses so that results are generalizable to those who are older or less healthy. Simply deleting cases in which missing data occur may result in serious listwide deletion problems in multivariate analyses and could compromise the generalizability of the findings. Some of the options for estimating missing data include use of the sample mean, use of the person mean (the mean of nonmissing items in the scale), regression estimates based on other data that are available, and multiple imputation (Little and Rubin, 1987; Raymond, 1986).

The extent to which data quality and psychometric problems occur in older populations is controversial and depends on the content of the questions being asked as well as the method of administration. For example, Colsher and Wallace (1989) found that although the percent of "don't know" responses increased with age, the extent depended on the nature of the items. It is important to determine not only whether data quality problems increase with age, but also whether the problem is of sufficient magnitude to seriously affect the interpretation of results. Some studies suggest that although data quality is negatively related to age, it may still be acceptable, even in the older age groups (Colsher and Wallace, 1989). For example, although time to complete self-administered questionnaires and rates of missing data were higher among older respondents, the percentage of those who had missing data for all items in multiple-item scales tended to be relatively low for all age groups (Sherbourne and Meredith, 1992).

Summarizing Health into a Single Index or Score

Despite the considerable agreement on the multidimensional nature of health, there continues to be a demand for a single summary score that can be used to describe overall health. There are two basic approaches to this—the use of some type of general health rating and the aggregation of health profiles (e.g., Sickness Impact Profile, SF-36) into indexes that summarize the profile scores. Summary scores and profiles fulfill different purposes; thus, we do not debate the use of one approach over the other, although this has been addressed (Patrick and Erickson, 1993). Instead, we discuss here some of the merits and difficulties that have been observed with respect to each approach as they apply to older adults.

Sometimes a measure of general health perceptions is used as a summary indicator. The most commonly used measure for this purpose is a single-item measure of self-rated health (rating of health as excellent, very good, good, fair, or poor). The popularity of this item as a summary measure is based on its consistent ability to predict future health and mortality in a variety of studies of older adults, over and above other measures of health status (Idler, Kasl, and Lemke, 1990; Mossey and Shapiro, 1982; Wolinsky and Johnson, 1992). However, general health ratings may be affected by different factors in older persons than younger persons, because of differences in expectations. In an analysis of determinants of health perceptions, older persons rated their health as better than did younger persons even though they had poorer health as indicated by measures of physical functioning, role functioning, energy, and fatigue (Mangione et al., 1993). The investigators noted as a result of these findings that global ratings may not adequately reflect other differences in health. Other research also suggests that general health perceptions are not adequate as a summary health status indicator. A British study found that women reported poorer health than men on all SF-36 scales except general health perceptions (Jenkinson, Coulter, and Wright, 1993). In addition, general health perceptions of epilepsy patients relative to patients with hypertension, diabetes, heart disease, or depressive symptoms were higher than were specific dimensions of health-related quality of life (Vickrey et al., 1994). Although the predictive ability of general self-rated health is clear, and its usefulness from that perspective is unquestioned, general health items/scales may be a poor choice as summary measures because of the lack of metric equivalence across age groups.

Another approach for obtaining a single score is to aggregate measures of the various domains of health (health profiles) into summary indexes. Numerous methods exist for doing so including summation of scales into higher-order indexes, utility methods, and nonutility methods such as derivation of integrated scores. For example, factor-analytically derived physical and mental health composite scores have been developed for the SF-36, also known as the RAND 36-item Health Survey 1.0 (Hays, Sherbourne, and Mazel, 1993; Ware, Kosinski, and Keller, 1994). In addition, overall summary scores for health-related quality of life measures have been derived by regressing criterion variables on scale scores to obtain scale weights (Bozzette et al., 1994).

Utility and preference approaches attempt to derive a single score that summarizes overall health such that the score reflects the value or preference for the overall health state. Utility scores typically range from 0 to 1, with 0 representing death and 1 perfect health. The values for the possible health states are determined either by obtaining normative value preferences (e.g., through use of a group of judges) or by methods that determine the values or preferences of each respondent. For example, the Quality of Well-being (QWB) Index is a preference measure in which normative preference weights are applied to each possible combination of levels of health on four domains (mobility, physical activity, role functioning, and symptoms) (Kaplan et al., 1989). There are several standard scaling methods for obtaining preference or value weights such as category rating, time tradeoff, standard gamble, and willingness to pay (Mulley, 1989). When information on utility and length of life is combined, the product is often referred to as quality-adjusted life years (QALYs) or well-years (Kaplan and Bush, 1982; Loomes and McKenzie, 1989). Such tools are considered useful for making policy decisions about allocation of scarce resources, where the goal is to maximize collective well-being (Mulley, 1989).

Despite the desirable features of utility measures, concerns have been expressed about how value or preference scores are obtained and how these summary measures are applied (Llewellyn-Thomas et al., 1984; Loomes and McKenzie, 1989). Questions have also been raised regarding the reliability, validity, and responsiveness of utility measures (Mulley, 1989; Patrick and Bergner, 1990). Standard gamble and time-tradeoff methods are often not feasible to employ with older adults because frail, older persons often have sensory and cognitive deficits. For example, in one recent study, only fifteen out of forty-one nursing home residents who were approached provided complete and usable preference data using the standard gamble, time tradeoff, category scaling, and rank-order methods (Patrick et al., 1994).

Practical Issues in Measuring Health in Older Persons

There appears to be variation in the extent to which older subjects consider completion of surveys as burdensome. Although respondent burden may be a considerable problem for the oldest-old and those with multiple health problems, some investigators have found that older adults enjoy interviews and even wish to prolong them (Rodgers and Herzog, 1992). Because many older adults are not accustomed to elaborate paper and pencil tests, a long self-administered survey may seem tedious. If questionnaires must be long, respondents should be encouraged to complete them a little at a time. Similarly, telephone interviews can be conducted in more than one phase (Carp, 1989), although this can result in increased rates of noncompletion of the second part (Rodgers and Herzog, 1992). Pretesting in a population similar to the one being studied can help determine the acceptable burden.

Most commonly used measures of health use multiple-item Likert scales because of their many advantages in terms of reliability, validity, sensitivity, ability to derive scores for persons with missing data, and tendency to minimize acquiescent response bias. Anecdotally, older individuals seem to be less tolerant of being asked a series of similar items, a belief confirmed by Wallace, Kohout, and Colsher (1992), who reported that older adults consider redundant questions as demeaning and irritating. They suggested that abbreviated forms of some of the more commonly used scales be developed. They further noted that the high internal consistency of many multiple-item scales is to some extent due to consistency bias, suggesting that many scales could be shortened without compromising their validity.

The formatting of the questions and the questionnaires both need to take into account the special needs of less advantaged segments of the older adult population. Guidelines for formatting are available (Aday, 1991). To the extent that recognition memory can be used rather than recall memory, data quality will be improved. For example, rather than asking respondents to write in the number of days or events, it is preferable to provide a set of predetermined categories (e.g., none, 1–5, 6–10) and require only that the respondent select the most appropriate category. The response options provide a context that in part determines the responses elicited from participants in the study (Schwarz et al., 1985).

Questionnaires need to be readable by those who may have vision problems. Allowing sufficient space on the page helps prevent confusion due to crowding of questions, reducing the chance that questions will be missed. Selection of light background colors to obtain the highest possible contrast facilitates this, as does use of a large type size (e.g., a 14-point font).

Determining the optimal number of response choices is somewhat controversial. Some believe that dichotomous response choices are best for the very old. The Geriatric Depression Scale is based on this premise and provides statements to which respondents answer yes or no (Yesavage et al., 1983). However, others have found that dichotomous items were disliked by most respondents because the restriction to two choices makes it difficult to adequately respond (Carp, 1989). In a study of older respondents' preferences for different formats, five-point scales were best liked and had the best distributions (Carp, 1989). There is evidence that the reliability of measurement plateaus around five response options (Cicchetti, Showalter, and Tyrer, 1985). Some have found that responses to five-point items more closely approximate continuous response data (Bollen and Barb, 1981; Johnson and Creech, 1983). However, in a study of different types of response formats for evaluative items in a sample of older adults, items with 10 response choices tended to yield the best data quality, whereas items with four response choices yielded the worst (Rodgers, Herzog, and Andrews, 1988).

Methods of Administration

Several methods of administration are available including self-administration, personal or telephone interview, proxy report, subjective ratings by trained observers or clinicians, and performance-based testing. Performance-based assessments are those in which individuals actually perform specific physical, self-care, or cognitive tasks (e.g., walk a specified distance, put on a shirt, count backwards from some number) and are assigned scores by trained observers according to a standardized scoring scheme. Selection of a method that will provide data of the highest quality for the particular population being studied requires an understanding of the comparability of each method. For some segments of older populations, such as those with cognitive problems or sensory limitations, the choices among methods may be more limited.

Self-administration is the least expensive and offers respondents the most privacy. However, it can be difficult for those with vision, reading, or language problems, as evidenced by the increased missing data when self-administration is used (McHorney, Kosinski, and Ware, 1994). Thus, use of self-administration may require extensive follow-up of missing and inconsistent responses. Personal or telephone interviews may be good alternatives. Although they are more costly and time consuming than self-administration, the savings in time needed to follow up on missing data and nonreturned forms may somewhat offset these costs. When personal interviews are used, the use of cards with response choices written out have proven helpful (Kutner et al., 1992).

For measures of physical functioning, self-care, and self-maintenance activities, performance-based measures allow assessment of those who are cognitively impaired and who thus could not easily complete a self-reported instrument. Disadvantages of performance-based measures include their cost and time, the need for special equipment and training of examiners, and the fact that they tend to assess individuals outside of their own familiar environment which may result in atypical scores (Guralnik and LaCroix, 1992).

The use of mixed modes of data collection combines the advantages of different modes to obtain the highest response rate and the best data quality. To do so requires an understanding of the equivalence of the various methods of data collection in terms of reported data. Herzog and Rodgers (1988) recommend a combination of telephone and face-to-face interviews because of the general demonstrated equivalence of these two methods. However, Weinberger et al. (1994) found relatively low correlations, among eight measures, between these two methods (correlations ranged from .33 to .77, median .61) in a sample of older adults. There is some evidence that self-administration is associated with higher reporting of dysfunction and illness, suggesting that it may yield more accurate (less socially desirable) information than face-to-face administration (Cook et al., 1993; McHorney et al., 1994). Another option is to begin with self-administration and provide help for those who have difficulty. For example, McHorney et al. (1994) found that a mailed questionnaire followed by a telephone interview yielded the best overall response rate in a general population, although they did not report these findings specifically for older adults. The equivalence of different methods may vary depending on the content of the questions (Cook et al., 1993; Rodgers and Herzog, 1987), thus future studies need to examine the equivalence of a variety of domains across methods.

Proxy Respondents

Often when cognitive impairment or frailty prevents older persons from responding for themselves, a spouse or family member may be asked to respond as a proxy on their behalf in order to obtain a representative sample. However, the need for proxies in general population settings may be relatively minimal. For example, in the EPESE studies of a general population of older adults, proxy reports were needed (at baseline) in only 2.0 to 6.8 percent of the cases across the four sites (Cornoni-Huntley et al., 1993).

Results of studies on proxy respondents suggest that some bias is introduced by using proxies, but the magnitude and nature of the bias depends on a variety of factors. These include the relationship of the proxy to the respondent, the amount of time spent with the subject, the nature of the questions, and the health, cognitive, and affective status of the person being evaluated (Epstein et al., 1989; Magaziner et al., 1988). The nature of the bias appears to be reasonably consistent across studies, with proxies tending to report poorer health and functioning than subjects themselves (Dorevitch et al., 1992; Magaziner et al., 1988; Rubenstein et al., 1984). Most studies focus on the ability of proxies to rate somewhat objective facets of the person's life, such as functioning or behavior. Less agreement might be expected with regard to more subjective information such as perceived health or feelings of well-being. Indeed, in a study of 292 individuals with epilepsy and their self-designated proxies, agreement was good for more observable measures of function (e.g., physical functioning), but relatively poor for more subjective, internal perceptions such as emotional well-being (Hays, Vickrey, Herman et al., 1995).

Selecting Appropriate Measures in Research Studies

When faced with choosing an appropriate set of health status measures, selection of a widely used tool can minimize the task and allow comparability to existing data sets. To the extent that the instrument has known reliability and validity and has been applied in various populations and settings, the likelihood that it might be useful in a new setting is good. However, such an instrument may not adequately focus on areas of special importance to the study, may not have measures that are sufficiently responsive to change in an area in which change is anticipated, and may include concepts that are not important to a particular study.

To be sure of adequately addressing the needs of a particular study, a more systematic approach for selecting measures should be taken. The selection of appropriate measures depends upon a variety of factors such as the purpose of the study, the setting, and the nature of the population. If the purpose of measurement is descriptive or to identify individuals in need of care or services, the type of approach may differ from a situation in which the purpose is evaluation of an intervention. Unfortunately, there are only a few general guidelines for doing so (Aday, 1991; Bergner and Rothman, 1987; Ware et al., 1981). However, investigators can examine methods of large studies with similar purposes and populations for guidelines and suggestions regarding measurement.

Perhaps the most common application of health status measures is to evaluate a health care or health-promotion intervention. In such studies, there are several steps that could be taken to select an appropriate set of health outcomes measures:

1. Develop a conceptual framework of the particular study including specification of the population, disease or condition, treatment or intervention, and relevant disease and health-related quality of life outcomes. The definition of each concept should include content areas and response dimensions that are likely to be affected either positively or negatively by the intervention. Sources of information

can include health professional focus groups, expert advisors, panels or focus groups of patients with the disease or condition, and reviews of the literature pertaining to the condition and its treatment. In addition, general impacts of a particular disease are sometimes identified by reviewing published disease-specific instruments.

2. Identify and review candidate measures of each health concept to determine the extent to which each one reflects the definition (has content validity). If there are several that might well represent a concept, further selection criteria could include psychometric adequacy (variability, reliability, construct validity, responsiveness to known change). Liang and colleagues (1985) discuss how to select measures with the best efficiency for detecting differences of the size expected to occur.

3. Select available measures fulfilling criteria. The challenge in this step is to integrate the best measures into the instrument or battery. Because many so-called disease-specific instruments include both disease-specific concepts as well as generic ones that are appropriate to that disease, this step may involve examination of possible redundancy and selection of the optimal measure among many.

4. Develop new measures as needed to fill gaps in framework.

5. Pretest entire instrument in a small sample of 5 to 30 patients similar to those in the main study to determine feasibility, acceptability, understanding.

6. Pilot-test entire instrument in sample (N = 100) of patients similar to those in main study; examine extent of missing data, variability (i.e., possible floor/ceiling effects), internal-consistency reliability, content validity, and construct validity. Evaluate test-retest reliability on a subset of patients. Revise instrument as needed.

The FICSIT study provides an example of this process. It is a multiple-site collaborative study of a variety of interventions to reduce frailty and fall-related injuries in selected target groups of older adults (Ory et al., 1993). The samples varied and ranged from community-dwelling to institutionalized persons who were frail and/or at risk of falls. The health measures were selected based on the following considerations: (a) importance of variable to the study purpose; (b) reliability and validity of measures over a range of health states including nursing home patients and healthy community-dwelling elderly; (c) sensitivity of the measures to change; and (d) burden to participants and staff (Buchner et al., 1993).

In studies of patients with particular conditions, a modular approach is increasingly being advocated (Aaronson, Bullinger, and Ahmedzai, 1988). In this approach, a standard comprehensive generic instrument is selected that best addresses the concepts of interest, and additional measures are included to supplement it that focus on concepts that are missed or inadequately assessed with the standard instrument. These supplements are often referred to as disease-targeted or disease-specific measures (Patrick and Deyo, 1989).

The large variability in health in older persons presents a problem when attempting to select measures that are appropriate for individuals at both ends of the continuum. A measure that will capture the variation at the low end of functioning (e.g., basic activities of daily living) may be limited by ceiling effects in the group of individuals at the healthy end of the continuum. If a large proportion of the sample scores near the ceiling (highest possible score), it decreases one's ability to detect change in the positive direction. For example, measures of ability to perform basic self-care activities (e.g., bathe, dress) in an active, healthy, older population would have ceiling effects.

Thus, comprehensive assessment of functioning in older populations requires a good representation of content at both ends of the spectrum as well as in the midrange. The MacArthur Foundation Research Network on Successful Aging has developed a battery intended to measure high-level physical and cognitive functioning in order to characterize the full range of functioning in heterogeneous older populations (Berkman et al., 1993). For example, the tests assessing cognitive function were designed to focus on aspects of higher cortical function necessary to perform complex cognitive activities. Tests were selected that were difficult enough to detect even mild impairment. This study focused on performance-based measures administered in the home; thus, the measures may be less practical for public health studies.

One strategy that might prove useful when assessing a broad population is to use a short screening questionnaire followed by more comprehensive assessment for those "at risk" (e.g., report some limitations). For example, the COOP charts developed as part of the Dartmouth Primary Care Cooperative Information Project and many comprehensive geriatric assessment strategies depend on this approach (Lachs et al., 1990; Nelson and Berwick, 1989).

Issues in Analyzing Change and Age Trends

A particular issue of interpretability of scores assessed at repeated points in time is that of changing referent points. As people observe others their own age becoming ill and frail, or as they experience more negative extremes of various health states, they may begin to modify their referent points for optimal or desired health, becoming more satisfied with less than optimal health (Heidrich and Ryff, 1993). This phenomenon has been referred to as "response shift" (Breetvelt and VanDam, 1991). If measures are administered over time, one might observe no change in satisfaction level or perceived health despite substantial change in measures of functioning. Some have even argued that the "retrospective pre-post assessment" is preferable to a prospective design, because of the likelihood of change in the frame of reference (Howard et al., 1981).

It is becoming increasingly apparent that the way in which health changes with age depends on socioeconomic status. Using a variety of health indicators in two large national data bases (Americans' Changing Lives, National Health Interview Survey), House and colleagues showed that health scores across age groups decline more rapidly for those in the lower socioeconomic strata than for those in higher strata (House et al., 1990, 1992). They also showed that the association between socioeconomic status and health is greater in older age groups. Thus, to appropriately interpret age differences, stratification by socioeconomic status is helpful. Similarly, the way in which health changes over time depends on gender (Maddox and Clark, 1992; Rahman et al., 1994; Verbrugge, 1989). Controlling for gender, therefore, may result in different associations or trajectories.

To understand how health changes over time with age, cross-sectional data of health scores by age group are often analyzed. The main problem with this approach is that health differences across the age groups reflect a combination of cohort effects (differences in generations and history), age effects, and survivor effects (health scores for older age groups reflect survivors to those ages), although it is plausible that age is explaining the bulk of the differences (House et al., 1990).

Cohort effects pertain to the substantial differences across age cohorts in life experiences, attitudes, education, economic experiences, and the nature of the health care available that could affect health (Bengston et al., 1985; Manton, Corder, and Stallard, 1993; Rowe and Binstock, 1987). Because the average age group (cohort) scores are based on the survivors, survivor effects can bias cross-sectional data by attenuating the strength of the decline. For example, findings that women have poorer functioning than men based on cross-sectional studies of the prevalence of functioning across age groups may be due in part to selective mortality (women with functional limitations are more likely to survive than men with functional limitations at any given age) (Manton, 1988). Manton found that these apparent gender differences did not exist when longitudinal studies of the onset of disability were conducted. Two studies have found general health ratings to be higher (better) in old-old age groups compared to young-old (Ferraro, 1980; Linn and Linn, 1980), suggesting that survivor effects are being manifested. Studies comparing age cohorts need to control for these other important differences to the extent possible.

Studies of within-group changes over time may more closely approximate true age changes. However, longitudinal studies of older adults also suffer from selective dropout. That is, those who are healthiest (physically or mentally) are more likely to remain in a study and complete all study forms, whereas those with problems tend to drop out or die. Thus, trends over time are reported for the most healthy portion of the original sample. This problem is more likely to occur in older age groups. Siegler and Botwinick (1979) found that among those aged 64 to 74, those who dropped out between the first and the second annual assessment had significantly lower scores on intellectual ability (WAIS) than those who remained over the entire 20-year portion of the study. When examining those aged 60 to 64, this selective dropout was not observed.

Summary

Health status is best defined from the perspective of the individual rather than the clinician, because generic concepts of health reflect the final common pathway of multiple chronic conditions and treatments. Although health is generally defined similarly for older and younger persons, definitions need to account for the diversity in health status in older populations and should incorporate positive as well as negative aspects of health. Consideration of the dynamic nature of health and of the way in which individuals evaluate their current health state can enrich understanding of the health status of an individual. The increasing diversity in health among older adults may be limited to the more physical domains of health status; psychological domains may be more stable across age groups.

Because of potential data quality problems, it is important to monitor psychometric features of measures in all studies of older adults. In particular, attention should be paid to floor and ceiling effects when measures are applied in diverse populations in order to assess the ability of a study to detect change. Pretesting of measures can determine to some extent in advance if the selected measures will have sufficient variability and data quality to meet the needs of the study. Missing data can serve as a clue that measures are presenting some difficulty to respondents, thus leading to selection of alternative measures or modification of the measures. General health perceptions measures yield summary evaluations of health status, but previous research indicates that interpreting these measures may be problematic in older adult studies.

Finally, adopting an existing set of measures should be possible for most situations, as a number of appropriate measures exist for studying older adults. However, we encourage investigators to continue to test existing measures and modify them when necessary to assure optimum data quality. It would be beneficial if studies of older adults routinely incorporated methodological components to allow for accumulation of knowledge about how well the measures work in these populations.

References

Aaronson, N. K., Bullinger, M., and Ahmedzai, S. 1988. A modular approach to quality of life in cancer clinical trials. *Recent Results in Cancer Research* 101:231–49.

Aday, L. A. 1991. *Designing and Conducting Health Surveys: A Comprehensive Guide.* San Francisco: Jossey-Bass.

Bengston, V. L., Cutler, N. E., Mangen, D. J., and Marshall, V. W. 1985. Generations, cohorts, and relations between age groups. In Binstock, R. H., and Shanas, E., eds., *Handbook of Aging and the Social Sciences* (2nd ed., pp. 304–38). New York: Van Nostrand Reinhold Company.

Bergner, M., and Rothman, M. L. 1987. Health status measures: An overview and guide for selection. *American Review of Public Health* 8:191–210.

Berkman, L. F., Seeman, T. E., Albert, M., Blazer, D., Kahn, R., Mohs, R., Finch, C., Schneider, E., Cotman, C., McClearn, G., Nesselroade, J., Featherman, D., Garmezy, N., McKhann, G., Brim, G., Prager, D., and Rowe, J. 1993. High, usual, and impaired functioning in community-dwelling older men and women: Findings from the MacArthur Foundation Research Network on Successful Aging. *Journal of Clinical Epidemiology* 46:1129–40.

Bindman, A. B., Keane, D., and Lurie, N. 1990. Measuring health changes among severely ill patients: The floor phenomenon. *Medical Care* 28:1142–52.

Bollen, K. A., and Barb, K. H. 1981. Pearson's R and coarsely categorized measures. *American Sociological Review* 46:232–39.

Bombardier, C., and Raboud, J. 1991. A comparison of health-related quality-of-life measures for rheumatoid arthritis research. *Controlled Clinical Trials* 12:S243–56.

Bozzette, S. A., Hays, R. D., Berry, S., and Kanouse, D. 1994. A perceived health index for use in persons with advanced HIV disease: Derivation, reliability, and validity. *Medical Care* 32:716–31.

Breetvelt, I. S., and VanDam, F. S. A. M. 1991. Underreporting by cancer patients: The case of response shift. *Social Science and Medicine* 32:981–87.

Buchner, D. M., Hornbrook, M. C., Kutner, N. G., Tinetti, M. E., Ory, M. G., Mulrow, C. D., Schechtman, K. B., Gerety, M. B., Fiatarone, M. A., Wolf, S. L., Rossiter, J., Arfken, C., Kanten, K., Lipsitz, L. A., Sattin, R. W., DeNino, L. A., and The FICSIT Group. 1993. Development of the common data base for the FICSIT trials. *Journal of the American Geriatrics Society* 41:297–308.

Carp, F. M. 1989. Maximizing data quality in community studies of older people. In Lawton, M. P., and Herzog, A. R., eds., *Special Research Methods for Gerontology* (pp. 93–122). Amityville, NY: Baywood Publishing Co.

Cassileth, B. R., Lusk, E. J., Strouse, T. B., Miller, D. S., Brown, L. L., Cross, P. A., and Tenaglia, A. N. 1984. Psychosocial status in chronic illness: A comparative analysis of six diagnostic groups. *New England Journal of Medicine* 311:506–11.

Chambers, L. W., Haight, M., Norman, G., and MacDonald, L. 1987. Sensitivity to change and the effect of mode of administration on health status measurement. *Medical Care* 25:470–80.

Chirikos, T. N., and Neste, G. 1985. Longitudinal analysis of functional disabilities in older men. *Journal of Gerontology* 40:426–33.

Cicchetti, D. V., Showalter, D., and Tyrer, P. J. 1985. The effect of number of rating scale categories on levels of interrater reliability: A Monte Carlo investigation. *Applied Psychological Measurement* 9:31–36.

Colsher, P. L., and Wallace, R. B. 1989. Data quality and age: Health and psychobehavioral correlates of item nonresponse and inconsistent responses. *Journal of Gerontology* 44:P45–52.

Cook, D. J., Guyatt, G. H., Juniper, E., Griffith, L., McIlroy, W., Willan, A., Jaeschke, R., and Epstein, R. 1993. Interviewer versus self-administered questionnaires in developing a disease-specific health-related quality of life instrument for asthma. *Journal of Clinical Epidemiology* 46:529–34.

Cornoni-Huntley, J., Ostfeld, A. M., Talor, J. O., Wallace, R. B., Blazer, D., Berkman, L. F., Evans, D. A., Kohout, F. J., Lemke, J. H., Scherr, P. A., and Korper, S. P. 1993. Established populations for epidemiologic studies of the elderly: Study design and methodology. *Aging: Clinical and Experimental Research* 5:27–37.

Cronbach, L. J. 1951. Coefficient alpha and the internal structure of tests. *Psychometrika* 16:297–334.

Davies, A. R., and Ware, J. E. 1981. *Measuring Health Perceptions in the Health Insurance Experiment.* Santa Monica, CA: The Rand Corporation.

Deyo, R. A., and Centor, R. M. 1986. Assessing the responsiveness of functional scales to clinical change: An analogy to diagnostic test performance. *Journal of Chronic Disease* 39:897–906.

Deyo, R. A., Diehr, P., and Patrick, D. L. 1991. Reproducibility and responsiveness of health status measures [Supplement]. *Controlled Clinical Trials* 12:S142–58.

Dorevitch, M. I., Cossar, R. M., Bailey, F. J., Bisset, T., Lewis, S. J., Wise, L. A., and MacLennan, W. J. 1992. The accuracy of self and informant ratings of physical functional capacity in the elderly. *Journal of Clinical Epidemiology* 45:791–98.

Epstein, A. M., Hall, J. A., Tognetti, J., Son, L. H., and Conant, L., Jr. 1989. Using proxies to evaluate quality of life: Can they provide valid information about patients' health status and satisfaction with medical care? [Supplement]. *Medical Care* 27:S91–98.

Feinson, M. C. 1989. Are psychological disorders most prevalent among older adults? Examining the evidence. *Social Science and Medicine* 29:1175–81.

Ferraro, K. F. 1980. Self-ratings of health among the old and the old-old. *Journal of Health and Social Behavior* 21:377–83.

Guralnik, J. M., and LaCroix, A. Z. 1992. Assessing physical function in older populations. In R. B. Wallace and R. F. Woolson, eds., *The Epidemiologic Study of the Elderly* (pp. 159–81). New York: Oxford University Press.

Guyatt, G. H., Deyo, R. A., Charlson, M., Levine, M. N., and Mitchell, A. 1989. Responsiveness and validity in health status measurement: A clarification. *Journal of Clinical Epidemiology* 42:403–8.

Hays, R. D., and Hadorn, D. 1992. Responsiveness to change: An aspect of validity, not a separate dimension. *Quality of Life Research* 1:73–75.

Hays, R. D., and Stewart, A. L. 1990. The structure of self-reported health in chronic disease patients. *Psychological Assessment: A Journal of Consulting and Clinical Psychology* 2:22–30.

Hays, R. D., Anderson, R., and Revicki, D. A. 1995. Psychometric evaluation and interpretation of health-related quality of life data. In Shumaker, S., and Berzon, R., eds., *The International Assessment of Health-Related Quality of Life: Theory, Translation Measurement and Analysis* (pp. 103–14). Oxford: Rapid Communications.

Hays, R. D., Sherbourne, C. D., and Mazel, R. M. 1993. The RAND 36-item health survey 1.0. *Health Economics* 2:217–27.

Hays, R. D., Sherbourne, C. D., and Mazel, R. M. 1995. *User's manual for the medical outcomes Study (MOS) Core Measures of Health-Related Quality of Life (MR-162-RC).* Santa Monica, CA: The Rand Corporation.

Hays, R. D., Vickrey, B., Hermann, B., Perrine, K., Cramer, J., Meador, K., and Spritzer, K., and Devinsky, O. 1995. Agreement between self- and proxy-reports of health-related quality of life in epilepsy patients. *Quality of Life Research* 4:159–68.

Heidrich, S. M., and Ryff, C. D. 1993. The role of social comparisons processes in the psychological adaptation of elderly adults. *Journal of Gerontology: Psychological Sciences* 48:P127–36.

Herzog, A. R., and Rodgers, W. L. 1988. Interviewing older adults: Mode comparison using data from a face-to-face survey and a telephone resurvey. *Public Opinion Quarterly* 52:84–99.

House, J. S., Kessler, R. C., Herzog, A. R., Mero, R. P., Kinney, A. M., and Breslow, M. 1990. Age, socioeconomic status, and health. *Milbank Quarterly* 68:383–411.

House, J. S., Kessler, R. C., Herzog, A. R., Mero, R. P., Kinney, A. M., and Breslow, M. J. 1992. Social stratification, age, and health. In Schaie, K. W., Blazer, D., and House, J. S., eds., *Aging, Health Behaviors, and Health Outcomes* (pp. 1–32). Hillsdale, NJ: Lawrence Erlbaum Associates.

Howard, G. S., Millham, J., Slaten, S., and O'Donnell, L. 1981. Influence of subject response style effects on retrospective measures. *Applied Psychological Measurement* 5:89–100.

Idler, E. L., Kasl, S. V., and Lemke, J. H. 1990. Self-evaluated health and mortality among the elderly in New Haven, Connecticut, and Iowa and Washington Counties, Iowa, 1982–1986. *American Journal of Epidemiology* 131:91–103.

Jenkinson, C., Coulter, A., and Wright, L. 1993. Short Form 36 (SF 36) Health Survey Questionnaire: Normative data for adults of working age. *British Medical Journal* 306:1437–40.

Jette, A. M., and Branch, L. G. 1981. The Framingham Disability Study: II. Physical disability among the aging. *American Journal of Public Health* 71:1211–16.

Johnson, D. R., and Creech, J. C. 1983. Ordinal measures in multiple indicator models: A simulation study of categorization error. *American Sociological Review* 48:398–407.

Kaplan, R. M., and Bush, J. W. 1982. Health-related quality of life measurement for evaluation research and policy analysis. *Health Psychology* 1:61–80.

Kaplan, R. M., Anderson, J. P., Wu, A. W., Mathews, C., Kozin, F., and Orenstein, D. 1989. The Quality of Well-Being Scale: Applications in AIDS, cystic fibrosis, and arthritis [Supplement]. *Medical Care* 27:S27–43.

Kessler, R. C., Foster, C., Webster, P. S., and House, J. S. 1992. The relationship between age and depressive symptoms in two national surveys. *Psychology and Aging* 7:119–26.

Kutner, N. G., Ory, M. G., Baker, D. I., Schechtman, K. B., Hornbrook, M. C., and Mulrow, C. D. 1992. Measuring the quality of life of the elderly in health promotion intervention clinical trials. *Public Health Reports* 107:530–39.

Lachs, M. S., Feinstein, A. R., Cooney, L. M., Drickamer, M. A., Marottoli, R. A., Pannill, F. C., and Tinetti, M. E. 1990. A simple procedure for general screening for functional disability in elderly patients. *Annals of Internal Medicine* 112:699–706.

Liang, M. H., Larson, M. G., Cullen, K. E., and Schwartz, J. A. 1985. Comparative measurement efficiency and sensitivity of five health status instruments for arthritis research. *Arthritis and Rheumatism* 28:545–47.

Linn, B. S., and Linn, M. W. 1980. Objective and self-assessed health in the old and very old. *Social Science and Medicine* 14A:311–15.

Little, R. J. A., and Rubin, D. B. 1987. *Statistical Analysis with Missing Data.* New York: Wiley.

Llewellyn-Thomas, H., Sutherland, H. J., Tibshirani, R., Ciampi, A., Till, J. E., and Boyd, N. F. 1984. Describing health states: Methodologic issues in obtaining values for health states. *Medical Care* 22:543–52.

Loomes, G., and McKenzie, L. 1989. The use of QALYs in health care decision making. *Social Science and Medicine* 28:299–308.

Maddox, G. L., and Clark, D. O. 1992. Trajectories of functional impairment in later life. *Journal of Health and Social Behavior* 33:114–25.

Magaziner, J., Simonsick, E. M., Kashner, T. M., and Hebel, J. R. 1988. Patient-proxy response comparability on measures of patient health and functional status. *Journal of Clinical Epidemiology* 41:1065–74.

Mangione, C. M., Marcantonio, E. R., Goldman, L., Cook, E. F., Donaldson, M. C., Sugarbaker, D. J., Poss, R., and Lee, T. H. 1993. Influence of age on measurement of health status in patients undergoing elective surgery. *Journal of the American Geriatrics Society* 41:377–83.

Manton, K. G. 1988. A longitudinal study of functional change and mortality in the United States. *Journal of Gerontology: Social Sciences* 43:S153–61.

Manton, K. G., Corder, L. S., and Stallard, E. 1993. Estimates of change in chronic disability and institutional incidence and prevalence rates in the U.S. elderly population from the 1982, 1984, and 1989 National Long Term Care Survey. *Journal of Gerontology: Social Sciences* 48:S153–66.

Markides, K. S., and Mindel, C. H. 1987. *Aging and Ethnicity.* Newbury Park, CA: Sage Publications, Inc.

McHorney, C. A., Kosinski, M., and Ware, J. E. 1994. Comparisons of the costs and quality of norms for the SF-36 health survey collected by mail versus telephone interview: Results from a national survey. *Medical Care* 32:551–67.

McHorney, C. A., Ware, J. E., Lu, R., and Sherbourne, C. D. 1994. The MOS 36-item Short-Form Health Survey (SF-36): III. Tests of data quality, scaling assumptions, and reliability across diverse patient groups. *Medical Care* 32:40–66.

McNeil, J. K., Stones, M. J., and Kozma, A. 1986. Subjective well-being in later life: Some issues concerning measurement and prediction. *Social Indicators Research* 18:35–70.

Miles, T. P., and Bernard, M. A. 1992. Morbidity, disability, and health status of black American elderly: A new look at the oldest-old. *Journal of the American Geriatrics Society* 40:1047–54.

Mirowsky, J., and Ross, C. E. 1992. Age and depression. *Journal of Health and Social Behavior* 33:187–205.

Mossey, J. M., and Shapiro, E. 1982. Self-rated health: A predictor of mortality among the elderly. *American Journal of Public Health* 72:800–8.

Mulley, A. G. 1989. Assessing patients' utilities: Can the ends justify the means? *Medical Care* 27:S269–81.

Nelson, E. C., and Berwick, D. M. 1989. The measurement of health status in clinical practice. *Medical Care* 27:877–90.

Nelson, E. C., Hays, R. D., Arnold, S., Kwoh, K., and Sherbourne, C. 1989. *Age and Functional Health Status* (P-7570-RC). Santa Monica, CA: The Rand Corporation.

Nunnally, J. C. 1978. *Psychometric Theory* (2nd ed.). New York: McGraw-Hill.

Ory, M. G., Schechtman, K. B., Miller, J. P., Hadley, E. C., Fiatarone, M. A., Province, M. A., Arfken, C. L., Morgan, D., Weiss, S., Kaplan, M., and The FICSIT Group. 1993. Frailty and injuries in later life: The FICSIT trials. *Journal of the American Geriatrics Society* 41:283–96.

Patrick, D. L., and Bergner, M. 1990. Measurement of health status in the 1990s. *Annual Review of Public Health* 11:165–83.

Patrick, D. L., and Deyo, R. A. 1989. Generic and disease-specific measures in assessing health status and quality of life. *Medical Care* [Supplement] 27:S217–32.

Patrick, D. L., and Erickson, P. 1993. *Health Status and Health Policy: Quality of Life in Health-Care Evaluation and Resource Allocation.* New York: Oxford University Press.

Patrick, D. L., Starks, H. E., Cain, K. C., Uhlmann, R. F., and Pearlman, R. A. 1994. Measuring preferences for health states worse than death. *Medical Decision Making* 14:9–18.

Rahman, O., Strauss, J., Gertler, P., Ashley, D., and Fox, K. 1994. Gender differences in adult health: An international comparison. *The Gerontologist* 34:463–69.

Raymond, M. R. 1986. Missing data in evaluation research. *Evaluation and the Health Professions* 9:395–420.

Rodgers, W. L., and Herzog, A. R. 1987. Interviewing older adults: The accuracy of factual information. *Journal of Gerontology* 42:387–94.

Rodgers, W. L., and Herzog, A. R. 1992. Collecting data about the oldest old: Problems and procedures. In Suzman, R. M., Willis, D. P., and Manton, K. G., eds., *The Oldest Old* (pp. 135–56). New York: Oxford University Press.

Rodgers, W. L., Herzog, A. R., and Andrews, F. M. 1988. Interviewing older adults: Validity of self-reports of satisfaction. *Psychology and Aging* 3:264–72.

Rowe, J. W., and Binstock, R. H. 1987. Aging reconsidered: Emerging issues and policy issues. Unpublished manuscript.

Rowe, J. W., and Kahn, R. L. 1987. Human aging: Usual and successful. *Science* 237:143–49.

Rubenstein, L. Z., Schairer, C., Wieland, G. D., and Kane, R. 1984. Systematic biases in functional status assessment of elderly adults: Effects of different data sources. *Journal of Gerontology* 39:686–91.

Schaie, K. W. 1994. The course of adult intellectual development. *American Psychologist* 49:304–13.

Schaie, K. W., and Willis, S. L. 1986. Can decline in adult intellectual functioning be reversed? *Developmental Psychology* 22:223–32.

Scholes, D., LaCroix, A. Z., Wagner, E. H., Grothaus, L. C., and Hecht, J. A. 1991. Tracking progress towards national health objectives in the elderly: What do restricted activity days signify? *American Journal of Public Health* 81:485–88.

Schwarz, N., Hippler, H., Deutsch, B., and Strack, F. 1985. Response scales: Effects of category range on reported behavior and comparative judgments. *Public Opinion Quarterly* 49:388–95.

Sherbourne, C. D., and Meredith, L. S. 1992. Quality of self-report data: A comparison of older and younger chronically ill patients. *Journal of Gerontology* 47:S204–11.

Siegler, I. C., and Botwinick, J. 1979. A long-term longitudinal study of intellectual ability of older adults: The matter of selective subject attrition. *Journal of Gerontology* 34:242–45.

Siu, A. L., Ouslander, J. G., Osterweil, D., Reuben, D. B., and Hays, R. D. 1993. Change in self-reported functioning in older persons entering a residential care facility. *Journal of Clinical Epidemiology* 46:1093–1102.

Starfield, B. 1974. Measurement of outcome: A proposed scheme. *Milbank Memorial Fund Quarterly* 52:39–50.

Stewart, A. L. 1992. A framework of health concepts. In Stewart, A. L., and Ware, J. E., Jr., eds., *Measuring Functioning and Well-Being: The Medical Outcomes Study Approach* (pp. 12–24). Durham, NC: Duke University Press.

Stewart, A. L., and King, A. C. 1994. Conceptualizing and measuring quality of life in older populations. In Abeles, R. P., Gift, H. C., and Ory, M. G., eds., *Aging and Quality of Life* (pp. 27–54). New York: Springer Publishing Company.

Stewart, A. L., Hays, R. D., and Ware, J. E., Jr. 1992a. Methods of constructing health measures. In Stewart, A. L., and Ware, J. E., Jr., eds., *Measuring Functioning and Well-Being: The Medical Outcomes Study Approach* (pp. 67–85). Durham, NC: Duke University Press.

Stewart, A. L., Hays, R. D., and Ware, J. E., Jr. 1992b. Methods of validating health measures. In Stewart, A. L., and Ware, J. E., Jr., eds., *Measuring Functioning and Well-Being: The Medical Outcomes Study Approach* (pp. 309–324). Durham, NC: Duke University Press.

Stewart, A. L., Sherbourne, C. D., Hays, R. D., Wells, K. B., Nelson, E. C., Kamberg, C. J., Rogers, W. H., Berry, S. D., and Ware, J. E., Jr. 1992. Summary and discussion of MOS measures. In Stewart, A. L., and Ware, J. E., Jr., eds., *Measuring Functioning and Well-Being: The Medical Outcomes Study Approach.* Durham, NC: Duke University Press.

Tugwell, P., Bombardier, C., Bell, M., Bennett, K., Bensen, W., Grace, E., Hart, L., and Goldsmith, C. 1991. Current quality-of-life research challenges in arthritis relevant to the issue of clinical significance. *Controlled Clinical Trials* 12:S217–25.

Verbrugge, L. M. 1989. The twain meet: Empirical explanations of sex differences in health and mortality. *Journal of Health and Social Behavior* 30:282–304.

Vickrey, B. G., Hays, R. D., Rausch, R., Sutherling, W. W., Engel, J., and Brook, R. H. 1994. Quality of life of epilepsy surgery patients compared with outpatients with hypertension, diabetes, heart disease, and/or depressive symptoms. *Epilepsia* 35:597–607.

Wagner, E. H., LaCroix, A. Z., Grothaus, L. C., and Hecht, J. A. 1993. Responsiveness of health status measures to change among older adults. *Journal of the American Geriatrics Society* 41:241–48.

Wallace, R. B., Kohout, F. J., and Colsher, P. L. 1992. Observations on interview surveys of the oldest old. In Suzman, R. M., Willis, D. P., and Manton, K. G., eds., *The Oldest Old* (pp. 123–34). New York: Oxford University Press.

Ware, J. E., Jr., and Sherbourne, C. D. 1992. The MOS 36-Item Short-Form Health Survey (SF-36): I. Conceptual framework and item selection. *Medical Care* 30:473–83.

Ware, J. E., Jr., Kosinski, M., and Keller, S. D. 1994. *SF-36 Physical and Mental Health Summary Scales: A User's Manual.* Boston: The Health Institute.

Ware, J. E., Jr., Snow, K. K., Kosinski, M., and Gandek, B. 1993. *SF-36 Health Survey: Manual and Interpretation Guide.* Boston: The Health Institute, New England Medical Center.

Ware, J. E., Jr., Brook, R. H., Davies, A. R., and Lohr, K. 1981. Choosing measures of health status for individuals in general populations. *American Journal of Public Health* 71:620–25.

Weinberger, M., Nagle, B., Samsa, J. P., Schmader, K., Landsman, P. B., Uttech, K. M., Cowper, P. A., and Feussner, J. R. 1994. Assessing health-related quality of life in elderly outpatients: Telephone versus face-to-face administration. *Journal of the American Geriatrics Society* 42:1295–99.

Weissman, M. M., Leaf, P. J., Tischler, G. L., Blazer, D. G., Karno, M., Bruce, M. L., and Florio, L. P. 1988. Affective disorders in five United States communities. *Psychological Medicine* 18:141–53.

Wolinsky, F. D., and Johnson, R. J. 1992. Perceived health status and mortality among older men and women. *Journal of Gerontology: Social Sciences* 47:S304–12.

World Health Organization. 1948. World Health Organization Constitution. In *Basic Documents.* Geneva: World Health Organization.

Yesavage, J. A., Brink, T. L., Rose, T. L., Lum, O., Huang, V., Adey, M., and Leirer, V. O. 1983. Development and validation of a geriatric depression screening scale: A preliminary report. *Journal of Psychiatric Research* 17:37–49.

11

Heterogeneity and Multiple Risk Factors in Aging Populations: Implications for Research

Pearl S. German, Sc.D., and Sam Shapiro, B.S.

The diverse character of individuals 65 years of age and older includes health status, as well as psychosocial, cultural, ethnic, and economic descriptors. Diversities in these areas have been presented and examined in several chapters of this text. The implications of heterogeneity have been observed, for example, epidemiologically (Salive and Guralnik; Wallace), behaviorally (Kaplan), and organizationally (Balsam and Bottum). This chapter extends the focus on heterogeneity more specifically into its meaning in public health theory and practice—particularly in research, interventions, and their evaluations.

The mandate of public health is to monitor the health of the community at every level and to devise interventions that are aimed at preserving, repairing or improving the well-being of the community. Clinical medicine, on the other hand, primarily treats individuals. While individuals are part of the community, and the community is important when considering the treatment of individuals, the paradigms of public health and clinical medicine differ. Therefore, the importance and utility of variability have a different focus in public health than they do in direct clinical care, although there are many important overlaps in research and teaching. For public health, heterogeneity in the population is a crucial consideration in design, method, and the ultimate application of findings.

The Public Health Perspective and Heterogeneity

The existence of differences among those 65 years and older can be observed from health statistics (U.S. Bureau of the Census, 1992) and is attested to in almost any presentation of research or report on an intervention. Some of the important ways in which diversity is observed and in which consideration of diversity is essential when these factors serve as independent variables to explain or predict outcome are age, subpopulations, ill health, functional status, social networks, nature of environmental exposures, and settings (Abeles, Gift, and Ory, 1994). There is diversity as well among dependent variables, which serve as the goal of intervention strategies. For example, an intervention in a frail elderly Swedish population (a group considerably more homogeneous than the older population in this country) had as its objective the postponement of decline. The results demonstrated differences in response, behaviors, and the level of change possible in this population (Svanborg, 1993).

With such broad and varied areas in which population differences exist, ways of organizing these areas into a more parsimonious and utilitarian grouping are essential. Description and measurement are the first steps in any research and service activity in public health. Areas crucial to public health in which targeted descriptions of heterogeneity are essential include:

1. Prevalence and incidence of disease, disability and chronic conditions for tracing the natural history of disease and for planning and organizing services and interventions and their assessment.

2. Characteristics associated with prevalence and incidence that identify appropriate target groups and appropriate interventions including preventive strategies.

3. Realistic goals for intervention based on the nature and degree of diversity within the target population.

4. Predicting manpower needs and planning for necessary training.

5. Cultural and ethnic diversity as an added and increasing concern relevant to all of the above.

The data in Table 11.1 illustrate the variability in the prevalence of disease and associated population characteristics. Death rates for the leading causes of death, heart disease, and cancer show important variability by age, sex, and race. Heart disease and cancer comprise about two-thirds of deaths in each of the race and sex

TABLE 11.1. Death Rates for Diseases of the Heart and Malignant Neoplasm, by Race, Age, and Sex, United States, 1989–1990 (Rate per 100,000)

Race and Age	Diseases of the Heart		Malignant Neoplasm	
	Male	Female	Male	Female
White				
55–64	538	198	512	375
65–74	1,278	605	1,083	671
75–84	3,067	1,954	1,854	996
85+	7,661	6,711	2,604	1,348
Black				
55–64	881	470	841	759
65–74	1,700	1,054	1,621	769
75–84	3,192	2,380	2,437	1,030
85+	6,368	5,899	3,041	1,383

Source: Fried and Wallace, 1992.

groups. With advancing age, both heart disease and malignancies increase as causes of death, although in recent years there has been a decline of deaths from heart disease. Heart disease is more likely to cause death in men than women at every age, with differentials greatest at younger ages. Black men in younger age groups have the highest death rates for both heart disease and cancer. While both diseases increase with increasing age, there continues to be a difference by sex and race. Table 11.2 shows that the prevalence of chronic disease also increases with age and all of these factors contribute to decisions about appropriate goals and appropriate target groups.

Differences in other health data follow this same pattern. In Table 11.3, mean differences in life expectancy can be seen between men and women, both black and white. It should be noted that there was no increase in life expectancy for black males between 1950 and 1991, a fact that is not true for white males and females and black females.

Further differences among racial groups are illustrated in reported need for assistance in everyday activities. For example, the percentage of persons age 65 and older who reported needing assistance with everyday activities varies considerably by race. While only 15 percent of the older white population reported needing such assistance, 25 percent and 19 percent of black and Hispanic older adults reported such need (U.S. Bureau of the Census, 1986).

In a female population chosen for indications of moderate to severe disability as subjects for a current study, there still exists evidence of variation and increased

TABLE 11.2. Increase in the Prevalence of Selected Chronic Diseases with Increasing Age, United States, 1985 (Rates per 1,000)

Condition	Age 45–64	Age 65–74	Age >75
Arthritis	268	459	495
Hypertension	259	427	395
Heart disease	129	277	349
Hearing impairment	159	262	347
Deformity or orthopedic impairment	161	168	176
Chronic sinusitis	185	151	160
Visual impairment	44	76	129
Diabetes	52	109	96
Cerebrovascular disease	18	54	73
Emphysema	15	50	39

Source: Fried and Wallace, 1992.

decline with increasing age. Table 11.4 shows data from the Women's Health and Aging Study (Guralnik, personal communication, 1993). This population was categorized into four specific disability functions or domains—upper extremity, mobility domain, higher functioning domain (IADLs) and self-care domain (ADLs). Those women chosen as study subjects had deficits in two or more domains. Table 11.4 gives the distribution of deficits by age in each of four functional domains at screening. As can be seen from the table, considerable variation (heterogeneity) in disability exists between functional domains and age groups.

TABLE 11.3. Life Expectancy at 65 Years of Age, by Race and Sex, 1950 and 1991

Race	1950	1991
White		
Male	13	15
Female	15	19
Black		
Male	13	13
Female	15	17

Source: National Center for Health Statistics, 1994.

TABLE 11.4. Disability Patterns in Four Domains of Functioning, by Age, Women's Health and Aging Study

Difficulty in Domain	Total	Age		
		65–74	75–84	85+
Upper extremity	33%	28%	35%	48%
Mobility domain	47	39	51	65
Higher-functioning domain (IADL)	22	14	24	46
Self-care domain (ADL)	21	14	22	43

Source: Personal communication, Jack Guralnik, September 1993.

Note: Includes only women with two or more disabilities. Each domain is a summary of several individual functions in the specific area noted.

The data presented above are examples of diversity in the oldest age group. These data represent the basis for essential epidemiological descriptions of the population, which serves as the foundation for the design of research including interventions and their evaluation.

Other Dimensions Related to Diversity

The organization of various aspects of heterogeneity is a beginning and basic approach. There are other important factors to be considered in how diversity is used. One factor is the aspect of design and analyses and whether the approach should be cohort or cross-sectional. A second factor is cumulative risk, which is important when estimating the role of certain risk factors for undesirable outcomes. It becomes essential to know the nature of the exposure to the behavior, environment, and other risks, as well as the length of time of that exposure.

Cohort Analysis

The importance of a cohort view of the older population and the need for clarity when examining differences that occur by age has been of particular interest to epidemiologists and social scientists. Cohorts—groups of individuals born within a specified number of years of each other—are generally examined as an entity as the group moves through life. These individuals are held to be affected by social, cultural, and economic environments that may differ from the environments of cohorts that precede and follow them. These influences include changes in the understanding and treatment of disease conditions and/or disabilities and will affect the natural history of adaptation to aging. The importance of cohort study has received consistent attention and was emphasized pointedly by Riley (1994) in a recent American Journal of Public Health editorial. "The full power of the cohort approach is still not fully utilized for understanding how lives might be changed to improve health, effective functioning and the quality of aging" (Riley, 1994, p. 1215). Cohort differences are stressed not only for importance in retrospectively evaluating research and history but for identifying and planning present and future public health strategies for interventions aimed at improving the lives of older individuals.

Cumulative Risk

The second factor to be considered when examining heterogeneity, particularly when older populations are under consideration, is that of cumulative risk. Length of life presents added risk, in part due to greater probability of exposure to a broad array of factors that increase the likelihood of developing a variety of diseases and conditions. In general, as shown earlier, increasing age is associated with increasing prevalence of chronic disease (Van Nostrand, Furner, and Suzman, 1993), although there are differences by sex and specific diseases. Reflected here are successes that have been achieved with some diseases. However, general disability and frailty can be demonstrated as increasing with age.

It has been suggested that the phenomenon of increased disease and conditions with age can be attributed to long latency periods of some diseases, physiological changes attendant on aging, and prolonged exposure to behavioral and environmental factors associated with disease. It is not entirely clear how much increased disease in older people is related to "aging per se and how much to prolonged risk factor exposure" (Kaplan, Haan, and Cohen, 1992). This is one dimension of cumulative risk—that is, the probability of developing a specific disease condition and/or disability because of a longer period of risk.

Another dimension of cumulative risk is reflected in the constant concern and attention to comorbidity (Fried and Wallace, 1992). Comorbid conditions present both the risk noted above (that is, a second condition develops as time passes because of those risks for the first condition), as well as the risk attendant on the presence of the condition that has been present for some period of time. A prevalent disease and/or condition can interact with other existing and prolonged risks to increase the probability of a second, third, or fourth condition than might be true for older individuals without an existing chronic disease.

Among the 85 percent of the 65 and older population who have at least one chronic disease, at least two-thirds have two or more other diseases (Van Nostrand, Turner, and Suzman, 1993). From another point of view, 49 percent of those 60 and older have two or more chronic conditions, 23 percent have 3 or more, and 8 percent have four or more. This increases with age so that at age 80 or older, 70 percent of women and 53 percent of men have two or more chronic conditions (Guralnik et al., 1989).

It is often unclear whether a new comorbid condition is secondary to an existing condition (such as hypertension leading to stroke) or has developed with the existing condition having contributed as a risk for the second condition (e.g., inactivity related to disability due to arthritis leading to circulatory problems) (Pope and Tarlov, 1991).

Ethnic and Cultural Minorities

Another important distinction in discussing heterogeneity, along with cohort and cumulative risk considerations, is the matter of ethnic and cultural differences and the meaning of these differences in the older population. There has been an accumulation over the years of information on other cultures and races making up part of the aged in the United States (Torres-Gil, 1986; Gibson, 1986; Jackson, 1993b; Green, Jackson, and Neighbors, 1993; Aday, 1993). We are collecting more information continually and have become sensitive to the special needs of these groups. As noted earlier in discussion of general heterogeneity, there are differences among ethnic racial groups in life expectancy and in reported need for assistance. Racial differences are reflected also in self-assessed health in Table 11.5, where at every age group, beginning at age 45, greater proportions of nonwhites reported poor or fair health.

Related to these group differences, we can anticipate that cohorts with different ethnic and cultural backgrounds will be coming to this country at a mature age. These individuals will require increased understanding of their differences. Cohorts

TABLE 11.5. Percentage Reporting Fair or Poor Health, by Race, Age, and Sex, United States, 1992

	Age		
	45–64	65–74	75+
Race			
White	16	24	32
Black	31	42	48
Sex			
Male	17	27	34
Female	18	25	33

Source: National Center for Health Statistics, 1994.

will include, for example, the recent immigration from Asia, Latin America, Mexico, and other countries.

Past exposures as well as specific ethnic and cultural factors need to be considered as do better understandings of the impact of abrupt and often traumatic displacements. More research is necessary in understanding the meaning of ethnic/cultural differences in order to shape intervention strategies for the appropriate delivery of health care and social, psychosocial, and economic services. Understanding the complicated interaction of the many different factors that influence the health and well-being of a population forms a good part of the public health mission.

Questions about diversity within a population are not limited to the older population. It is an important consideration in all investigations of basic public health knowledge and practice. There are, however, aspects of the older population that make understanding of its diversity particularly meaningful. These include demographic shifts, such as the increased numbers entering this age group and the increasing life expectancy of those 65 and over. This will increase the complexity of patterns of disease and disability and other areas of adaptation.

The field has witnessed rapid changes in policy and health care structures. For example, there has been an increasing emphasis on prevention as a strategy for dealing with the specific needs of older people. As research and interventions on and for older people continue to expand, appropriate uses of diversity and its role and impact assure greater substance and rigor to the work of public health.

A Typology of Heterogeneity

The broad array of perspectives from which the older population can be considered suggests that some order or typology for dealing with heterogeneity in older populations would assist in the application of public health strategies to the problems faced by this group. An operational orientation or typology intended as a guide through the maze of heterogeneity seeks to answer the following considerations: How can heterogeneity be structured parsimoniously and what are the implications of that structure? When is heterogeneity descriptive? When is it analytic and what are the goals of the analysis? The objective of any model of typology is to provide a guide for managing widely differing characteristics found in older populations and in subgroups of that population when investigating public health issues and when planning strategies of intervention. It is a guide to the research into health and welfare that aims to establish a firm knowledge base for the research and services undertaken to improve health and welfare. Such a tool should serve in the design and assessment of interventions (that is, public health action) to achieve these ends.

Attention to heterogeneity should focus on the objective of the evaluation. If relatively rare attributes are of concern, there will not be sufficient numbers required for understanding the meaning of these less-frequent attributes unless the population is very large and extensive. The level of knowledge, based on past work, of the importance of specific characteristics to health and health care guides the choice of which characteristics are to be measured. Evidence on the effect of various characteristics and the ease with which evidence can be gathered are issues to be addressed when planning studies.

Relatively Immutable Characteristics

There are characteristics of older populations that offer little or no scope for action aimed at their change. This includes, for example, gender, education, increasing age, and some past life experiences. These characteristics are important in research for their role in many areas; they are not subject to change but have an impact on outcomes. For example, increasing age has been demonstrated to be associated with increasing disease and disability (Hadley et al., 1993; Guralnik and Simonsick, 1993). At the same time, the level and rate at which this association appears in individuals differs greatly within an age group (U.S. Bureau of the Census, 1992). Though unchangeable, these factors are important both in research for establishing their influence and in intervention trials because of potential for acceptance and adaptation.

An example of the influence of fixed characteristics on health is reflected in the relationship of years of formal education to reported poor health and to the prevalence of selected chronic conditions (Tables 11.6 and 11.7). Lower education is associated with reports of poor health and with higher rates of chronic disease.

TABLE 11.6. Percentage Reporting Poor Health, by Age and Years of Schooling

	Age	
Years of Schooling	55–64	65+
<4	49	53
4–7	47	43
8–11	32	33
12	15	24
13–15	14	20

Source: Adapted from Preston and Taubman, 1990.

TABLE 11.7. Prevalence of Selected Chronic Conditions
(per 1,000), by Education, Age 65
and Older

Condition	Less than High School	High School and Above
Arthritis	519	426
Hearing impaired	312	267
Diabetes	100	77
Heart disease	300	264
Hypertension	398	370
Emphysema	45	28

Source: Adapted from Preston and Taubman, 1990.

Characteristics Accessible to Change

A second grouping of heterogeneous population characteristics are those that can be modified, ameliorated, or more readily changed and are factors often associated with effects on illness and health and the natural history of advancing years of life. These are factors accessible to strategies, although in varying degrees, aimed at achieving particular public health goals, and include changes in behaviors that can affect desired outcomes in health and well-being. Examples of such characteristics are:

1. Mortality and morbidity due to varied diseases (health risk behaviors such as use of tobacco and alcohol).

2. As a subset of the above, the course of chronic disease (health promotive behaviors such as activity, exercise, and diet).

3. Functional capacity, disability, and frailty.

4. The use of health care services, including access, quality, and type.

These characteristics often play several roles in research, such as outcomes to be understood in documenting the course of disease and disability. They are also factors that, in association with other variables, may influence outcomes as, for example, disability and age leading to the use of health services. These more changeable characteristics often are examined in conjunction with less amenable-to-change characteristics because of the hypothesized interaction or combined effect both sets may have on a specified outcome.

The role of these modifiable characteristics of prevention, particularly secondary and tertiary prevention (which is more appropriate to older individuals than to younger people), has been receiving increasing attention. A multiple-site study recently completed at Johns Hopkins University tested the effect of preventive services on the overall health and cost of care of older individuals. This study, a randomized clinical trial of a community population, offered preventive services from primary care physicians and evaluated the results of these services. Findings from this study, the Senior Health Watch, illustrate specific issues that arise from heterogeneity (German et al., 1994).

An effort was made in the Senior Health Watch to estimate the influence of various characteristics differentially distributed in this older population on the level of appeal that the offer of free preventive visits might have. The design of the study required individuals to make arrangements with their primary care clinicians to receive the preventive services. Response rates depended on the willingness of this older population to make the effort to secure these services. Table 11.8 gives the odds ratios of individuals in the experimental group who responded to the offer of preventive services. The variables used include both fixed characteristics and those considered accessible to change. Men and women were analyzed separately since some of the predictive variables were gender specific, such as having had a mammogram prior to baseline. Having a female provider, a factor subject to modification, had an influence on female patients, patient gender being fixed and not subject to modifi-

TABLE 11.8. Senior Health Watch Odds Ratios for Characteristics Associated with Preventive Visits

	Odds Ratio	C.I.
Men		
Married	1.52	(1.09, 2.08)
Type practice of provider*		
Solo	1.95	(1.38, 2.75)
Hospital	4.35	(0.92, 20.52)
Women		
Confidant	1.57	(1.16, 2.11)
Female provider	2.33	(1.45, 3.70)
Education†		
High school	1.75	(1.04, 1.69)
College	1.37	(0.937, 2.02)
Mammography‡	1.75	(1.37, 2.23)

*Comparison group was providers in group practices.
†Comparison group had 0–8 years of education.
‡Reported having mammography within two years of baseline.

cation. The result was an increase in receptivity to preventive services. For males this effect appeared to be associated with having a solo practitioner. This table demonstrates how different characteristics influence behavior, which in turn influences strategies for change.

Another example from this prevention intervention study demonstrates heterogeneity of change over time. An analysis was made of factors influencing health status. For this group, it was of interest to understand the factors that were related to relatively lower rates of decline in health status at the end of two years. A lesser rate of decline is a necessary consideration since, in an older group, a general decline is anticipated for the group as a whole. It was observed that the presence of Medicaid or Medigap insurance was one factor that was associated with a significantly lower decrease of decline in health status in the intervention group. Economic status is a heterogeneous characteristic across the 65 and over group and in this case seems to be a positive influence on a desired outcome.

Additional psychosocial and environmental characteristics show considerable heterogeneity in the older population and changeability of these characteristics is uncertain. These characteristics vary in the extent and nature to which they appear in the older population. There is less evidence of the nature and specificity of the influence of the characteristics. Although research and interventions in these areas have taken place and continue to be carried out with important results, problems of definition and measurement continue to challenge research and strategies for intervention. In addition, the ease of securing appropriate study populations with these characteristics or in designing appropriate interventions aimed at specific dimensions is always a concern. Examples of these factors include:

1. Psychosocial characteristics: mental status, coping mechanisms, beliefs, and attitudes.

2. Support networks: formal and informal.

3. Environmental exposure: *past and current*, occupational, and living arrangements.

4. Impact of occurrences and experiences: loss of status, income, and loved ones, and change of home.

When these kinds of hypothesized influences are examined for effect on some outcome, important factors surface that can have an impact on how public health programs are planned. In examining receptivity to preventive services, certain behaviors indicate specific attitudes toward prevention, and this influences desired outcomes. In the Senior Health Watch, women who had had a mammogram or Pap smear before baseline were more likely to embark on the prevention program being offered. Similarly, certain health attitudes together with the intervention in this study were associated with a lower decline in health status at the end of two years for the intervention group as compared to controls. Variables associated with lower decline in health included physical activity, reduction of cholesterol, and reduction of weight.

Heterogeneity in Research

Research has as one of its main goals increased knowledge of specific problems. For examination of conditions and diseases, epidemiologists describe and examine incidence and prevalence and the factors associated with them. The natural history of disease is approached in the same way. This strategy is observed in demographic studies and in various psychosocial and economic analyses of populations. The hypothetical approach to factors associated with the specific subject of the research is essential as a guide for information to be gathered. Past knowledge that the factor or factors of interest are distributed differently among populations assures the tagging of such factors whether or not they are hypothesized to influence different levels of disease or different outcomes in length and quality of life and use of services and their cost.

The choice of variables to be gathered through large national surveys represents the state of the art regarding characteristics thought to be both differentially distributed in the population and associated with specific outcomes. Associated with this identification of essential information is the constant and ongoing work being carried out to establish appropriate, reliable, and valid measures, such as managed care and disability. All of these factors play a role in the design of analysis and guide careful attention to the complications of diversity in populations during the analytic phase of research studies.

Heterogeneity in Interventions and Evaluation

The major goal of an intervention is to apply a strategy to an appropriate population aimed at improving or minimizing an identified problem. Evaluation assesses the success of the intervention, including the circumstances and characteristics of the target group that interact with the intervention to achieve different levels of success or failure.

Past work facilitates designing interventions, and this will be particularly true of work that has established the extent and nature of heterogeneity. There are many points in the flow of an intervention, beginning with its conception and design, in which the consequences of heterogeneity in a population play an essential role and must be considered.

Definition and measurement of the specifics of heterogeneity can identify study populations and provide the means for setting goals and establishing priorities for interventions. Understanding factors associated with the heterogeneity of a modifiable risk factor within the older population may provide a means for targeting an intervention. For example, an exercise health promotion program may be targeted for specific subgroups of older adults who are least likely to engage in regular physical activity or who are at greatest health risk from a lack of physical activity. In summary, a clear understanding of the nature of the heterogeneity helps to identify the problem around which the intervention is designed, and—equally important—the projected level of success that is sought.

Heterogeneity and cumulative risk have an important role related to the choice of a population and the projected level of success. Intervention target populations can be characterized by the level of achievement possible, and this in turn directs the choice of strategy and the way in which this strategy is to be implemented. Examples include the following:

1. There are populations where little pathology is identified but which are hypothesized by virtue of their characteristics to be at high risk for specific disease conditions and/or disability developing or even being present in early undiagnosed stages. This includes the identification of high risk based on past epidemiological work. Older women with a history of falls are at high risk for subsequent falls. This is a group where education in preventive measures and evaluation of environmental risk would be appropriate.

2. There are populations where existing disease conditions and/or disabilities have been established, but these conditions are identified at an early or moderate stage where a certain degree of disability and frailty are observable.

3. There are populations in which a high degree, in both numbers and severity, of disease, disability, and/or frailty is documented (including many comorbidities).

The nature and extent of the heterogeneity will define the intervention and the objectives. In the Senior Health Watch Study, care was taken to identify data to be collected that documents differences hypothesized to influence the impact of the intervention. An important issue was acceptance of the program, since it was necessary for older individuals to take action in order to receive waivered services. Prevention programs and services tend to be focused heavily on primary prevention (U.S. Department of Health and Human Services, Public Health Service, 1991), and there was concern that older populations would perceive preventive actions and services as less relevant for them. There were, of course, anticipated differences within the older group in individual responses to offers of free prevention services. The first wave of analysis revealed that those with the lowest health status and highest indicators of continuing severity of illness were the *least* likely to respond to the intervention by accepting the preventive services (German et al., 1994). In a bivariate analysis of the relationship of age and health status, as measured by the Quality of Well-Being Scale (QWB) (Kaplan and Anderson, 1988), with making a preventive visit, the highest rate of active participation was for those with a moderate health status and those at less advanced ages. This would suggest that in consideration of projected goals and interventions to achieve them, the existing heterogeneity in an older population will greatly influence success.

In an intervention assessment where an experimental group is compared to a control group, the heterogeneity of the two groups is of less concern if the population is a representative one and the design is a randomized trial. However, to the extent that the samples are large enough to support analysis of the internal differences within the experimental and the control group, then the existing heterogeneity within the groups is a potential for increasing the rigor of the assessment as well as for obtaining a clearer picture of the dynamics of the intervention. Of interest is the influence the specific heterogeneous characteristics have on the intervention and on outcome. Such understanding helps in the design of future intervention strategies and the role of specific characteristics that enhance interventions. There are, as well, differing characteristics that can influence dropout and cross-over rates during the course of the study. Thus, it would seem to be incontrovertible that heterogeneity has importance in interventions at several points and for various reasons.

Summary

Existing heterogeneity in the older population is amply demonstrated by data at all levels and encompasses health status, psychosocial factors, and cultural, ethnic and economic dimensions. This difference has a special meaning for public health programs because of the mandate of public health to care for the general population. Of concern in public health are differences in the prevalence and incidence of disease, in characteristics associated with these patterns, in varied goals addressing specific programs and specific populations, and in training the necessary work force. Methods of handling diversity include attention to cohort versus cross-sectional designs and analyses and to continued examination of cumulative risk. The last factor is of particular importance for the older population where the question remains of whether increasing disease with age is related to age per se, to long incubation periods, and/or to prolonged exposure and behaviors. A second dimension of cumulative risks is that of comorbidity, the presence of one disease related to the development of other diseases and/or disorders.

Ethnic and cultural differences pose challenges to public health, and health statistics document the influence of these factors on the health of older individuals. Older ethnic groups who have either aged in this country or have newly arrived represent an added complexity.

An approach to multiple and complex heterogeneity is consideration of the nature of the heterogeneity and its role in research and intervention. Varied characteristics can be immutable (age, sex, race), while others are more malleable (mortality/morbidity, access and use of health care, psychological status, support systems, and environmental exposure) and therefore relevant for intervention strategies. In research, all of these factors can be approached from the knowledge base of their effect on health. This guides the type of information to be gathered and the method of analyses. An understanding of heterogeneity can also be used to choose a population. Heterogeneous characteristics can describe subpopulations who by definition require development of different goals. The utility of heterogeneity in interventions and their assessment is heightened by an understanding of the role of the various descriptors, in setting realistic goals and in understanding the ultimate effect of an intervention when the heterogeneity of the population affects outcome.

For public health purposes, teaching, research, practice, and delivering direct services all demand a clear understanding of the broad differences that exist in the enormously varied 65 years of age and older population. Much work has been done and more is under way in which differences in a population are examined, interventions operationalized, and results evaluated. Heterogeneity of the older population has been and can continue to be an asset to public health. It will always be a challenge with which we must deal.

References

Abeles, R. P., Gift, H. C., and Ory, M. G. 1994. Introduction. In Abeles, R. P., Gift, H. C., and Ory, M. G., eds., *Aging and Quality of Life*. New York: Springer Publishing Company.

Aday, L. *At Risk in America: Vulnerable Populations in the United States*. 1993. San Francisco: Jossey-Bass.

Fried, L. P., and Wallace, R. B. 1992. The complexity of chronic illness in the elderly: From clinic to community. In Wallace, R. B., and Woolson, R. F., eds., *The Epidemiologic Study of the Elderly*. New York: Oxford University Press.

German, P. S., Burton, L. C., Shapiro, S., Steinwachs, D. M., Tsuji, I., Paglia, M. J., and Damiano, A. 1994. Extended coverage for preventive services: Response and results in an elderly population. *American Journal of Public Health*

Gibson, R. G. 1986. Blacks in an aging society. *Daedalus* 115(1):349–72.

Green, R. L., Jackson, R. S., and Neighbors, H. W. 1993. Mental health and health seeking behavior. In Jackson, J. S., Chatters, L. M., and Taylor, R. J., eds., *Aging in Black America*. Newbury Park, CA: Sage Publications.

Guralnik, J. M., and Simonsick, E. M. 1993. Physical disability in older Americans. *Journals of Gerontology: Special Issue. Physical Frailty: A Treatable Cause of Dependence in Old Age* 48.

Guralnik, J., LaCroix, A., Everett, D., and Kovar, M. S. 1989. Aging in the eighties: The prevalence of co-morbidity and its association with disability. *Advance Data from Vital and Health Statistics*, No. 170. Hyattsville, MD: National Center for Health Statistics.

Hadley, E. C., Ory, M. C., Suzman, R., and Weindruch, R. 1993. Foreword. In *Physical Frailty: A Treatable Cause of Dependence in Old Age. Journal of Gerontology: Special Issue* 48.

Jackson, J. S. 1993a. Foreword. In Jackson, J. S., Chatters, L. M., and Taylor, R. J., eds., *Aging in Black America*. Newbury Park, CA: Sage Publications.

Jackson, J. S. 1993b. Status and functioning of future cohorts of African-American elderly: Conclusions and speculations. In Jackson, J. S., Chatters, L. M., and Taylor, R. J., eds., *Aging in Black America*. Newbury Park, CA: Sage Publications.

Kaplan, R. M., and Anderson, J. P. 1988. A general health policy model: Update and applications. *Health Services Research* 23(2):203–36.

Kaplan, G. A., Haan, M. N., and Cohen, R. D. 1992. Risk factors and the study of prevention in the elderly: Methodological issues. In Wallace, R. B., and Woolson, R. F., eds., *The Epidemiologic Study of the Elderly*. New York: Oxford University Press.

National Center for Health Statistics. 1994. *Health, United States, 1993*. Hyattsville, MD: Public Health Service.

Pope, A. M., and Tarlov, A. R., eds. 1991. *Disability in America: Toward a National Agenda for prevention*, Chapter 6. Institute of Medicine. Washington, DC: National Academy Press.

Preston, S. A., and Taubman, P. 1990. *Demography of Aging*.

Riley, M. W. 1994. Changing lives and changing social structures: Common concerns of social science and public health. *American Journal of Public Health* 84(8):1214–17.

Svanborg, A. 1993. A medical-social intervention in a 70-year-old Swedish population: Is it possible to postpone functional decline in aging? *Journals of Gerontology: Special Issue: Physical Frailty, A Treatable Cause of Dependence in Old Age* 48:84–88.

Torres-Gil, F. 1986. The Latinization of a multigenerational population: Hispanics in an aging society. *Daedalus* 115(1):325–48.

U.S. Bureau of the Census. 1992. *Sixty-five Plus in America* (Current Population Reports, Special Studies, P23-178RV). Washington, DC: U.S. Government Printing Office.

U.S. Bureau of the Census. Current Reports, Series P-70, No. 19.

U.S. Department of Health and Human Services. 1991. *Healthy People 2000* (Pub. No. 91-50212). Washington, DC: Public Health Service.

Van Nostrand, J. F., Furner, S. E., and Suzman, R., eds. 1993. Health data on older Americans: United States, 1992. National Center for Health Statistics, *Vital Health Statistics* 3(27).

Chapter

12

On the Economic Analysis of Interventions for Aged Populations

Ronald J. Ozminkowski, Ph.D., and Laurence G. Branch, Ph.D.

Nearly every government-funded intervention designed to affect the health of an aging population comes with a mandate for evaluation. Some examples that will be discussed here are the Department of Veterans Affairs Adult Day Health Care Program, the National Long Term Care (Channeling) Demonstration Project, the Program of All-inclusive Care for the Elderly (PACE), and the New York Quality Assurance System. Many private-sector innovations, notably in the pharmaceutical market, are subject to evaluation as well, in efforts to convince regulators and/or purchasers that the product is safe, effective, and a worthwhile use of funds. Most of these evaluations contain an economic analysis designed to estimate the relative costs and benefits of the intervention compared to the status quo. Properly done, economic analyses of interventions recognize that a simple comparison of costs between the intervention and its alternatives may not be very useful for policy-making or investment decisions. Appropriate policy and investment decisions are more likely based on what one may get in return for his or her dollars. Selecting the least expensive program without consideration of its relative benefits or effectiveness is likely to lead to the waste of scarce economic resources.

The opinions expressed in this chapter are those of the authors; they do not necessarily represent the opinions of Abt Associates, Inc. We acknowledge sincere appreciation to Anna Aizer for her professional assistance in screening and summarizing some of the relevant literature.

With this context in mind, the following description of economic analyses of interventions for the health of the aged devotes a significant amount of energy to the methods required to estimate whether interventions work and how much impact they may have. As Weiss noted, evaluations are part of a larger set of problem-solving activities that reflect a research process. This process is designed to identify a problem, generate possible solutions, implement those solutions, evaluate the solutions, and use the results of the evaluation either to fine-tune the intervention or to affect public or private policy making (Shadish, Cook, and Leviton, 1991). This chapter describes the processes required to produce a good economic evaluation, noting, as Weiss did, that good evaluations require high-quality efforts in the other problem-solving activities as well.

What Is Evaluation and Why Do It?

Rossi and Freeman (1993) defined *evaluation* as "the systematic application of social research procedures for assessing the conceptualization, design, implementation, and utility of social intervention programs." In other words, evaluation researchers "use social research methodologies to judge and improve the ways in which human services policies and programs are conducted, from the earliest stages of defining and designing programs through their development and implementation" (p. 5). The research procedures involved in the evaluation of health interventions are the focus of this chapter, and, more importantly, of millions of dollars of public and private expenditures annually.

But why evaluate? Why not take those dollars and efforts and pour them directly into the programs being provided, thus expanding the capacity to improve the health of the aged and other members of society? The answer is that, without an evaluation, policy makers, patients, clients, or others affected by health interventions will not know whether they are getting their money's worth from the programs they invest or participate in, whether their limited funds could be better spent elsewhere, or whether (and how) those programs could be improved and patients or clients served better.

An example of the usefulness of evaluations for decision making is provided by Kelly (1993). He noted that research on Adult Day Health Care (ADHC) has had a fourfold impact on care offered by Department of Veteran Affairs (VA) providers. First, evaluation results have assisted in defining the health care focus of ADHC and shaped consequent program design at many VA medical centers. Second, evaluation results have encouraged integration of research and program development. A third effect includes education of clinical program staff in the importance of program evaluation in patient care delivery. Finally, Kelly reported that research on ADHC often heightened the sensitivity of clinical staff to issues of cost-effectiveness even beyond the ADHC program.

Planning the Evaluation, Identifying Outcomes and Hypotheses

The purpose of an impact analysis is to test a program hypothesis, generally stated as the notion that the program's activities will have some beneficial influence on its participants (Mohr, 1992). Successful impact analyses result from formal, intensive planning efforts. Black (1993) suggested that these efforts address every stage of the research process, including:

Problem specification for the population of interest

Generating a description of the program

Developing hypotheses to test about the program from an examination of theory, the literature, and program descriptions, memoranda, or reports

Choosing a research design that is adequate to test these hypotheses

Specifying analytic methods consistent with the design, and making contingency plans for analyses when the design breaks down

Collecting data

Conducting the analyses of interest

Reporting the results and their limitations

Generating recommendations for the program planners

All of these issues should be the focus of project meetings, site visits, and other efforts conducted before the full evaluation design is developed. Hedrick, Bickman, and Rog (1993) noted that carefully planned research is more likely to proceed smoothly, and that moving too quickly without a plan increases the likelihood that the evaluation will be unfocused, address the wrong questions, miss important concepts, collect incomplete data, and yield irrelevant, poor, or even unusable information.

The first two elements of the evaluation research process are perhaps the most important focuses of the evaluation plan. Failure to identify correctly the health problems faced by the aged population of interest may lead to irrelevant or at least second-best programing efforts. Failure to understand the design and actual workings of the program may lead to evaluations lacking validity, even if the rest of the technical research processes are exemplary. Recognizing these issues, many evaluation funders ask for detailed evidence of an understanding of the problems or issues to be addressed by the programs they wish to have evaluated when proposals for competitive evaluation projects are solicited.

Describing the Black Box and Developing the Evaluation Plan

A useful evaluation plan requires efforts to learn the inner workings of the program being evaluated. Efforts also should be expended to learn what happens to "control" or "comparison" subjects (those not exposed to the program). According to Weiss, evaluators should "trace the life course of the program" including "the structures set up for its implementation, the motivations and attitudes of its staff, the recruitment of participants, the delivery of services, the ways in which services and schedules and expectations change over time, the responses of participants and their views of the meaning of the program in their lives" (Shadish, Cook, and Leviton, 1991, p. 203).

Knowing the contents of the intervention "black box" has several advantages. For example, it:

> Helps focus the evaluation, reducing the chance that the evaluation will go off-track and thus reducing the likelihood that irrelevancies will dominate the evaluation activities and result in wasted resources and frustration (Hedrick, Bickman, and Rog, 1993);

> Allows one to generate specific and testable hypotheses about the impact of the intervention (Rossi and Freeman, 1993);

> Helps one to make clear statements about the causes of outcomes actually observed in the treatment and control groups (Shadish, Cook, and Leviton, 1991); and

> Gives information needed to help reviewers of the evaluation decide if its results may generalize to other cases not directly studied (Shadish, Cook, and Leviton, 1991).

A good program description often can be developed on the basis of formal documents such as legislation, administrative regulations and manuals, funding proposals, annual reports, project memoranda, brochures, and previous evaluations (Rossi and Freeman, 1993). Government clients often provide basic project descriptions in requests for proposals (RFPs), but respondents to the RFPs and their clients can gain much by obtaining access to internal documents that provide evidence of how the program really works. In addition, site visits to observe the intervention program and face-to-face interviews with program providers, participants, and funders can provide useful information not available from written sources. For the PACE project, both Branch, Collum, and Zimmerman (1995) and Kane, Illston, and Miller (1992) conducted visits to intervention sites and interviewed key staff persons. Follow-up telephone calls were made to develop a more complete understanding of the operations of that demonstration project.

In many instances, those who design the evaluation study are involved with the development of the program and its administration, thereby facilitating the investigation into its inner workings. Sometimes the evaluators include the providers themselves, but care must be taken to assure objectivity in this case. An example of a merging of intervention and evaluation staff and perspectives is Tougaard and colleagues' (1992) study of the economic benefits of teaching patients with chronic obstructive pulmonary disease about their illness.

After the program description is developed, an evaluation program model can be generated that notes the relationships between the program objectives, activities, and expected outcomes (Rossi and Freeman, 1993). This evaluation model should be reviewed by as many stakeholders as possible (i.e., by all who are significantly affected by the program or who express a strong interest in its evaluation and subsequent policy recommendations).

Most social programs have multiple stakeholders, including program beneficiaries, service providers, program managers, funders, political action groups, consumer groups, or other organizations. Often these stakeholders have conflicting agendas and desires for intervention programs and public policy. Some stakeholders may oppose evaluations or perceive them as a threat. These and other stakeholders may desire to influence the program components to be analyzed, the specific outcome measures addressed, the resources committed to the evaluation, the analytical methods chosen, and the plan for utilizing evaluation results (Rossi and Freeman, 1993). It is doubtful that agreement among the many stakeholders will be obtained about all such issues. However, discussions with stakeholders about the evaluation plan will be enlightening and are likely to lead to a greater degree of validity (and perceptions of validity) of the study's methods.

Program Outcomes and Hypotheses

A useful evaluation plan will include substantial efforts to identify appropriate outcome measures for the analyses. According to Rossi and Freeman (1993), a poorly conceptualized outcome measure is not likely to represent well the objectives of the program and may lead to validity problems. They also note that the selection of unreliable outcome measures may result in underestimates of the effectiveness of the program.

Mohr (1992) introduced the concept of the *outcome line*, which illustrates graphically the relationships among program activities (efforts exerted by program personnel) and subsequent, related outcomes. Mohr considers his concept of the outcome line as a causal chain; program activities lead to the accomplishment of some outcomes noted as subobjectives, and these subobjectives lead to the accomplishment of major outcomes of interest.

Mohr noted that the complete outcome line provides a visual representation of the program theory. He suggested continually asking the question "Why perform this activity?" to help extend and complete the line. The completed line can then be used to help identify the outcomes that should be the focus of the economic evaluation. Mohr suggested that the goal is to find the particular set of outcomes needed for a good judgment of the effectiveness or value of the program; he called these the "inherently valued" outcomes (p. 14). Mohr noted that an outcome is inherently valued if either of the following statements is true:

On the outcome line, if outcome X is attained, subsequent outcomes do not matter.

Or, if outcome X is attained, one can safely assume that subsequent outcome Y will also be attained at a satisfactory level.

In either case, outcome X should be the focus of the evaluation.

In general, the process of completing an outcome line will result in a good idea of hypotheses to be tested in the economic evaluation. These hypotheses can be obtained from several sources, such as economic or other discipline-based theory; the economic and health services literature on the subject of interest; meta-analyses; case histories and case studies; focus groups; Delphi techniques; or other interviews with program staff, care providers, targets of the intervention, funders, other stakeholders, or experts in the substantive area (Black, 1993; Hedrick, Bickman, and Rog, 1993; Luft, 1989; Rossi and Freeman, 1993).

Design Issues, Reliability and Validity Threats

The purpose of the impact analyses of the evaluation is to test the program theory (i.e., that the program has some beneficial effect on desired economic or other outcomes of interest). The means of determining whether the program theory is correct is called the *design* of the evaluation (Mohr, 1992). The main goal of the evaluation design is to isolate the effects of extraneous or mediating factors so that observed differences between program participants and comparison or control group members can be attributed with confidence to the intervention and not to other plausible rival interpretations (Rossi and Freeman, 1993). The term "control group" is typically used in randomized (experimental) designs; the term "comparison group" is typically used in nonrandomized, quasi-experimental designs. Designs that fail to isolate extraneous and mediating factors are likely to result in evaluation findings that are adversely influenced by validity threats.

The best way to minimize the probability that program participants and comparison group members differ is via random assignment to either of these two categories. *Random assignment* can be defined as the unbiased (i.e., random) allocation to either program participant or control group status. This notion is to be contrasted with *random sampling*, which precedes random assignment. In random sampling, those who are offered the option of participating in an intervention (with later assignment to intervention or control groups) are selected in an unbiased manner from a population of interest, with known probabilities of selection (Rossi and Freeman, 1993). The difference between random assignment and random sampling is important because, without random sampling, evaluations that use random assignment to treatment or comparison groups are still likely to have substantial validity problems.

Cook and Campbell (1979) stated that the case for random assignment can be made because it is the best means of reducing the likelihood of various threats to the internal validity and statistical conclusion validity of the evaluation. They defined *internal validity* as the extent to which conclusions can safely be drawn regarding cause-effect relationships between program participation and subsequent outcomes. They defined *statistical conclusion validity* as the extent to which one may detect statistically the effects that are present as a result of program participation. We note examples of threats to these and other types of validity below. First we present a discussion of the potential use of randomization and its design alternatives as a means of facilitating the interpretation of evaluation results.

Randomization and Design Alternatives

Cook and Campbell (1979) listed several situations that make randomized designs more feasible. These include:

When lotteries are socially acceptable as a way of distributing scarce intervention resources. This may be the case when the demand for the intervention exceeds the supply of resources to be devoted to it. A randomized evaluation is a type of lottery in which each participant has a known and equal chance of being assigned to intervention or control groups.

When the innovation cannot be delivered in all units at once. When it is impossible to introduce the intervention at the same time to all of its participants, one can randomly assign which times the intervention is received. When this is done, the first and last to receive the intervention are equivalent in a probabilistic sense and can be used in comparisons as intervention and control groups.

When those who may receive the intervention are separated geographically and communication between them is low.

When change from the status quo is mandated but solutions to the problem of interest are acknowledged to be unknown. In situations like this, there is a strong desire for change and a willingness to try alternative interventions to determine which accomplish the desired outcomes.

When persons express no preference among alternatives being considered.

When the evaluator has strong control over the participants in the evaluation. Random assignment is facilitated by strong links to the client, funder, or targets of interest and control over how resources are allocated to intervention and control group members.

Examples of health interventions for the aged that incorporated randomized designs include the Channeling project's examination of the benefits of case management services as a deterrent to institutionalization (Brown, 1989), another study of case management that compared a neighborhood team approach to a centralized individual model (Eggert et al., 1991), a study of the impact of a Geriatric Assessment Unit on health care expenditures (Applegate et al., 1991), and the first phase of the evaluation of the VA's Adult Day Health Care program as an alternative to nursing home placement (Hedrick et al., 1993).

Rossi and Freeman (1993) noted that randomization is difficult to apply or maintain when:

The intervention is in its early stages. Projects in early stages may need frequent changes in structure to perfect their operation or delivery.

The enrollment demand is minimal. When very few potential clients express an interest in the intervention, diversion of a subset of these potential clients to control status may be unacceptable to certain stakeholders.

Participants, providers, or other stakeholders have ethical qualms about denying treatment to those perceived to be in need. However, if the demand for the intervention exceeds the supply of resources one may devote to it, randomization may be viewed as the fairest way to allocate those resources.

Time and money are limited. Randomized controlled trials often require extensive management processes that tend to consume large amounts of time and money.

Stakeholders prefer generalizability over internal validity concerns. The tight controls on selection processes and program management required in randomized evaluations often mean that the randomized experiment must be small in size. Hence it is likely to be less generalizable to the population of interest.

The integrity of the evaluation may be threatened easily. This may occur by failure of intervention or control group members to follow protocols, morbidity or mortality, or other reasons for dropping out of the evaluation.

An example of a nonrandomized study of adult day health care is a Canadian effort described by Neufeld and Strang (1992). The authors cited the small scale of the program and the fact that it was still in its developing stages as the primary reasons random assignment was deemed infeasible.

When randomization is not feasible, quasi-experimental designs may be used to make inferences about the effect of the intervention. The usefulness of a quasi-experimental design depends on the ability to find a comparison group of subjects who are similar to those who obtain the intervention. Finding an appropriate comparison group can be done in a variety of ways, such as:

by using generic comparisons. In this instance, established outcome norms are used as a basis for comparison to intervention subjects;

by matching. In this case, comparison groups are established by finding subjects who are identical in relevant respects (e.g., demographics, preferences, socioeconomic factors) to persons in the intervention group;

by using a regression-discontinuity design. This is appropriate when the selection procedure used to establish eligibility for the intervention is known and consistently and accurately applied; and

by statistical processes. Multivariate statistical procedures such as regression analysis are used to account for differences between intervention and comparison group members so that observed outcomes may be attributable to the intervention program (Rossi and Freeman, 1993).

Cook and Campbell (1979) noted that statistical processes dominate program evaluation research, with the most common mode of causal inference resulting from the treatment of intervention status as a binary (yes or no) variable in a multiple regression analysis. Thus, we will focus on this type of design.

When multiple regression techniques are used to rule out differences between treatment and comparison group members as reasons for observing outcomes of interest, the effect of the intervention is inferred from the size and statistical significance of the regression coefficient for the binary intervention status indicator. An example from the National Long Term Care Demonstration (the Channeling project) evaluation illustrates this (Brown, 1989). The purpose of that demonstration was to assess whether nursing home placement could be avoided or delayed by the provision of case management services in the community. For the evaluation of the demonstration, intervention participants were assigned to a control group or to one of two intervention groups that differed according to the amount of case management services received. Relationships between outcome measures of interest, the two case management intervention types, and other factors were modeled in a linear regression equation as follows:

$$(1) \; Y = \alpha_1 + \alpha_2 B + \alpha_3 F + \alpha_i \Sigma S_i + \alpha_j \Sigma X_j + \epsilon$$

where Y represents an outcome of interest (e.g., total health care expenditures), B and F are binary indicators for membership in the two case management intervention groups, S_i reflects a group of binary indicators to account for the fact that multiple sites across the country were included in the intervention, and X_j represents a group of confounding factors that influence outcomes. The inclusion of the S_i and X_j factors adjusts for differences in the two intervention groups and the control group. A critical issue, of course, is the extent that X_j accounts for *all* the confounding factors, a point that we will return to later.

In equation (1), the alphas represent factors that have to be estimated statistically. These factors illustrate the impact of the relevant variable on the outcome of interest. For example, α_2 and α_3 represent the relative impact on the outcome variable of membership in each of the two case management intervention groups, compared to membership in the control group.

Validity and Reliability in Economic Analyses of Health Interventions

Two types of validity—internal validity and statistical conclusion validity—were defined earlier. Below we describe several threats to the internal validity and statistical conclusion validity of an evaluation. We also define construct validity and external validity and describe problems in those areas that may compromise the quality of the evaluation. Cook and Campbell (1979) devoted several pages of their text to validity threats, so we restrict our offering to the more problematic ones often encountered in economic analyses of health interventions for aged populations.

Internal Validity

Threats to internal validity make it more difficult to infer causal relationships between the intervention in question and the outcomes observed in the sample of aged persons who are studied. Several internal validity threats are described by Cook and Campbell (1979). Of these, perhaps the most pervasive in health services research is selection bias. *Selection bias* refers to systematic, uncontrolled differences between participants in the evaluation and the population from which they came, or between those who receive the intervention and those who do not.

Random sampling and random assignment can minimize the threat of the two most common types of selection bias. The first type of selection bias is the possibility that those who decline to participate in the evaluation of the intervention are systematically different from those who do participate, resulting in differences between those in the evaluation and those in the aged population of interest. Participants who volunteer for the evaluation may be more highly educated, be more motivated to try new approaches to care, be less risk-averse, have greater exposure to advertisements of the intervention, or be different in other unmeasured ways than those who decline to participate. If the factors that determine participation in the evaluation also influence the outcomes of interest, observed differences in outcomes between intervention subjects and the comparison group members may be due to those factors, not just to the intervention itself (Rossi and Freeman, 1993).

To adjust for this type of selection bias without random sampling, one must attempt to estimate the influence of factors that determine the desire to participate in the evaluation, and then incorporate the predicted probability of participation for each individual into the impact assessment. Usually, multiple regression techniques are used for this purpose. Heckmann (1976) and Olsen (1980) described these techniques and their underlying theory in detail. It should be noted that the successful implementation of these techniques often requires reliable survey data about the decision whether to participate in the evaluation, and always requires a good statistical model of how the predictors of participation affect that decision. Cook and Campbell (1979) argued that, without these attributes, regression-based corrections for selection bias may produce misleading results.

Many evaluations solicit participation from a population of interest and then randomly assign participants either to receive the intervention or to a control group that receives no treatment or usual treatment. If random assignment fails to produce equivalent intervention and control groups, or if serious attrition from either group occurs, the systematic differences that result between the groups will lead to the second type of selection bias. Initial attempts at random assignment may fail if intervention providers do not support the need for randomization or make conscious (nonrandom) decisions to assign participants to intervention or control groups. Attrition may be problematic if intervention subjects who are not affected much by the intervention become disgruntled and leave the experiment, or if the intervention or control group subjects die, move, or fail to comply with the study protocol at different rates (Rossi and Freeman, 1993).

Brown (1989) tested for these problems in the evaluation of the Channeling project. In that project, applicants were selected from demonstration sites and, after verification of functional eligibility, were subsequently randomly assigned to a control group or either of two demonstration interventions relatively early during the application process. The interventions varied according to the extent of case management activities for elderly who were at risk of nursing home placement. To address whether the randomization scheme resulted in similar intervention and control groups before the intervention took place, Brown examined 53 demographic, socioeconomic, functional status, and previous health care utilization measures collected at initial screening. Only a few significant differences were found, no more than one would expect from chance alone, and there was no pattern to the differences (i.e., neither treatment nor control groups had consistently higher or lower values on these variables).

An example in which random assignment failed was a study by Menard and colleagues (1992) of systolic hypertension in elderly patients. In the study, 4,736 subjects were randomly divided into an active treatment or placebo group. After five years of follow-up, treatment was terminated in 13 percent of those in the active group because of side effects. In addition, the authors reported that application of the protocol rules meant that active treatment was necessary for 44 percent of those in the placebo group when systolic blood pressure reached a critical point. These problems led to significant differences in treatment and control groups that may not be attributable to the intervention per se.

Statistical Conclusion Validity

Threats to statistical conclusion validity make it more difficult to detect important relationships between the intervention and observed outcomes. Cook and Campbell (1979) provided a detailed description of several threats to statistical conclusion validity. We limit our focus to threats that are often problematic in economic evaluations of health interventions for aged populations. These include low reliability of outcome or other measures, low statistical power to detect important relationships between the intervention and outcomes, and violated assumptions of statistical tests.

Low Reliability. When outcomes or other variables of interest are measured with low reliability, the result may be an underestimation of the effects of the intervention on the outcomes of interest (Rossi and Freeman, 1993). *Reliability* can be defined in a practical sense as the degree of consistency between two measures of the same thing. These "two measures" could result from any of the following (Black, 1993):

Splitting the sample used in the evaluation into two parts and applying the same test or measure to each part

Performing repeated tests on the same sample members

Having two scorers use the same test on the same sample members

Applying two different but related tests on the same sample members (this also can be done to assess construct validity, which is described later)

Similar results for measures obtained from these techniques provide evidence of reliable measures. Black (1993) noted that reliability also can be measured in terms of "internal consistency," which is the degree of homogeneity of items on a test or questionnaire (i.e., the relative degree to which the responses to individual items correlate with the total test score). Rossi and Freeman (1993) noted that reliability will increase as the number of related questions asked about a concept increases. They also noted that single questions are rarely adequate to measure important concepts or outcomes of interest.

Internal consistency measures have been developed by Cronbach (1951) and Kuder and Richardson (1937). These measures are more closely related to classical test theory than are the reliability techniques obtained from two measures as described above. However, Nunnally (1978) showed that reliability estimates obtained from internal consistency techniques and multiple tests tend to be highly correlated. The advantage of the internal consistency measure is that there is no need to split the evaluation sample, use multiple scorers, or perform more than one test.

Technically, reliability refers to the *use* of a measure; it is not an inherent feature of the measure. Therefore, even standard, well-known scales should be assessed for reliability in every evaluation in which they are used (Carmines and Zeller, 1979). Requests for evaluation proposals should state that reliability estimates are part of the scope of work of the project, and responses to RFPs should note how reliability may be assessed.

Ozminkowski, Supiano, and Campbell (1991) provided an example of reliability estimation for a scale of satisfaction among volunteers who performed enrichment activities in nursing homes in two Michigan counties. For that project, volunteers were recruited from local areas to work in eight nursing homes in Washtenaw County or Wayne County. Volunteers were trained to help social workers provide memory training groups, creative writing groups, and life history-taking sessions in the homes. Part of the evaluation of the volunteers' experience was assessed with an eight-item scale that addressed positive and negative dimensions of the nursing home experience (e.g., was the experience happy, rewarding, worthwhile, fun, depressing, anxiety producing, scary, or frustrating?). Reliability of each dimension was assessed using Chronbach's alpha method and found to be high (0.87 and 0.84, respectively). With Chronbach's alpha method, as with most measures of internal consistency, reliability may vary from 0.0 to 1.0, with 0.0 illustrating no internal consistency and 1.0 illustrating complete consistency.

Low Statistical Power. Low statistical power to detect important relationships between interventions and observed outcomes usually results from having too few subjects in the intervention and comparison groups. Power can be defined as the ability to detect a real program effect (Rossi and Freeman, 1993). Power is usually measured in terms of a percentage, with 80 percent power to detect a program effect as a popular objective to attain. A priori, one can estimate the power one is likely to attain from a given evaluation sample size, or one can estimate the sample size required to obtain a given level of power. Cohen (1977) and Kraemer and Thiemann (1987) provided methods for conducting such power analyses. To strengthen the design of the evaluation, these analyses should be required by clients and/or offered by those responding to requests for evaluation proposals.

The power of a proposed evaluation design must be considered with a competing demand in mind. Without increasing the sample size for the evaluation, one may increase statistical power, but this would occur at the expense of increasing the probability of making a Type-I (alpha) error (i.e., concluding that the intervention has an effect when it really does not). Conversely, one can avoid concluding that the program is effective when it is not by choosing a more stringent level for statistical testing (e.g., 0.01 instead of the more customary 0.05 probability for making an alpha error). However, doing this will decrease the power to detect a program effect unless the sample size is increased. Rossi and Freeman (1993) suggested that evaluators, clients, and other stakeholders decide a priori which type of error (low power to detect a program effect versus incorrectly concluding that the program is effective) is more important to avoid for policy or decision-making purposes, and then design the study accordingly.

The potential for low power and Type-I error was considered in the evaluation of the Channeling project. Researchers considered: (1) the pattern of findings in several analyses, (2) the magnitude of the regression coefficients that measured the impact of the two forms of case management, and (3) the statistical significance of the estimated impacts of Channeling case management (Brown, 1989). The hypothesis was that consistency across multiple analyses with respect to the direction, size, and statistical significance of the estimates of Channeling's impact would provide evidence that the evaluators avoided problems with statistical power and limited the odds of making incorrect conclusions about program effectiveness. This approach is recommended for evaluations with multiple outcomes of interest because the likelihood of finding at least one statistically significant relationship increases with the number of tests conducted. If only a few significant results are obtained, or if the results are not consistent with expectation, chance (rather than the intervention) may have been the determining factor for the observed outcomes.

Violated Assumptions. Statistical tests are used in most evaluations to make inferences about the impact of the intervention on outcomes of interest. The validity of these tests often depends upon the likelihood that their underlying assumptions are met. For example, some tests for differences in means between intervention and control group members are predicated upon the equality of variances between the two groups (i.e., that the distribution of scores for a given measure is comparable between the two groups). Other procedures, such as multiple regression techniques, are based upon normal distributions in the outcome measures, low correlations between intervention status and confounding measures, constant variances among regression residuals, and the appropriate specification of linear or nonlinear relationships between outcomes and their determinants (Kennedy, 1992). The degree of robustness of the statistical tests to their underlying assumptions varies. Even so, as a matter of course, evaluators should consider the underlying assumptions of the tests they propose to use. They also should note how violations of those assumptions might influence the ability to detect significant relationships between the intervention and outcomes of interest, and adjust the testing strategy or the design of the evaluation to avoid problems.

Appropriately used, statistical tests will contribute to an understanding of the relationships between the intervention and outcomes of interest. As the results of statistical tests are considered, the researcher should note in particular whether estimates of the effects of the intervention are important in a practical sense, not just in a statistical sense (meaningful as well as significant). For example, one should consider whether the effects are great enough in magnitude to suggest a worthwhile public policy or to contribute to decision-making processes about the intervention. If the effects are small but statistically significant, one should consider whether policy changes would be worth their cost to stakeholders.

Construct Validity

Construct validity refers to the extent to which facets of the conceptual framework are operationalized successfully in the evaluation (Hedrick, Bickman, and Rog, 1993). Black (1993) noted that, to be valid, a questionnaire must be logically consistent and cover comprehensively all of the aspects of the concept to be studied. This is sometimes referred to as content validity as well as construct validity. If the concepts employed in the evaluation have construct validity, they also are likely to be useful for classifying intervention and comprison group members accurately according to the phenomenon of interest, and for predicting their behavior in the future. For example, valid measures of depression in the elderly will accurately classify most elderly people as either high, medium, or low in terms of their depression level.

Cook and Campbell (1979) described several threats to construct validity. Examples include the lack of a theoretical base for developing concepts measured in the evaluation, a failure to consult theory and previous work for guidance regarding the expected relationships between outcomes and the intervention, the use of a single measure or method for characterizing a concept of interest, and interactions between testing methods and treatment processes. Measures have construct validity if they measure what they are intended to measure. Consistent with the spirit of Cook and Campbell, Freeman and Rossi (1993) noted that construct validity is likely if the measures chosen by the evaluators:

are consistent with past work on the concept (i.e., do not contradict the usual ways that the concept has been used in the past);

produce results that are similar to those found in previous uses; and

have internal consistency. In this respect, valid measures first must be reliable ones. If many items are used to measure a concept, each item should produce roughly similar results if used independently.

The Channeling project research team was worried that two issues may have compromised the construct validity of the evaluation (Brown, 1989). These issues were the use of proxy respondents for up to 45 percent of elderly persons who were meant as the subjects of the evaluation, and the use of different methods for collecting some data between intervention and control group members. Both of these methods might have interacted with the interventions to produce the outcomes observed.

To deal with the proxy respondent issue, the Channeling researchers looked for significant differences in outcomes when proxies were used versus when they were not used. For most outcome measures, differences were small and not significant. The exception to this pattern was the measure of global life satisfaction, which was significantly higher on average among Channeling subjects when proxies were used. For this measure, one cannot tell whether the use of the proxies produced the observed results, or whether those who underwent the intervention were more satisfied with their life situation (Brown, 1989).

Because of a lack of resources, the Channeling project used two different data collection methods. Some data for those who received case management intervention services were collected by case managers, while data for control group members were collected by the evaluators. This risky but unavoidable strategy could have resulted in observed outcomes that were due to the data collection strategy instead of the intervention.

To address this possibility, the evaluators compared intervention and control group members on several baseline variables that were collected by researchers and case managers after the initial screening but before the intervention took place. As noted above, the researchers already had evidence from the screening data that random assignment produced equivalent intervention and control groups, so differences in the baseline measures that consistently favored one group could be attributable to the data collection strategy. The researchers found that about half of the baseline variables were measured similarly by case managers and evaluators. The remaining variables appeared to have been measured differently and were excluded as adjustors for confounding influences in subsequent analyses. This strategy led to a specification error in the regression equations (i.e., important confounding variables were omitted from the analyses). This specification error limited the statistical conclusion validity of the tests of the impact of case management.

External Validity and Generalizability

External validity is defined as the extent to which one can generalize from the evaluation data and context to other populations and settings (Cook and Campbell, 1979; Hedrick, Bickman, and Rog, 1993). To be generalizable, the evaluation must be conducted on a sample that was selected in an unbiased manner from the population at risk or the population at need (Rossi and Freeman, 1993).

Generalizability may be compromised in a number of ways. For example, extremely motivated (or not), or otherwise high- (or low-) quality staff may produce an intervention leading to results that are not generalizable to other settings or populations (Rossi and Freeman, 1993). Also, interactions between the treatment and its timing may reduce generalizability. Interventions held only on weekends when people are relatively less active or in a state of relaxation may produce different results than if offered at various times and days throughout the week. Similarly, interventions offered in an institutional setting such as a nursing home may not produce the same result as when offered outside the nursing home or in an alternative setting such as a hospital swing bed. Finally, interventions for the young-old (e.g., aged 65–74) may not produce results that are generalizable to the old-old (above age 85). To avoid these problems, large samples may be required and interventions may be provided at various times and places.

Tradeoffs among Validity Threats

It is readily apparent that many factors can influence the validity of an economic evaluation of a health intervention. Researchers and stakeholders are well advised to consider the potential for biases as alternative evaluation designs are considered. Cook and Campbell (1979) noted that random assignment is no guarantee of high-quality research, but it does help minimize the influence of confounding factors on outcomes of interest. However, random assignment does not prevent threats to external validity or construct validity, nor does it prevent all of the internal validity or statistical conclusion validity threats. When random assignment is not possible, quasi-experimental designs are required, but these may be more susceptible to validity threats (Rossi and Freeman, 1993). How does one decide what tradeoffs to make?

Hedrick, Bickman, and Rog (1993) suggested that, for analyses that focus heavily on the impact of an intervention, statistical conclusion validity and internal validity may be more important. In such evaluations, the ability to detect a real program effect and the confidence with which one assumes causality between the program and observed outcomes are important. Cook and Campbell (1979) noted that the interests of internal validity are more important (and hence should have more influence on the design of the evaluation) when the cost of being wrong about a causal inference is high. If an ineffective policy may be implemented on a wide scale or an effective program may be reduced or eliminated as a result of the evaluation, internal validity considerations should be paramount. This is because threats to internal validity reduce the ability to make appropriate inferences about causal relationships between the intervention and outcomes of interest.

A good general strategy for evaluators is to engage stakeholders in several conversations or meetings to obtain agreement (or at least air their differences) about their priorities. Would they prefer a less rigorous evaluation that uses a larger sample and produces more generalizable results, or would they prefer a more rigorous one that is smaller in scale but produces better estimates of the impact of the intervention? Which is more important for good policy or responsible decision making? Cook and Campbell stated that jeopardizing the ability to make causal inferences for the sake of increasing the generalizability of a study "usually entails minimal gain for a considerable loss" (p. 84), but this reflects a value judgment on their part.

Data Issues and Sources

As the economic evaluation is being planned and design issues are addressed, researchers will give careful thought to potential data sources. Ideally, data considerations would not have much influence over the design of the study, as one could design the optimal scientific way to proceed and collect data accordingly. This rarely happens however, because most primary data collection efforts are time consuming and they can be extraordinarily expensive. As a result, instead of asking the question "What data do I need to implement this optimal design and how do I collect them?" researchers are often forced to face up to their limited funding and time constraints and ask "If these are the only data available, what valid work can I do with them?" The answer often suggests a much more limited scope than one would like to take, and it may require many caveats about the limitations of the evaluation. Decisions regarding which data collection efforts and analyses to forgo should be made in conjunction with the client and other stakeholders. Omitting part of the desired evaluation framework increases the potential to produce biased or misleading results (Hedrick, Bickman, and Rog, 1993).

When time and money permit, primary data collection (i.e., that which is new and specifically tailored to the intervention being evaluated) may be preferable, because this approach keeps a strong tie between the design of the analysis and measurement of the concepts one really cares most about. To contrast, when dealing with secondary data (i.e., data collected originally for some other purposes), evaluators often must use the data in unintended ways. Thus, variables included in the secondary data sets may not really represent what the researchers wish to measure (Hedrick, Bickman, and Rog, 1993).

The use of secondary data was problematic in the assessment of the New York Quality Assurance System (NYQAS), which was a new survey-based method for certifying the quality of nursing homes in New York State. For that evaluation, the major data source included information on only the few medical conditions or problem types that were necessary to assign nursing home residents to a Resource Utilization Group-II (RUGs-II) category (Schwartz et al., 1994). These data were collected for reimbursement purposes; reimbursement was based upon the average RUGs-II score for elderly in the nursing home. Because of this, the evaluators did not have enough information to assess whether services provided matched service needs. As a result, the evaluation focused on only a few important outcomes. These included whether NYQAS resulted in a change in the rate of deterioration in physical functioning, and whether it was associated with the prevalence of selected adverse outcomes that could be measured with secondary data.

Luft (1989) and Hedrick, Bickman, and Rog (1993) offered some tips for dealing with secondary data:

Find out where data were assembled and how they were collected. Establish a liaison with data set developers or programmers who can offer consultation on the nature and contents of the data and how data change over time.

Print the first 100 or so observations from the data set. Carefully screen the contents of the data fields to make sure the data set does not suffer from many missing values that would make important fields unusable.

Conduct logical tests of the items in the data set (e.g., compute age from date of birth, compute lengths of stay from admission and discharge dates, etc.). Note questionable values (extremely long lengths of stay, age over 100, gynecological use by males, etc.).

Sort the questionable values from the logical tests according to the source of the data. Then determine whether some observational units (e.g., physicians, hospitals, nursing homes) seem to have a large number of problematic observations. Investigate further whether problematic observations should be dropped; often the liaison noted above may be helpful in this regard.

When regression analyses are run, use options in the statistical programs to check for observations with heavy influence on the coefficients of policy-relevant variables. Identify the influential observations and sort according to source to see if the influential ones tend to come from the same sources. Rerun the regressions with and without the influential observations and note the change in the policy-relevant variable coefficients.

If one is lucky enough to have multiple, independent data sets that allow measurement of the same concepts, compare measures from the two data sets for consistency. Evidence from outside sources may suggest that one data set should be the preferred one for analysis.

Despite the caveats and concerns one might have to make when secondary data sets are used, they are often the only available data that can be used to study questions of interest. It has been noted that data collected for reimbursement purposes (e.g., to facilitate proper payment for health care services) tend to be quite reliable and valid (Hendrick, Bickman, and Rog, 1993). This bodes well for economic studies.

Conducting Data Analysis

After the design of the economic intervention has been established and the data have been collected, analyses of relationships between the intervention and outcomes of interest may begin. The analyses to be collected depend entirely upon the outcomes of interest and the hypotheses derived during the evaluation planning and design stages.

In most economic evaluations, quantitative analyses are conducted using statistical tests. In a randomized experiment, differences in mean outcome levels between the treatment and control groups are often used to measure the impact of the evaluation. Analyses also may be conducted for subgroups of interest (e.g., comparing males to females or comparing racial or ethnic groups) if the design allows, again usually based upon differences in means. The size of the intervention effect is often expressed as the difference in means between the intervention and control groups, divided by a pooled standard deviation of the outcome values. This "effect size" is a unitless measure that can be noted for comparisons to other studies (as in meta-analyses) or for comparisons among subgroups of interest.

Effect size estimates can be generated for randomized or quasi-experimental studies. With quasi-experimental designs, regression analyses or other techniques are often used to adjust for the impact of confounding variables when the impact of the intervention is estimated. Several good textbooks of quasi-experimental methods or econometric methods are available to help estimate program impact (e.g., Cook and Campbell, 1979; Rossi and Freeman, 1993; Kmenta, 1986; Kennedy, 1992). We have already noted several issues to consider during the planning and design stages; successfully addressing those issues increases the likelihood of conducting useful data analyses.

So far we have not differentiated program costs, health expenditures, or other monetary measures from other outcomes of interest. This is because the planning, design, and analytical issues raised above should be considered regardless of the outcome of interest. However, in the last thirty years or so, techniques for cost-benefit analysis, cost-effectiveness analysis, and cost-utility analysis have been perfected and become popular for investment decision making and program evaluation. Because there are several good textbooks describing these techniques (Gramlich, 1981; Warner and Luce, 1982; Drummond, Stoddart, and Torrance, 1987), we provide just a brief review of some issues relevant to those techniques here.

Cost-Benefit, Cost-Effectiveness, and Cost-Utility Analyses

Cost-benefit analysis (CBA) refers to a set of techniques used to estimate the lifetime dollar costs and dollar benefits that would be received as a result of the innovation. Costs and benefits in out-years of the program are discounted at a specified rate, so they may be measured in current dollars. Discounting is used to adjust for the fact that dollars spent or received in the future are less valuable than those spent or received in the present. Discounted costs are subtracted from discounted benefits, to calculate the net present dollar value of the innovation. Alternatively, if one is unsure about the appropriate discount rate to use, an internal rate of return can be calculated. The internal rate of return equals the discount rate necessary to achieve a net present value of zero dollars. High rates of return correspond to higher net present values; both indicate economically worthwhile programs.

Cost-benefit analysis was developed to facilitate comparisons between alternative programs whose costs and benefits could be monetized. The program with the higher net present value or rate of return would be preferable. When costs and benefits accrue at different times throughout the life of the programs being compared, the discount rate chosen can influence the difference between the net present values that are estimated. Krahn and Gafni (1993) noted that the decision of which discount rate to use should not be taken lightly, since changes in the rate chosen can dramatically reorder funding priorities. High discount rates favor short-term interventions that tend to be therapeutic in nature. Low rates favor long-term programs that are typically preventive in nature. The appropriate choice of the discount rate depends on whose perspective the analysis is based. If the perspective is an individual's, his or her time preference rate for money should be used as the discount rate. If the perspective is the government's or society's, a social discount rate should be used (e.g., the real long-term growth rate in the economy over the last generation, usually measured since the end of World War II). Analysts often estimate net present values using a variety of discount rates. This is one form of sensitivity analysis often conducted.

Cost-benefit analysis requires that all program costs (direct and indirect) and benefits be estimated in dollar terms. There is often controversy about assigning dollar values to program benefits (e.g., how does one place a dollar value on a year of life saved, if that is the benefit of the program?). When it is impossible, or at least controversial, to assign dollar values to benefits, *cost-effectiveness* or *cost-utility analysis* are preferred techniques.

Cost-effectiveness and cost-utility analyses are useful for comparing interventions with similar outcome measures or objectives (e.g., to reduce morbidity or mortality). In cost-effectiveness analysis (CEA) and cost-utility analysis (CUA), program costs are monetized but program benefits are noted in the appropriate outcome units, such as years of life saved, quality-adjusted years of life saved, cancers detected, and the like. The results of the CEA or CUA are arrayed in terms of cost per unit of benefit; lower cost-per-unit-of-benefit programs are preferred.

Cost-utility analysis differs from cost-effectiveness analysis in that an explicit attempt is made to estimate the value of the benefits obtained. Subjects are asked to value the benefits, usually on a scale from 0 to 1, with 1 indicating a higher value or utility. For example, subjects may be asked how valuable one extra year of life may be, or may be asked to value a specified number of reduced days of disability or illness. The analysts then adjust the amount of each benefit obtained from the intervention by the value estimates (Drummond, Stoddart, and Torrance, 1987). Cost-utility analysis is still a relatively new analytic technique; hence its use is controversial. For example, Gill and Feinstein (1994) noted that quality of life is "a uniquely personal perception" (p. 619). They said this makes it difficult for investigators to characterize quality of life for their study populations, and that many researchers fail to give reasons for selecting the quality of life measures they use. In addition, they noted that health-related quality of life is usually not distinguished from overall quality of life. Construct validity threats are problematic.

Another issue in CEA or CUA is whether to discount nonmonetary benefits, and, if so, which discount rate to use. Many researchers are uncomfortable with the notion that future lives, for example, are less valuable than present lives. However, arguments for discounting benefits do not require such assumptions. Keeler and Cretin (1983) showed that a lower (or zero) discount rate for benefits than costs means that every health program can be made more economically attractive by delaying it indefinitely! This is because delays reduce the present value of costs needed to achieve the benefits of the program, but, without discounting, the benefits, remain the same. Thus, the longer we wait, the better the cost-effectiveness ratio ap-

pears. Krahn and Gafni (1993) suggested that the appropriate discount rate for benefits reflects how stakeholders feel about buying future as opposed to present health
benefits with today's dollars. To avoid double-discounting, they also noted that discounting in a CUA should be done carefully. This is because many popular utility
measurement procedures already are based upon estimates of time preferences for
the benefits being considered.

There are several issues to consider when performing a CBA, CEA, or CUA.
The appropriate discount rate and the decision regarding which stakeholder's views
should drive the analysis have already been mentioned. Others to consider were suggested by Rossi and Freeman (1993), Drummond, Stoddart, and Torrance (1987),
and Warner and Luce (1982); these include:

> The limits to efforts to identify costs and benefits. Mohr (1992) suggested ap-
> plying the concept of the outcome line to identify benefits for consideration.

> Whether benefits for different categories of respondents should be weighted dif-
> ferently (e.g., should benefits to those with more severe access problems or to those
> with greater needs for service be weighed more heavily than benefits to others?).

> Which assumptions are/are not selected as the basis of sensitivity analyses.

> The marginal costs per unit of benefit of the program (i.e., how much more
> one unit of benefit costs in each program being compared). This gives insight
> into which programs should be expanded first, and at what point to stop ex-
> pansion. Theory suggests expanding the program with the lower marginal cost,
> and to stop expanding when the marginal costs per unit of benefit of each pro-
> gram are equal.

> How the results of the analysis should be used in subsequent decision-making
> processes. Warner and Luce (1982) noted that CBA and CEA are simply tools
> that facilitate decision-making processes. They should not be the only sources
> of information for the decision-making processes, and often have not been the
> driving forces in those processes.

These issues should be considered in the evaluation planning and design stages.
The rationale for decisions made, and the results of the accompanying analyses,
should be described in detail in the project report.

Reporting the Evaluation

The evaluation report may be the only document that many stakeholders see.
Whether or not the report is used as the basis for subsequent policy, it will add to

the knowledge base and cast impressions on its audience. Black (1993), Hedrick, Bickman, and Rog (1993), and Luft (1989) noted that the evaluation report should contain:

a clear statement of the research question;

a discussion of relevant outcomes and program activities;

a list of hypothesized relationships among program activities and outcomes, supported by theory, literature, program documents, or qualitative studies;

a description of the evaluation subjects, the population they were selected from, and the sampling procedure used to select subjects for analysis;

an account of the conditions under which data were collected;

a description of measurement instruments and the reliability and validity of their use in the evaluation;

a discussion of analytic design and methods and associated validity threats;

a presentation of the results of the analyses conducted for the evaluation, and a comparison of these results to previous studies;

the rationale for sensitivity analyses chosen and the results of those analyses;

a thorough discussion of the limitations of the evaluation's scope, design, methods, and generalizability; and

conclusions and recommendations.

In short, the complete history of the evaluation should be documented, along with concerns about its usefulness to stakeholders and for subsequent policy. Hedrick, Bickman, and Rog (1993) noted that the impact of resource constraints on the evaluation should be discussed. They say the researchers should state explicitly what would be necessary for a comprehensive study and how the research either meets or does not meet those requirements. Luft (1989) suggested sending a draft of the evaluation report to intervention site personnel. They will often help find and correct errors and can help interpret unexpected results.

Discussion and Recommendations

Economic evaluations of interventions may be used to help sell a program model to other settings, to help make informed decisions about program refinement, or to alter public policy. If one examines the literature, however, it is difficult to cite many examples of the influence of program evaluations on decision making for several reasons (Shadish, Cook, and Leviton, 1991):

Program managers and providers may resist changes suggested by the evaluation.

The wide variety of stakeholders may include those who feel threatened by an evaluation and work to suppress its conduct or use in policy making.

Policy evolves gradually, over a long period, from implicit rules about what can be done, improvisation in new situations, negotiation of conflicts, opportunities that arise, countermoves when bargaining breaks down, and other reasons. The evaluation may have little impact over these.

As Weiss noted, "evaluations often are not used to make decisions because they require an unusual concatenation of circumstances. Among the requisite conditions appear to be: research directly relevant to an issue up for decision, available before the time of decision, that addresses the issue within the parameters of feasible action, that comes out with clear and unambiguous results, that is known to decisionmakers, who understand its concepts and findings and are willing to listen, that does not run athwart of entrenched interests or powerful blocks, and that is implementable within the limits of existing resources" (Shadish, Cook, and Leviton, 1991, p. 191).

Regardless of these issues, Weiss went on to say that stakeholders and policy makers *do* pay attention to the quality of the evaluation and may use its results to add to the knowledge base they draw upon when decisions are made. Moreover, evaluation research continues to pass the market test: If it were not desirable and useful for important purposes, funders would not continue to devote hundreds of millions of dollars to it annually. Thus, it is important to pay attention to the factors that can determine how well the evaluation takes place. We conclude with several recommendations for consideration.

Spend the time to prepare a good evaluation plan. Failure to do so risks addressing the wrong question.

To keep the focus of the evaluation on track and generate useful findings, get to know the black box of the intervention. Generating an outcome line will help.

Talk to stakeholders frequently.

Consider random sampling and random assignment to treatment and control groups.

Generate contingency plans for the failure of the evaluation design.

Collect information on the determinants of the decisions made whether to participate in the evaluation.

To enhance reliability, derive multiple measures of important concepts.

Assess the reliability of outcome measures or other important variables.

Consider the threats to the validity of the evaluation design and plan the project to avoid as many threats as possible.

If possible, do not violate the assumptions under which statistical tests are to be conducted.

Conduct a power analysis to assure that sample sizes are appropriate for analyses of interest.

Vary the time and place of the intervention, if possible, to enhance the generalizability of the evaluation results.

Look for problems or inconsistencies in secondary data sets. Conduct an investigation to determine whether some observations should be discarded.

Conduct sensitivity analyses to assess the impact of important assumptions on the evaluation results.

Send a draft report to multiple stakeholders and address their concerns.

As Weiss noted, "evaluation is a rational enterprise that takes place in a political context" (Shadish, Cook, and Leviton, 1991, p. 187). No evaluation is perfect and good ones are not easy to do, but the better ones pay attention to the scientific research process as well as to the politics of the situation at hand.

References

Applegate, W. B., Graney, M. J., Miller, S. T., and Elam, J. T. 1991. Impact of a Geriatric Assessment Unit on subsequent health care charges. *American Journal of Public Health* 81:1302–6.

Black, T. R. 1993. *Evaluating Social Science Research: An Introduction.* London: Sage Publications, Inc.

Branch, L. G., Coulam, R. F., and Zimmerman, Y. A. 1995. The PACE evaluation: Initial Findings. *The Gerontologist.* 35:349–59.

Brown, L. 1989. The evaluation of the National Long Term Care Demonstration: 2. Estimation Methodology. In Defriese, G. H., Ricketts, T. C., and Stein, J. S., eds., *Methodological Advances in Health Services Research.* Ann Arbor, MI: Health Administration Press.

Carmines, E. G., and Zeller, R. A. 1979. *Reliability and Validity Assessment.* Beverly Hills, CA: Sage Publications, Inc.

Chronbach, L. J. 1951. Coefficient alpha and the internal structure of tests. *Psychometrika* 16:297–334.

Cohen, J. 1977. *Statistical Power Analysis for the Behavioral Sciences* (rev. ed.). New York: Academic Press.

Cook, T. D., and Campbell, D. T. 1979. *Quasi-Experimentation: Design and Analysis Issues for Field Settings*. Boston: Houghton Mifflin Co.

Drummond, M. F., Stoddart, G. L., and Torrance, G. W. 1987. *Methods for the Evaluation of Health Care Programmes*. Oxford: Oxford University Press.

Eggert, G. M., Zimmer, J. G., Hall, W. J., and Friedman, B. 1991. Case management: A randomized controlled study comparing a neighborhood team and a centralized individual model. *Health Services Research* 26:471–507.

Gill, T. M., and Feinstein, A. R. 1994. A critical appraisal of the quality of quality of life measurements. *Journal of the American Medical Association* 272:619–26.

Gramlich, E. M. 1981. *Benefit-Cost Analysis of Government Programs*. Englewood Cliffs, NJ: Prentice-Hall, Inc.

Heckmann, J. J. 1976. The common structure of statistical models of truncation, sample selection, and limited dependent variables, and a simple estimator for such models. *Annals of Economic and Social Measurement* 5:475–92.

Hedrick, S. C., Rothman, M. L., Chapko, M., and Connia, R. T. 1993. Summary and discussion of methods and results of the Adult Day Health Care Evaluation Study. *Medical Care* 31:SS94–103, Supplement.

Hedrick, T. E., Bickman, L., and Rog, D. L. 1993. *Applied Research Design: A Practical Guide*. Newbury Park, CA: Sage Publications, Inc.

Kane, R. L., Illston, L. H., and Miller, N. M. 1992. Qualitative Analysis of the Program of All-Inclusive Care for the Elderly (PACE). *Gerontologist* 36:771–80.

Keeler, E. B., and Cretin, S. 1983. Discounting of life-saving and other non-monetary benefits. *Management Science* 29:300–310.

Kelly, J. R. 1993. The Adult Day Health Care Evaluation Study: Impact on VA Programs. *Medical Care* 31:SS116–21.

Kennedy, P. 1992. *A Guide to Econometrics* (3rd ed.). Cambridge, MA: MIT Press.

Kmenta, J. 1986. *Elements of Econometrics* (2nd ed.). New York: Macmillan Publishing Co.

Kraemer, H. C., and Thiemann, S. 1987. *How Many Subjects?* Newbury Park, CA: Sage Publications, Inc.

Krahn, M., and Gafni, A. 1993. Discounting in the economic evaluation of health care interventions. *Medical Care* 31:403–18.

Kuder, G. F., and Richardson, M. W. 1937. The theory of the estimation of test reliability. *Psychometrika* 2:151–60.

Luft, H. S. 1989. Health services research as a scientific process: The metamorphosis of an empirical research project from grant proposal to final report. In Defriese, G. H., Ricketts, T. C., and Stein, J. S., eds., *Methodological Advances in Health Services Research*. Ann Arbor, MI: Health Administration Press.

Menard, J., Day, M., Chatellier, G., and Laragh, J. 1992. Some lessons from the systolic hypertension in the elderly program (SHEP). *American Journal of Hypertension* 5:325–30.

Mohr, L. 1992. *Impact Analysis for Program Evaluation*. Newbury Park, CA: Sage Publications, Inc.

Neufeld, A., and Strang, V. 1992. Issues in the evaluation of small-scale adult day care programs. *International Journal of Nursing Studies* 29:261–73.

Nunnally, J. C. 1978. *Psychometric Theory*. New York: McGraw-Hill.

Olsen, R. J. 1980. A least squares correction for selectivity bias. *Econometrica* 48:1815–21.

Ozminkowski, R. J., Supiano, K. P., and Campbell, R. 1991. Volunteers in nursing home enrichment: A survey to evaluate training and satisfaction. *Activities, Adaptation and Aging* 15:13–43.

Rossi, P. H., and Freeman, H. L. 1993. *Evaluation: A Systematic Approach* (5th ed). Newbury Park, CA: Sage Publications, Inc.

Schwartz, C. E., Ozminkowski, R. J., Hoaglin, D., Cella, M. A., and Branch, L. G. 1994. Can a survey influence quality of care in nursing homes? The influence of the New York Quality Assurance System on resident deterioration and adverse outcomes. *Journal of Aging and Health* 6:549–72.

Shadish, W. R., Cook, T. D., and Leviton, L. C. 1991. *Foundations of Program Evaluation: Theories of Practice*. Newbury Park, CA: Sage Publications, Inc.

Tougaard, L., Krone, T., Sorknaes, A., and Ellegaard, H. 1992. Economic benefits of teaching patients with chronic obstructive pulmonary disease about their illness. *Lancet* 339:1517–20.

Warner, K. E., and Luce, B. R. 1982. *Cost-benefit and Cost-effectiveness Analysis in Health Care: Principles, Practice, and Potential*. Ann Arbor, MI: Health Administration Press.

Part

IV

Challenges
for Intervention
and Services

Chapter

13

Postponing Disability: Identifying Points of Decline and Potential Intervention

S. Jay Olshansky, Ph.D., and Mark A. Rudberg, M.D., M.P.H.

For most of the last one hundred thousand years, humans have been exposed to a particularly hostile environment in which forces external to our biology—primarily infectious and parasitic diseases and predation—have been the primary causes of death. As humans gained control over the environment during the past two hundred years, it soon became evident that these nonbiological forces of natural selection, which have been operating on our species for thousands of years, could be modified. The process of senescence and the expression of senescence-related diseases and disorders is, therefore, a relatively new phenomenon, experienced only recently by humans and animals raised by humans in protected environments.

In the late nineteenth and early twentieth centuries, the early stages of our mortality transition from high to low death rates produced extremely rapid increases in life expectancy at birth. However, these gains in longevity were attributable almost entirely to reductions in death rates, at younger ages, from infectious and parasitic diseases and maternal mortality. The population saved from dying from these nonbiological forces of mortality then lived for several more decades, only to succumb at much later ages to what are now referred to as senescence-related diseases (principally vascular diseases and cancer). It is clear that the trade-off of a large gain in life expectancy at birth (of about twenty-eight years) for a redistribution of death from the young to the old was worthwhile.

In the latter part of the twentieth century an unexpected phenomenon occurred: The risk of death at middle and older ages began declining. The declines were attributable almost entirely to reductions in the risk of death from vascular diseases, a cause of death associated with the process of senescence. This recent mortality transition has been so widespread throughout the nations of the developed world that it has been referred to as a new stage in our epidemiological transition (Olshansky and Ault, 1986; Rogers and Hackenberg, 1989).

What trade-offs might be expected if the current trend toward declining death rates from vascular diseases continues or if the historical trend toward increasing total cancer mortality is reversed? For example, it is not clear how the health of future generations of older people might be affected by modern medicine and lifestyle modifications that succeed in prolonging life.

One school of thought—based on the concept of a compression of morbidity—maintains that the lifestyle changes and medical advances that bring forth a reduced risk of death from fatal diseases will simultaneously lead to a postponement in the onset of the nonfatal diseases that are major contributors to frailty and disability among those who survive to older ages (Fries, 1989). The underlying premise of this theory is that there is a fixed biological limit to life toward which populations are progressing. As improved lifestyles simultaneously postpone the onset and expression of fatal diseases, as well as nonfatal but highly disabling diseases and disorders, more people will be pushed toward their biological limits, and morbidity and disability will be compressed into a shorter duration of time before death.

A second school of thought—based on the concept of an expansion of morbidity—maintains that the forces that influence the onset and age-specific increase in the expression of the nonfatal diseases associated with senescence (such as Alzheimer disease, osteoarthritis, sensory impairments, etc.) are largely independent of the forces that influence the risk of death from fatal diseases (Brody and Miles, 1990; Olshansky et al., 1991; Rudberg and Cassel, 1993; Verbrugge, 1984). Thus, further reductions in death rates from fatal diseases could expose the saved population to a longer duration of time during which nonfatal but highly disabling diseases and disorders have the opportunity to be expressed. Implicit in this theory is the etiological independence of the fatal and nonfatal diseases and the premise that there is no genetic program for death.

A considerable debate has taken place in the literature regarding these two important hypotheses (Crimmins, Saito, and Ingegneri, 1989; Mathers, 1991; Robine and Ritchie, 1991; Rogers, Rogers, and Belanger, 1989, 1990; Wilkins and Adams, 1983). Although the evidence to date tends to favor the expansion of morbidity hypothesis, there are reasons why ongoing research in this area should be interpreted with caution. The empirical studies addressed to this debate have focused on health transitions observed only during the past twenty years, with emphasis placed on the decade of the 1980s. It is difficult to draw conclusions about the possible future compression or expansion of morbidity from studies based on such short time periods.

Additionally, it should be recognized that cohorts surviving through older ages today are a highly selected subgroup of their original birth cohort—a product of over 65 years of mortality selection. For example, in the United States the proportion of the 1900 birth cohort that survived to ages 65 and 85 were 52.2 percent and 18.2 percent, respectively (Figure 13.1). Based on middle-range assumptions about the future course of mortality made by the Social Security Administration (Bell, Wade, and Goss, 1992), the birth cohort of 1990 can expect to have 85.2 percent survive past age 65 and 45.1 percent survive past age 85. These are extremely large increases in cohort survival observed over short time periods. One consequence of extended survival will certainly be increases in demographic and genetic heterogeneity of future cohorts of older people relative to the more selected cohorts surviving to older ages today. Thus, caution should be exercised when interpreting extrapolations into the future, of findings about health transitions observed for highly selected cohorts over very short time periods.

More appropriate tests of the expansion and compression hypotheses require difficult-to-obtain data on secular trends in the age-at-onset and age progression of both fatal and nonfatal senescent diseases. Until such data are obtained and analyzed, it is not possible to determine with certainty whether recent declines in the risk of death from vascular diseases have had a positive or negative impact on the

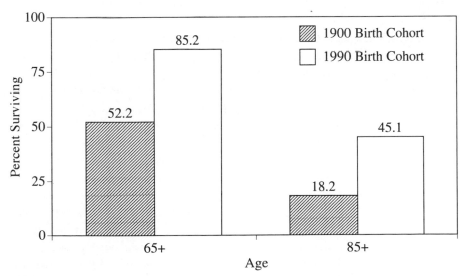

FIGURE 13.1 Cohort survival for U.S. birth cohorts, 1900 and 1990.
Source: Social Security Administration.

overall health status of the older population. In any case, the major forces of medicine and medical technology are proceeding with efforts to reduce the risk of death from currently fatal diseases without an answer to the important question of whether their success will improve or make worse the overall health status of the older population.

Evolutionary Perspectives

The compression and expansion of morbidity hypotheses have been analyzed within the conceptual framework of a relationship between changes in death rates from fatal diseases and their possible effects on health status. Scientists involved in this debate have expertise in one or more of the following: epidemiology, demography, medicine, and statistics. It is proposed here that theoretical and analytical studies involving the discipline of evolutionary biology can contribute to this debate.

Consider the evolutionary explanation for why senescence exists. According to evolutionary theory, natural selection is highly efficient at eliminating individuals with deleterious genes before puberty, but it declines as a force of influence on the gene pool as soon as reproductive maturation begins, and becomes a negligible force by the end of the reproductive period. This apparently simple concept holds the key to why senescence occurs and why survival into and beyond the reproductive period is necessary in order to observe its expression. According to Medawar (1952), senescence can be revealed "only by the most unnatural experiment of prolonging an animal's life by sheltering it from the hazards of its ordinary existence." As previously noted, conditions of extended survival into and beyond the reproductive period have been experienced only recently in our history by humans and other species raised by humans in protected environments.

What are the implications of this theory for the compression and expansion of morbidity hypotheses? If the expression of genes in the postreproductive period is beyond the reach of natural selection, then senescence and its related disabling disorders cannot be a result of the direct action of selection. Senescence-related diseases and disorders observed in organisms surviving into and beyond their reproductive period may therefore be an inadvertent consequence of selection operating uniformly on some other characteristic of the life history—such as reproduction (Medawar, 1952; Carnes and Olshansky, 1993; Williams, 1957). If this is the case, then the biochemical machinery necessary to maintain the biological integrity of an organism should diminish as the reproductive potential of individuals is achieved.

The implication of the evolutionary model is that as survival extends farther beyond the end of the reproductive period, it should become progressively more difficult to modify the expression of senescent diseases and disorders that lead to disability and death. This phenomenon has been referred to as biologically based entropy in the life table (Carnes and Olshansky, 1993; Olshansky and Carnes, 1994).

Three implications of evolutionary theories of senescence address the compression and expansion of morbidity hypotheses. One implication is that if progress continues to be made in modifying the expression of fatal senescent diseases, then the saved population will inevitably face other fatal disorders—with a frailty distribution of unknown character relative to prevailing conditions. For instance, individuals saved from dying of heart disease may live longer—only to face other diseases and disorders at later ages like stroke (McGovern et al., 1992) or dementia.

The second implication is that as survival improves at younger and middle ages, the genetic heterogeneity of future older cohorts is expected to increase. This means that individuals who, in earlier time periods, would never have had the opportunity to live so long will be surviving into older ages. These individuals will carry with them into older ages genes that never before have had the opportunity to be expressed in the form of senescent diseases and disorders. It is possible that increased genetic heterogeneity among future cohorts of older people could lead to the expression of new or infrequently observed senescent diseases and disorders. For example, children who would ordinarily die at young ages from phenylketonuria (PKU) and early-onset diabetes, will now survive to older ages for the first time.

The third implication is that because senescence did not evolve under the direct force of selection, its expression is inherently modifiable without manipulating the genome. Thus, it is possible to manipulate the environment and lifestyles in order to achieve improvements in health at any age. Although the extent to which such modifications can continue is uncertain, there are points of intervention that can already be identified.

Identifying Points of Decline and Intervention

Although it is imperative that scientists develop and test hypotheses regarding the possible expansion or compression of morbidity for populations, geriatricians have the difficult and immediate task of addressing the daily needs of older persons. In this section, we first provide a definition of disability, then discuss various methods used by physicians and other caregivers to intervene in its onset and progression.

Definition of Disability

The World Health Organization (WHO) defined disability as any restriction or lack of ability to perform an activity in the manner or within the range considered normal for a person (World Health Organization, 1980). The WHO developed a simple schema to conceptualize disability: Disease can lead to impairment, which can lead to disability (referred to as the disablement process). An impairment is a loss or abnormality of a structure or function. An example is arthritis of the knee, which can cause a decrease in range of motion of the knee. This can be of such a degree that a person may lose the ability to walk. Since walking is considered a normal activity, individuals with this impairment may be considered disabled in walking. Disability does not happen de novo, but rather is thought to be one step in the progression of disease manifestation.

Physicians are trained to diagnose and treat the many different medical conditions affecting persons. Understanding why these conditions arise can provide insight into how to postpone and treat disability. In the past, treatments were focused on the major medical conditions resulting in death, which include primarily heart disease, cancer, and stroke. The fact that life expectancy at middle and older ages has risen considerably in the past quarter century in the United States is a testament to the influence of both modern medicine and lifestyle modifications (including changes in dietary habits) on the risk of death from fatal diseases.

Medical science has also begun to focus increasingly on the major medical conditions not associated with mortality, but associated with disability and quality of life. These include, among others, the sensory impairments, dementia, arthritis, and osteoporosis. These conditions are increasingly becoming a public health problem as the population ages. Before exploring the relationship among these two categories of conditions and disability, it is instructive to explore what we know about these fatal and nonfatal conditions associated with aging from the public health model of prevention.

The currently fatal conditions will continue to be associated with death in the future. Although it appears that the average age at death from heart disease has been postponed, heart disease still remains the leading cause of death. Efforts to decrease the overall death rate from cardiovascular disease appear to invoke not only changes in risk factor modification, such as hypertension treatment, but other important factors, such as promoting healthy life styles. As for cancer, the age-adjusted death rates are continuing to increase. This may be due to increased survival among individuals with cardiovascular diseases, who then live into an age range where their relative risk of dying from cancer increases. Preventing specific kinds of cancer also has been difficult. Even the most easily modifiable form of cancer, lung cancer from smoking, has been impossible to prevent and is expected to continue to be a public health problem in the future. It has not been possible to prevent strokes, although risk factors are known. It may be that the best we can do for now is to postpone these fatal conditions into later stages of life.

With survival continuing to increase into the 65 and older age range, individuals are at increasing risk for the many different nonfatal conditions common among older persons. What is the current state of knowledge about how to prevent or postpone major nonfatal disabling conditions? Dementia is one common nonfatal disease with a prevalence that rises dramatically with advancing age—affecting up to 50 percent of those over age 85 (Evans et al., 1989). There is no clear etiology and there are no primary preventive measures for dementia despite the considerable amount of ongoing research on this disease. Hip fractures also increase exponentially with age (Brody, 1985), as a result of the two major risk factors—osteoporosis and falls. Although much is known about both of these factors, implementing preventive strategies on a population basis is difficult. For osteoporosis, it may be that progress in reducing subsequent hip fractures is most effective if therapy begins in the pediatric and young adult population rather than in older-age groups. Losses of hearing and sight (sensory impairments) are also prevalent problems among those who survive to older ages. Hearing impairments affect up to 40 percent of those persons over age 65 (Rich, 1990). Although excessive noise is a known risk factor for hearing loss, this disorder is also thought to have a strong genetic component—making prevention difficult in some cases. Visual disorders are widely prevalent in older age groups. Macular degeneration is the leading cause of blindness among older people in the United States: Primary prevention does not exist and few treatments are effective. Glaucoma, the second leading cause of blindness in the elderly population, can be treated if diagnosed early. Cataracts are a common condition that cannot be prevented but can be treated (tertiary prevention) with surgery. Finally, at present, it is possible to ameliorate some symptoms of arthritis with medication and surgery—but it is not possible to prevent or even delay its occurrence. In the next section, we describe how these conditions can be addressed in terms of preventing and postponing disability in the older age groups.

Disability is an abstract concept that has many different domains. In reality, a person can have a disability in one or more domains simultaneously—including physical, cognitive, and social domains. Each domain taps into a different area of functioning; even within a domain, different measures can be used. For example, the physical domain can be measured in terms of difficulty with basic physical activities such as Activities of Daily Living (ADLs), including bathing, dressing, transferring from bed to chair, toileting, eating, and maintaining continence (Katz et al., 1963), and Instrumental Activities of Daily Living (IADLs), which are less standardized and include shopping, managing money, housecleaning, and using the telephone, among others. Thus, disability must be operationalized within a particular domain in order to be measured effectively.

Although the WHO schema is linear, the development of disability rarely follows such a simple pattern. Disability does not necessarily follow impairment, and many persons who have impairments never develop a disability. As an example, arthritis of the knee may be painful but not necessarily disabling. Also, many persons have multiple impairments or comorbidities (Guralnik et al., 1989) that, only in combination, lead to disability (Furner, Rudberg, and Cassel, 1995). For example, the combination of arthritis and visual impairment may lead to a person being unable to walk, while having only one of these impairments may not lead to disability. Multiple conditions that lead to disability may be thought of as a web of causality for disability, and are among the most difficult challenges facing the geriatrician treating disability in older persons.

The WHO schema also treats disability within a domain as a dichotomous function when, in fact, it is not. The level or degree of disability can vary considerably. For instance, a disability in dressing (one of the ADLs) can range from the most severe state in which total personal help is required for a person to get dressed, to a milder state in which a person is still able to accomplish the task, but with difficulty. Although both of these situations can be considered a disabled state (each person is not able to perform an activity within the normal range), each situation has different implications for care. The former requires assistance in dressing while the latter may require simple modification of clothing (e.g., replacing buttons with Velcro closures).

Finally, because the level of disability is often subjective, individuals with the same physical complication may have entirely different needs, experiences, and interpretations. This occurs not just because of subjective interpretations of need, but also because the level of disability is heavily influenced by the extent to which normal daily activities are disrupted. As an example, a knee injury can be severely disabling to an athlete but only mildly disabling to his or her coach. The degree of social and medical care is influenced heavily by the domain of a disability, subjective interpretations, and the extent to which routine activities are disrupted.

Age at the Onset of Disability

The onset of disability is difficult to define and measure for several reasons. First, the onset is gradual for many disabilities. For example, a person with arthritis of the knee may first walk slower and then walk with a cane or a walker. Learning to compensate for impairments occurs routinely as people modify their behaviors and environments in ways that mitigate their impairments—thus blurring the age at onset of disability. The age at which a person is first defined as disabled is therefore unclear at best and, in part, depends on the goals of measurement. In general, the process of disablement tends to be insidious in its origin rather than acute, especially in older populations.

Second, it is important to recognize that disability is dynamic. A person can improve, stay the same, or become worse with time (Rudberg, Parzen, Leonard, and Cassel, 1996; Verbrugge and Balaban, 1989). For example, a person with arthritis of the knee who cannot walk may have surgery and then regain the ability to walk independently. Furthermore, since many conditions associated with disability are chronic (Furner, Rudberg, and Cassel, 1995) and can fluctuate in their severity, changes in the level of disability should also be expected. For scientists involved in research on evaluating population trends in health expectancy, measuring the onset and level of disability is therefore one of the most difficult tasks.

Postponing or Preventing Disability

Is it possible to intervene in order to postpone or prevent disability? Although there is considerable debate on this issue (Rudberg and Cassel, 1993), some methods of intervening in the disablement process have proven successful while the health benefits of other methods are questionable. To clarify these issues for the reader, we will distinguish among What We Know, What We Think We Know, and What We Would Like to Know about postponing or preventing disability. The discussion will occur within the context of the public health model of disease prevention—modified for disability. Specific examples will be provided, although this is not intended to be a complete list. In so doing, some of the most important issues in geriatrics will be emphasized. An abbreviated summary of the diseases and disorders that are known to be amenable to modification, or that may be amenable to modification, is provided in Table 13.1.

What We Know

It is possible to prevent some forms of disability in old age. One example of primary prevention is providing immunizations for pneumococcal pneumonia and influenza—both of which are common among the aged and can often lead to disability, hospitalization, and death (Lavizzo-Mourey and Diserens, 1989). Immunizations for these infectious diseases are effective, and their expanded use would certainly reduce disability associated with these diseases. Unfortunately, many elderly persons even in developed nations do not get immunized, in spite of the fact that immunizations are covered by most national health care programs for those over age 65.

An example of secondary prevention of disability is screening and treating high blood pressure. There is good evidence to indicate that treating hypertension in old age decreases the likelihood of disabling strokes (SHEP Cooperative Research Group, 1991). We emphasize the importance of both screening and treating because there are diseases such as prostate cancer that can be screened but for which the treatments may not necessarily extend survival (Chodak et al., 1994) or improve function.

Many forms of tertiary prevention of disability are known, mostly in the form of rehabilitation services. Specific examples include physical therapy for arthritis of

TABLE 13.1. Prospects for Primary, Secondary, and Tertiary Prevention of Fatal and Nonfatal Conditions

Condition	What We Know			What We Think We Know		
	1°	2°	3°	1°	2°	3°
Diabetes	0	0	+	+	+	+
Depression	0	0	+	0	+	+
Hearing impairment	0	0	+	+	+	+
Alzheimer's disease	0	0	+	+	0	+
Vascular dementia	+	0	+	+	0	+
Cataracts	0	0	+	+	0	+
Glaucoma	0	0	+	+	+	+
Macular degeneration	0	0	+	0	0	+
Arthritis	0	0	+	+	0	+
Hip fracture	+	0	+	+	+	+
Osteoporosis	0	+	+	+	+	+
Stroke	+	0	+	+	0	+
Coronary heart disease	+	0	+	+	+	+
Lung cancer	+	0	+	+	0	+
Colon cancer	0	+	+	+	+	+
Breast cancer	0	+	+	0	+	+
Prostate cancer	0	0	+	0	+	+

1° = primary prevention, 2° = secondary prevention, 3° = tertiary prevention; + = Yes, 0 = No.

the knee, assistive devices for vision such as glasses and surgery for cataracts and glaucoma, assistive devices for hearing such as hearing aids, and adaptive devices such as canes and grabbers to help navigate one's environment. Although some interventions may alter the course of a disability, canes and grabbers, for example, alter the balance between the environment and the person—which also can make independent living possible. In geriatrics it is often equally important to modify the environment as it is to modify disease processes.

What We Think We Know

There is evidence to indicate that manipulating the environment or behaviors can delay the onset, or possibly even prevent some forms, of disability, but definitive proof as to the effectiveness of manipulation is lacking. One form of primary prevention believed to reduce disability is weight reduction, which is thought to alter, among other age-related problems, the progression of knee arthritis (Felson et al., 1992). However, many individuals at their "optimum" weight still experience knee arthritis and the disability associated with it. The definition of optimum weight in older persons still remains a subject of debate (Andres et al., 1985). This example illustrates that it is not essential to prevent a disease such as osteoarthritis of the knee in order to prevent the disability associated with it. Delaying the progression of a disease can be equally effective as long as the disability is postponed beyond the observed survival time (Brody and Miles, 1990).

Screening for cancer is an example of secondary prevention. Cancer in older age groups is associated with the development of disability. Also, we think we know that cancer screening is effective in older persons—a conclusion often based on the extrapolation of data from younger age groups. Unanswered issues include: At what age or level of comorbidity should screening for cancers stop? Are treatments as effective in older age groups as they are in younger age groups? And what are the barriers to implementing widespread use of cancer screening? The practical problem is how to provide these services efficiently to a diverse group of older persons who have various health beliefs, goals, and comorbid conditions.

An example of tertiary prevention is geriatric assessments—a process by which older persons are evaluated for medical and social problems, all with a focus on improvement of function and lessening disability. There is some evidence that geriatric evaluations work (Landsfeld et al., 1995), but it is not conclusive (Reuben et al., 1995). For instance, it is possible that researchers evaluating the benefits of geriatric assessments are selecting persons who are not at risk or who may not otherwise benefit from this kind of intense, expensive intervention. This brings up the issue of how to target an intervention. Should interventions be provided to everyone over a given age, or should they be provided only to those most likely to benefit? Determining who is most likely to benefit from an intervention is an ongoing area of research.

What We Would Like to Know

What are some of the avenues that researchers are presently investigating to prevent disability? Hormone manipulations may be one example. For instance, growth hormone has been shown to increase muscle and visceral organ mass (Rudman et al., 1994). Other interventions include exercise (Fiatarone et al., 1993; Hickey et al., 1995) and diet (Masoro, 1993). It is thought that making people less frail and more robust may decrease the likelihood of future disability. The questions that remain are: (1) Do these interventions decrease disability? (2) Who actually benefits from these interventions and at what moment in an individual's life should interventions begin? and (3) How should these interventions be implemented on a population basis?

Screening for dementia is another example of what we want to know more about. Although methods of screening for this disease exist, they are used only when it is already symptomatic. With new evidence on the genetics of dementia (Corder et al., 1994), it may be possible to screen for the disease well before it is symptomatic, perhaps at or even before birth. This information may help individuals and their families plan for the consequences associated with having dementia. More important, understanding the genetics of dementia may lead to therapy to postpone its onset or progression—a development that may not come without hazards. For example, it is not unreasonable in the present era to think that the identification of a genetic predisposition for specific diseases and disorders could also be used to determine insurance risk, a potential form of genetic discrimination.

An example of treating the complications of conditions and their related disability is the improvement of the continuum of long-term care services. As health care reform changes, creativity is required in order to provide effective and efficient long-term care services necessary to prevent the complications of conditions and disability (Kane and Kane, 1991). Previously, it was stated that hospitalization is associated with disability for many older persons; conversely, the myriad of long-term care services following posthospitalization is associated with improvement in disability for some. Understanding the factors associated with improvement in function and making this system more user-friendly and efficient is another example of what we want to know more about.

Conclusions

Only within the last two hundred years have humans been able to profoundly modify selection pressures such that survival into older ages has become a common event. Although gains in life expectancy in this century are largely a result of reductions in death rates at younger ages, recent trends in old-age mortality indicate that it is possible to modify the expression of fundamental senescent processes. What is uncertain at this time is whether modifying the temporal expression of senescent mortality will have a positive, negative, or neutral effect on the health of future cohorts of older persons. Two schools of thought have emerged on this issue—one predicting a compression of morbidity into a shorter duration of time before death, and the other predicting an expansion of morbidity. The data required to test these hypotheses appropriately are difficult to obtain, and the data that do exist do not provide definitive evidence supporting either view. Furthermore, recent changes in population heterogeneity are likely to have an influence on future trends in the health of the older population—the impacts of which have yet to be fully understood. It is argued here that both theoretical and methodological developments in the field of evolutionary biology may prove useful in addressing these important public policy issues.

The conclusion from evolutionary biology that the expression of senescent diseases and disorders is inherently modifiable is supported by the day-to-day efforts of geriatricians and their patients. Identifying common points of age-related declines in the physical functioning of older persons permits the appropriate targeting of interventions for their related disabilities. Interventions in the disablement process include primary prevention such as immunizations, secondary prevention such as cancer screening, and tertiary prevention such as geriatric assessments, among many other examples. Scientists are continuing their efforts to verify what we think we know, and identifying what we would like to know about continuing to modify the disablement process. There is reason to be optimistic that further gains will be made in increasing life expectancy and expanding the portion of the life span that is free from major disability. These will occur by understanding the mechanisms involved in the expression of senescence-related diseases and disorders, and identifying new and more innovative methods of altering senescence itself and/or manipulating our environments to lessen the adverse health impacts associated with existing conditions.

References

Andres, R., Elahi, D., Tobin, J. D., Muller, D. C., Brant, L. 1985. Impact of age on weight goals. *Annals of Internal Medicine* 103(6, Part 2):1030–33.

Bell, F. C., Wade, A. H., and Gross, S. C. 1992. Life Tables for the United States Social Security Area, 1900–2080. Actuarial Study No. 107. SSA Publication No. 11–11536. Washington, DC: Social Security Administration.

Brody, J. 1985. Prospects for an aging population. *Nature* 315:463–66.

Brody, J. A., and Miles, T. P. 1990. Mortality postponed and the unmasking of age-dependent non-fatal conditions. *Aging* 2(3):283–89.

Carnes, B. A., and Olshansky, S. J. 1993. Evolutionary perspectives on human senescence. *Population and Development Review* 19(4):793–806.

Chodak, G. W., Thisted, R. A., Gerber, G. S., Johansson, J. W., Adolfsson, J., Jones, G. W., Chisholm, G. D., Moskovitz, B., Livne, P. M., and Warner, J. 1994. Results of conservative management of clinically localized prostate cancer. *New England Journal of Medicine* 330(4):242–48.

Corder, E. H., Saunders, A. M., Risch, N. J., Strittmatter, W. J., Schmechel, D. E., Gaskell, P. S. Jr., Rimmler, J. B., Locke, P. A., Conneally, P. M., Schmader, K. E., et al. 1994. Protective effect of apolipoprotein E type 2 allele for late onset Alzheimer disease. *Nature Genetics* 7(2):180–84.

Crimmins, E., Saito, Y., and Ingegneri, D. 1989. Changes in life expectancy and disability-free life expectancy in the United States. *Population and Development Review* 15(2):235–67.

Evans, D. E., et al. 1989. Prevalence of Alzheimer's disease in a community population of older persons. *Journal of the American Medical Association.* 9262:2551–2556.

Felson, D. T., Zhang, Y., Anthony, J. M., Naimark, A., and Anderson, J. J. 1992. Weight loss reduces the risk for symptomatic knee osteoarthritis in women: The Framingham Study. *Annals of Internal Medicine* 116(7):535–39.

Fiatarone, M. A., O'Neill, E. F., Doyle, N., Clements, K. M., Roberts, S. B., Kehayias, J. J., Lipsitz, L. A., and Evans, W. J. 1993. The Boston FICSIT Study: The effects of resistance training and nutritional supplementation on physical frailty in the oldest old. *Journal of the American Geriatrics Society* 41(3):333–37.

Fries, J. F. 1989. The compression of morbidity: Near or far? *Milbank Quarterly* 67(2):208–323.

Furner, S. E., Rudberg, M. A., and Cassel, C. K. 1995. Medical conditions differentially affect the development of IADL disability: Implications for medical care and research. *Gerontologist* 35(4):444–50.

Guralnik, J., LaCroix, A. Z., Everett, D. F., and Kovar, M. G. 1989. Aging in the Eighties: The prevalence of comorbidity and association with disability. Advance Data from Vital and Health Statistics, No. 170, Hyattsville, MD: National Center for Health Statistics.

Hickey, T., Wolf, F. M., Robins, L. S., Wagner, M. B., and Harik, W. 1995. Physical activity training for functional mobility in older persons. *Journal of Applied Gerontology* 14(4):357–371.

Kane, R. L., and Kane, R. A. 1991. A nursing home in your future? [editorial; comment]. *New England Journal of Medicine* 325(6):360–61.

Katz, S., Ford, A. B., Moskowitz, R. W., Jackson, B. A., and Jaffee, M. W. 1963. Studies of illness in the aged. The Index of ADD: A standardized measure of biological and psychosocial function. *Journal of the American Medical Association* 185:94.

Landsfeld, C. S., Palmer, R. M., Kresevic, D. M., Fortinsky, R. H., and Kowal, J. 1995. A randomized trial of care in a hospital medical unit especially designed to improve the functional outcomes of acutely ill older patients. *New England Journal of Medicine* 332:1338–44.

Lavizzo-Mourey, R., and Diserens, D. 1989. Preventive care in the elderly. In Lavizzo-Mourey R. et al., eds., *Practicing Prevention for the Elderly*. Philadelphia: Hanley & Belfus, Inc.

Masoro, E. J. 1993. Dietary restriction and aging. *Journal of the American Geriatrics Society* 41(9):994–99.

Mathers, C. 1991. *Health Expectancies in Australia, 1981 and 1988*. Canberra: Australian Institute of Health Publications.

McGovern, P. G., Burke, G. L., Sprafka, J. M., Xue, S., Folsom, A. R., and Blackburn, H. 1992. Trends in mortality, morbidity, and risk factor levels for stroke from 1960 through 1990. *Journal of the American Medical Association* 268(6):753–59.

Medawar, P. B. 1952. *An Unsolved Problem of Biology*. London: Lewis.

Olshansky, S. J., and B. Ault. 1986. The fourth stage of the epidemiologic transition: The age of delayed degenerative diseases. *Milbank Quarterly* 64:355–91.

Olshansky, S. J., and Carnes, B. A. 1994. Demographic perspectives on human senescence. *Population and Development Review* 20(1):57–80.

Olshansky, S. J., Rudberg, M. A., Carnes, B. A., Cassel, C. K., and Brody, J. 1991. Trading off longer life for worsening health: The expansion of morbidity hypothesis. *Journal of Aging and Health* 3, No. 2:194–216.

Reuben, D. B., Borok, G. M., Wolde-Tsadik, G., Ershoff, D. H., Fishman, L. K., Ambrosini, V. L., Liu, Y., Rubenstein, L. Z., and Beck, J. C. 1995. A randomized trial of comprehensive geriatric assessment in the care of hospitalized patients. *New England Journal of Medicine* 332:1345–50.

Rich, L. F. 1990. Ophthalmology. In: Cassel, C. K., Riesenberg, D. E., Sorensen, L. B., and Walsh, J. R., eds. *Geriatric Medicine* (2nd ed., pp. 394–404). New York: Springer-Verlag.

Robine, J. M., and Ritchie, K. 1991. Healthy life expectancy: Evaluation of a new global indicator of change in population health. *British Medical Journal* 302:457–60.

Rogers, R., and Hackenberg, R. 1989. Extending epidemiologic transition theory: A new stage. *Social Biology* 34(3-4):234–43.

Rogers, R., Rogers, A., and Belanger, A. 1989. Active life among the elderly in the United States: Multistate life-table estimates and population projection. *Milbank Quarterly* 67(3-4):370–411.

Rogers, R., Rogers, A., and Belanger, A. 1990. Longer life but worse health?: Measurement and dynamics. *Gerontologist* 39(5):640–49.

Rudberg, M., and Cassel, C. 1993. Are death and disability in old age preventable? *Facts and Research in Gerontology* 7:191–202.

Rudberg, M. A., Parzen, M. I., Leonard, L., and Cassel, C. K. 1996. Functional limitation pathways and transitions in community-dwelling older persons. *Gerontologist* 36(4):430–440.

Rudman, D., Drinka, P. J., Wilson, C. R., Mattson, D. E., Scherman, F., Cuisinier, M. C., and Schultz, S. 1994. Relations of endogenous anabolic hormones and physical activity to bone mineral density and lean body mass in elderly men. *Clinical Endocrinology* 40(5):653–61.

SHEP Cooperative Research Group. 1991. Prevention of stroke by antihypertensive drug treatment in older persons with isolated systolic hypertension. *Journal of the American Medical Association* 265:3255–64.

Verbrugge, L. M. 1984. Longer life but worsening health?: Trends in health and mortality of middle-aged and older persons. *Milbank Quarterly/Health and Society* 62:475–519.

Verbrugge, L. M., and Balaban, D. J. 1989. Patterns of change in disability and well-being. *Medical Care* 27(3):S128–47.

Wilkins, R., and Adams, O. B. 1983. Health expectancy in Canada, late 1970s: Demographic, regional and social dimensions. *American Journal of Public Health* 73(9):1073–80.

Williams, G. C. 1957. Pleiotropy, natural selection and the evolution of senescence. *Evolution* 11:398–411.

World Health Organization. 1980. *International Classification of Impairments, Disabilities, and Handicaps*. Geneva: World Health Organization.

Chapter

14

Aging, Bioethics, and Public Health: Issues at the Intersection of Three Multidisciplinary Fields

Rosalie A. Kane, D.S.W.

Gerontology is a broad and multifaceted field that overlaps with public health in many ways. Similarly, bioethics as a field has commented broadly on policies, programs, and choices that relate to the health status and health care of people of all ages. This chapter focuses on ethical issues and themes that are specific to *both* public health and aging. Even then, the chapter makes no attempt to enumerate all ethical issues relevant to the confluence of public health and aging. Rather, it raises a range of illustrative topics organized according to major intellectual and practice streams in public health. In part, the goal is to show how attention to biomedical ethics would influence the establishment of public health goals, research, and programs for older people.

An introductory section discusses the intersection of the three fields—public health, gerontology, and bioethics—with an emphasis on characteristic approaches to problem solving in bioethics. The remainder of the chapter is organized according to substantive areas in public health, namely: (1) prevention, (2) epidemiology/health services research, (3) public information/health education, (4) environmental health, and (5) public health regulation and quality assurance.

In each of the subareas of public health, general ethical issues and dilemmas arise. Ethical issues in public health are more often identified in relation to younger people than to people over age 65, the concern of this book. When addressing older people, bioethicists have tended to concentrate on matters of health care delivery— for example, determining appropriate decisions about life-prolonging treatments or medical choices as they are worked out in the relationships between patients and health care professionals (sometimes called "bedside ethics") and in setting policies regarding fair allocation of health resources among elderly groups and between older people and younger people (distributional justice).

This chapter takes a different tack. As much as it is possible to make such distinctions, the chapter concentrates on ethical issues related to the public health endeavor rather than to health care delivery itself. To anticipate the conclusions, the various sections of the chapter argue that public health should adopt the following stances as part of an ethics agenda related to older people:

1. In its *prevention* capacity, (a) work toward prevention of dysfunction and psychological distress that result both from failure to detect problems, and from iatrogenic complications of overtreatment or inappropriate service plans, and (b) consider carefully the ethical issues around primary prevention and secondary prevention (disease screening) for older people, rather than dismissing older people as inappropriate candidates for such interventions because of shorter remaining life expectation.

2. In its *epidemiological and health services research* capacity, guard against framing problems, defining variables, and specifying outcomes in a way that devalues older people, or stereotypes the roles and functions appropriate for people in their later years.

3. In its *public information* capacity *and health education* capacity, fulfill a moral imperative to articulate meaningful goals and to specify meaningful problems related to the elderly in a way that will do good rather than harm.

4. In its *environmental health* capacity, examine noxious decision-making environments and residential environments that are associated with poor health outcomes for older people who need long-term care.

5. In its *licensure, regulatory, and quality assurance* roles (which are roles often fulfilled by public health departments at federal, state, and local levels), reexamine the importance of maximizing physical safety and minimizing risks that might befall older people compared to the importance of creating circumstances where older people with disabilities can lead normal lifestyles and purchase care at relatively low costs.

In general, one can distinguish three types of decisions that are made by and on behalf of older people: medical treatments, life-change decisions (such as residential moves), and everyday decisions. The chapter argues that public health pay more attention to the last type of decision. It also argues for making explicit the values that each older person holds and for attempting to develop individual plans and options within systems of care that accord with values. Finally, it holds that public health officials have an obligation to speak out as a public health responsibility when there are obvious discrepancies between widely held human values and the kinds of health care programs embodied in public policy. Nursing homes are classic examples of settings that fail to conform to the way people prefer to live their lives and, arguably, the way nursing homes have been regulated increases the problem. If so, the issue is a public health matter.

Three Intersecting Fields

The charge for this chapter requires examination of the intersection of three interrelated fields: public health, gerontology, and bioethics. As stated above, numerous ethical issues in public health are not particularly specific to aging, and numerous ethical issues in aging fall outside the purview of public health. The attempt here is to zero in on this three-way intersection. To set the stage, let us briefly consider elements of each field.

Public Health

The ultimate concern in public health is health of populations, with health broadly defined to include psychological and social well-being and positive health, not just absence of illness. Public health is both a scholarly field and a practice field. In the United States, its major endeavors include:

1. Epidemiological studies to identify determinants of the incidence and prevalence of disease and disability, including social determinants

2. Health services research to identify the determinants, including social determinants, of health care utilization and outcomes

3. Disease prevention and health promotion efforts

4. Development of environmental health programs and policies

5. Public health practice at federal, state, and local levels, including:
   a. direct services (e.g., public health nursing)
   b. screening
   c. public education on health matters
   d. regulation and inspection
   e. quality assurance

Gerontology/Aging

Gerontology is directed at understanding human aging in society. Its practical arm, aging services, is directed at developing programs and policies that promote successful aging. Like public health, gerontology is multidisciplinary and has a scholarly and an applied side.

Advocacy for older people is a hallmark of programs funded under the Older Americans Act (OAA). In fulfilling that mission, professionals in the aging field are conscious of tensions among multiple goals: advocating for programs that benefit the elderly, particularly those with greatest needs; combating ageist stereotypes that depict older people as inevitably frail and decrepit; and creating age-neutral programs, which sometimes benefit an older constituency and sometimes penalize it. Settling on a stance with regard to these issues requires ethical analysis, and sometimes these topics are also the concern of public health.

Gerontology deals with both the aging process and the old. *Old* is hard to define, however. Chronological age is a poor marker of functional status. Life expectancy and onset time for age-related changes differs across ethnic groups and disability groups. The OAA focuses on age 60+. Fiscal aging in terms of many retirement and health benefits, such as Social Security, private pensions, and Medicare, starts around age 65. Geriatricians and long-term care experts typically think of age 75+ as the age when health-related problems for the elderly begin. Regardless of how they define "old," however, gerontologists must take the needs of the whole population into consideration in recommending services and programs for the elderly. First, older people are part of families and communities, and the interests of older people are inevitably intertwined with those of younger people. Second, policies that affect younger people bear a direct relationship to the circumstances of those same people in their old age.

Bioethics

Ethics is a branch of philosophy that concerns itself with the morality of conduct. Bioethics is an applied field that considers moral issues related to health, with health once again defined broadly to include psychological and even social well-being. It is a multidisciplinary endeavor, attracting people in philosophy, theology, law, social science, medicine, and nursing, as well as public health and gerontology. Like public health and gerontology, bioethicists engage in research (philosophical, legal, and empirical) and it also has an applied arm (with ethics committees and ethics consultation).

Most health professions, such as medicine, nursing, and social work, and some health occupations, such as case management (Geron and Chassler, 1994; National Association of Private Geriatric Care Managers, 1990) and nursing home administration (American Association of Homes and Services for the Aging, 1994), have fashioned codes of ethics. Such codes are intended to regulate the conduct of members of the occupational group. But bioethics deals much more broadly with dilemmas and uncertainties at both the individual and policy level.

Much work in bioethics has involved application of principles as a form of problem solving, especially the principles of *respect for autonomy, beneficence*, and *justice* (Beauchamp and Childress, 1994). The principle of respect for autonomy holds that each person has the right to direct his or her own life without interference from others, unless the person is harming others. Philosophers Collopy (1988) and Agich (1993) have made efforts to explore the operational meaning of respecting personal autonomy when an elderly person has substantial disabilities and dwindling capability for self-direction. Both suggest that the principle needs to be expanded to include positive ways to enhance the decision-making opportunities of older people (as opposed to merely refraining from interfering with their decisions). Similarly, commentators have reexamined the concept of beneficence (i.e., doing good) in light of the tensions that regularly occur in practice between the beneficent views of professionals about what is in the best interests of a client and the older person's own preferences (Collopy, 1993).

Another trend in bioethics is the exploration of virtuous or moral conduct attendant on various roles (e.g., patient, physician, nurse) and the analysis of the attributes of a "good" society in which the healthy and the well coexist. To take two examples in this vein of work by philosophers, Macklin (1990) explored the desirable nature of a nursing home as a social entity, and Jameton (1988) explored the responsibilities that older people receiving long-term care have toward others.

Although some bioethics issues have yielded substantive answers to substantive questions (e.g., when does death begin?), most questions do not lend themselves to absolute answers. However, decisions must be reached in individual cases, whether these cases entail treatment decisions for individuals or decisions about whether to adopt a public policy or regulation. Accordingly, *procedural ethics* has had an important role in establishing orderly ways to consider ethical issues. Ethics committees and commissions, institutional review boards, informed consent procedures, grievance procedures, dispute resolution mechanisms, mandatory disclosures—all such procedures are expected to enhance the likelihood of sound ethical solutions, but they do not in themselves propose answers.

Commonalities and Distinctions

The three fields (public health, gerontology, and biomedical ethics) are multidisciplinary, with both applied and research functions. All three labor for the public good at individual and societal levels, all emphasize fairness, and all have expressed official concern for those who are most vulnerable or needy in society. The distinctions relate to the predominant focus. Public health focuses on entire populations, regardless of age (and may not, in fact, give enough attention to elderly people). Gerontology focuses on older people and may, without vigilance, fail to recognize the interdependence of people of all ages. Bioethics is concerned with articulating moral issues and solving ethical problems related to health care on individual and policy levels; sometimes bioethicists touch on issues that affect aging, sometimes issues related to bioethics, and, occasionally, issues where these fields converge.

According to Beauchamp (1995), the philosophy of public health has four characteristics that converge with bioethics: a methodology that emphasizes community and scientific approaches to improving community health; a priority value placed on prevention; a communitarian focus on defining public good and making the public good the object of common action; and a balancing of the claims of individual autonomy against claims of society as a whole, which may justify overriding individual freedoms. In passing, public health actions also may alienate strong interest groups.

How these themes should play out regarding public health for an older public in an aging society merits scrutiny. The rest of this chapter deals with ethical issues that relate to aging according to major arenas in public health. Many of these areas are insufficiently explored at present.

Prevention

Prevention of disease and disability is perhaps the aspect of public health most identifiable to the general public. Much preventive effort deals with prevention of diseases, disability, and premature death among children, adolescents, and relatively young adults. In such instances the payoff of success can be many decades of productive life. The efficacy of preventive effort *begun* after age 65 is the subject of some controversy (Kane, Kane, and Arnold, 1985). Amid conflicting claims for efficacy, the public health field is challenged to establish a precise agenda for prevention aimed at people already old. Indeed, we argue that primary and secondary prevention undertaken on behalf of someone already in old age is often highly justified. Flu vaccination and smoking cessation are two examples of primary prevention that arguably should be pursued vigorously for older people, and some disease screening also seems justified because of the availability of efficacious treatments that prolong life and reduce illness. We also argue that tertiary prevention is of high importance for older people. The sections that follow identify illustrative ethical issues that arise around prevention activities for older people.

Population Screening and Access to Prevention

Screening, sometimes known as secondary prevention, is a key technique in early detection of disease, leading to more effective treatment and prevention of more serious morbidity. Such screening is often accompanied by health education. Public health officials can efficiently bring their programs to places where young people go to school or working-age people are employed. Elderly people are harder to find for both health education programs and health screening programs.

In the United States a variety of preventive and health screening procedures are not covered under Medicare, the usual source of funding for health care for the elderly. If public health authorities adhere to a philosophy that values prevention over treatment, they should surely lobby to change these incentives. On the other hand, some commentators might argue that relatively low costs of many health screening activities makes them a lower priority for insurance coverage than the more onerous expenses associated with disease treatment.

The major ethical questions concern the proportion of resources that should be expended, not only on screening as opposed to treatment (which is an ethical question related to public health in general), but also on outreach efforts to screen elderly populations as opposed to screening younger populations. For example, it would be possible to involve family physicians and other primary care providers in screening efforts, but these efforts might be relatively expensive compared to screening approaches for younger people. An even more expensive approach would involve in-home screening, such as is done by health visitors attached to some primary care practices or health departments in England (Williams, 1989).

Cost-Effectiveness Paradigms for Prevention

Prevention of some conditions affecting the elderly have a highly cost-effective payoff. For example, relatively inexpensive flu vaccines have high efficacy. Other preventive programs have the greatest payoff when started early (in order to alter risk factors that are mutable). Research is presently insufficient to predict the likely payoff for all preventive efforts, such as dietary changes and exercise, when begun in old age (Kane, Kane, and Arnold, 1985). Many ethical issues can be identified. For example, is it right to go ahead anyway for minimal or unclear results? How hard should one push, in the name of prevention, for very old people with limited pleasures to give up favored foods? Is such behavior change likely to make a difference for an 85-year-old? What about emphasizing smoking cessation, which we do know is good preventive policy at any age? Should no-smoking policies be enforced in nursing homes when they are not in other dwelling places?

Older people are systematically disadvantaged in almost all cost-effectiveness comparisons. The outcomes for success are often measured in terms of lifetime productivity saved, which Avorn (1984) argued systematically discriminates against older people who are not in the labor force. Knowing this, should we seek a new paradigm?

Obligation to Counter False Claims

Older people seem particularly vulnerable to "hard sells" on preventive miracles in the form of vitamins, minerals, and other alleged health-enhancing regimens. Does the public health enterprise have any obligation to declare limits to utility of preventive efforts? What if the particular products are believed to do no harm, but they erode limited retirement incomes?

After Screening, What?

Ethical issues abound if, through screening, problems are identified that have no corresponding ameliorative actions. In the mid-1990s, a genetic test became available to detect a trait for some forms of Alzheimer disease. This has led to questions about whether there is a duty to inform a young person that Alzheimer disease is in his or her future, questions complicated by the knowledge that the person may lead a long life and die of other causes without suffering Alzheimer symptoms.

To take a different example, screening is sometimes done in the community to detect elder abuse or other serious problems affecting older people's well-being. Once identifying a previously undiscovered situation of elder abuse (physical or financial), authorities have an obligation to intervene helpfully. What if the most common intervention—removing the older person to a nursing home—is perceived to be worse than the abuse? Does the older person have the right to choose what, in his or her opinion, is the lesser evil (Kane and Caplan, 1993)? Similar questions, though perhaps less dramatic, can be asked about other screening: for breast cancer or prostate cancer in old age, for depression, or for ADL impairment. Some prior understanding is needed about what will be done differently once the condition is identified and, in each case, ethical analysis would be useful.

What Should Be Prevented?

Perhaps the greatest potential for prevention for older people is prevention of dysfunction and disability secondary to disease and its treatment. This includes prevention of iatrogenic illnesses caused by medical treatments, bedrest, and hospitalizations. It includes preventing dysfunction through attention to prosthetic devices— from eyeglasses and hearing aids to walkers. It emphasizes good-fitting dentures, foot care, and the like. It encompasses appropriate rehabilitation and restorative treatments. It also includes avoiding the excess disability incurred when health professionals and family members cease holding expectations for a person who is sick. Much of this falls into the arena of tertiary prevention—prevention of excess disability or handicap through prompt and effective treatments. These programs may have a less satisfactory ring to them for prevention specialists than exercise and nutrition programs, although the latter are based on more dubious evidence of effects.

To the extent that prevention addresses problems of excess disability, educational campaigns will need to be targeted to physicians and health care professionals as much as to consumers. Physicians need to learn that incontinence can be alleviated and that medications can be reduced. But, how much money should be spent countering advertising claims about medications, aiming at both providers and consumers? Jerry Avorn, at Harvard University, has developed creative approaches, such as "un-ads" and "counter-detailing" (Avorn and Soumerai, 1983). This involves "fighting fire with fire" by using common promotional techniques to advertise the dangerous properties of various medicines that are overused for old people. Public health officials are unlikely to be able to muster enough resources to counteract the budgets of advertisers, however. Given finite resources, should resources be used for such campaigns, and if so, how much?

Epidemiology/Health Services Research

Epidemiology, the use of multifactorial designs to identify factors associated with the incidence and prevalence of disease and disabilities, is sometimes considered the core science of public health. Oversimplifying a bit, health services research uses a similar epidemiological paradigm to examine the factors associated with utilization or effectiveness of services. Epidemiological and health services research projects relating to the well-being of the elderly are, of course, numerous. At first glance, the dry issues of research methodologies have little to do with ethics. In fact, however, value judgments lurk in research designs and measures, and identification and discussions of values are legitimate concerns for bioethics. The way problems are framed and outcomes specified should be consistent with a view of a good old age in a just society.

Values Inherent in the Choice of Research Topics

The way epidemiological and health services research questions are framed influences societal perceptions about whether old people are a resource or a problem. To take an actual example, a national data set on assistance across the generations measured monetary assistance in two directions (young adults to older adults and vice versa) but measured in-kind assistance in a different way for younger older people; the only tangible assistance that older people could claim for younger people was child care, whereas younger people were asked about personal care and health-related assistance to their older relatives. This assumption made it impossible to measure and take adequate account of the help that older people give their children and other relatives who have physical disabilities requiring hands-on care.

Numerous examples could be given of assumptions built into research questions. Social well-being of older people could be studied by examining their participation in a wide range of organized leisure activities, while voluntary and civic leadership or self-improvement activities are ignored. Even the selection of topics worthy of study related to the health and well-being of older people presupposes some model of what is good and important in old age. For example, understudied topics include the prevalence of sexual dysfunction among the elderly and effective treatments; the effectiveness of group and individual psychotherapy; the prevalence and precursors of marital discord arising in later years and the effectiveness of marriage counseling; or how typical activity programs in nursing homes affect the perceived well-being and emotional health of nursing home residents with varying educational and social backgrounds and cognitive and functional abilities. Similarly, a review of three decades of research in long-term care revealed only one study that even examined whether the double occupancy that prevails in nursing homes is injurious to the health of older people. Rather, these room arrangements have been taken for granted as proper and benign.

Value Judgments May Underlie Definitions

Prevalence studies have shown extraordinarily high levels of mental health problems among frail elderly people, especially those using long-term care services. It may be possible, however, that we have too sensitive and all-encompassing measures of mental disorders in older people.

A related example concerns the common habit of measuring "behavior problems" of older people in nursing homes (Szwabo and Grossberg, 1993). We may be doing a disservice to older people by grouping together depressed affect, social withdrawal complaining behavior, and a wide range of behavior called "aggressive" as behavior problems. The high prevalence will be useful for those attempting to raise funds for services, yet some of the behaviors classified as problems may be descriptive of the normal range of behavior in any group (i.e., if younger people were observed in their daily lives, their anger, talkativeness, silence, and so on might not be classified as problems). Or, even worse, some reactions labeled as problem behaviors may be reasonable and even adaptive responses to stressful situations.

Another definition that perhaps needs new scrutiny is that of elder abuse and neglect. A host of categories exist beyond physical abuse and clear neglect of established duties. These include psychological abuse, financial abuse, neglect, and self-neglect. James Callahan has periodically wondered in print whether harm is sometimes done by proliferating elder abuse cases to be handled by adult protective services authorities for situations that, in younger age groups, would be handled in the criminal justice system (Callahan, 1982). The category of self-neglect is particularly problematic unless clear-cut standards and reliable measures are available to distinguish self-neglect from informed decisions not to accept professional advice.

Values Inherent in Outcomes Measured

Values are particularly apparent in the choice of outcome measures by which to evaluate programs. Measurement of functional status (ADL and IADL) has become standard, and appropriately so. However, in some studies of good and bad outcomes of programs for the elderly, the *only* outcomes examined are mortality (a hard outcome to use properly, when death is expected relatively soon for much of the population), morbidity, and functional abilities. If a range of social and psychological indicators are not used, this can result in misleading information. For example, people may seem better off in nursing homes based on ADL measures or some other "unmet need" measure (and, indeed, need is in some ways met by nursing home care) than at home, even though the older people themselves would assert that they believe life is better outside a nursing home.

To take another example, if we seek to measure socialization as a positive outcome (either as a valued end-point or as an intermediate variable signifying social involvement) should we count attendance at an adult day care center? Or rather, should we count such attendance only if the older person expressed enjoyment of the activity? Similarly, if only negative outcomes of family caregiving are measured, it will be possible to show greater or lesser burden, but it will be impossible to show any positive effects on family caregivers related to caring for an elderly family member (Kane, 1995a).

Summary measures also can be a problem. The well-known Quality Adjusted Life Years (QUALYs) approach and similar techniques could end up devaluing life with a severe impairment or life in a nursing home as the end of "active life expectancy." Yet, even if life in a nursing home for people with substantial disabilities seems not worth living, the solution may be to change the model of care rather than devalue survival. Furthermore, people who place an extremely negative valence on having a disability may well prefer life with that disability over death (Menzel, 1990).

In intervention studies, an outcome measure is sometimes chosen for its convenience or well-researched history without regard to whether it is even logical to use. Respite care programs for family caregivers is expected to produce greater happiness and well-being even if the respite is ordinarily used to enable caregivers to attend funerals, visit sick relatives, get hospital care, and so on (Montgomery, 1995). Sometimes programs such as meal programs or home improvement programs are expected to result in positive changes in life satisfaction or morale scales that measure, not immediate affective state, but perception of life accomplishment. A program may have value, yet not have this kind of effect. Finally, as already indicated, cost-effectiveness studies may systematically militate against older people if their worth is judged by productive years of life.

Objectifying Older People

Even as we strive to perform accurate multidimensional assessments of older people, we must guard against the ever-present danger that we lose sight of the abstraction involved in these assessments. We cannot conclude that we have depicted the older person accurately enough to prescribe life plans based on the sum of such answers.

One example is case-mix designations, which are used to identify the level of service needed by various long-term care clients and the amount of reimbursement received. Public health researchers need to be vigilant against easy assumptions that we can measure what is best for an older person in sweeping ways of measuring their disability levels and needs for services. In fact, even the usually unassailable idea of a continuum of care may be an ethical problem if it forces older people to shape their lives to some abstract view of where they fall on a continuum (Kane, 1993).

Heeding Values of Older People

Relatively little attention has been given, either in clinical or research contexts, to measuring the preferences and values of subgroups of older people and incorporating them into measures of desired outcomes. Comprehensive assessments used by case managers in long-term care ask about virtually everything else, but ignore preferences except, narrowly and recently, around end-of-life treatments. Yet care plans are very personal and intimate and should, therefore, be built on personal values. Then it would be possible to ask questions about the extent to which a particular program is consistent with the values and preferences of its users—in either its processes or outcomes (McCullough et al., 1993; Kane, 1995b).

In preliminary research at the University of Minnesota, we showed that when older long-term care users are asked, they can identify and express their values regarding a list of general topics—for example, privacy, daily routines, family involvement, preferred activities, attitude toward pain and discomfort, and preference to take risks or be protected. Moreover, they do so with variation within their individual response patterns (Kane, 1995b). Our sample also gave meaningful answers to the question: "What makes you feel most like yourself?" which was designed to tap a sense of identity. Case managers then became challenged to think of creative ways to use the information gleaned through this discussion of values and preferences.

Public Information and Health Education

Public health is an educational enterprise, involving professional, consumer, and citizen information. Public health authorities are charged with the responsibility for framing the issues related to health of the aged and aging public in a way that is clear and accurate. This may also entail responding to various ways that problems are framed and depicted in the media. For example, for the last several decades the expected increase of the elderly population resulting in a lowered proportion of wage-earning adults has been heralded in news accounts and congressional hearings as a crisis. Yet authorities in other countries confront similar statistics without such alarmist rhetoric. Commenting on population aging in Canada, Denton and colleagues (Denton, Li, and Spencer, 1987) point to the reduction in anticipated numbers of children who depend on the wage-earning segment of society as a countervailing force. They conclude that Canada should be able to cope readily with the expected growth in the elderly population without experiencing a crisis. Perhaps the mission of public health should be expanded to counteract the panicky nature of public dialogue about societal aging.

Similarly, public health authorities should help reshape the dialogue on specific points, especially when statistics are advanced that are amenable to several interpretations. For example, we constantly hear that a disproportionate amount of health care costs is spent on the 12 percent of the population over 65. Surely an organized response is needed to reframe the question. If only 12 percent of health care costs were spent on the 12 percent of Americans over age 65, surely that would be insufficient. We *expect* older people on average to use more health services than their younger counterparts, just as we expect people between age 5 and 20 to use educational resources way out of proportion to their representation in the population. More to the point, surely, is whether the current investment in the health of older people is achieving the best results that could be expected, given the state-of-the-art of health sciences. Thus, aging and public health officials might come together to clarify that they see nothing inappropriate in older people consuming a relatively large fraction of the health care dollar.

In yet another example, intergenerational conflict is a favored topic of many politicians, who suggest that young wage earners are unfairly saddled with payment for entitlement programs for older people. Public health officials can set such records straight with a fact-based presentation of the way public and private transfers of wealth and services flow up and down and across the generations. In fact, an extraordinary amount of support is given by older people to their younger relatives, much more than flows in the opposite direction.

Environmental Health

Most issues related to environmental toxins and pollutants are not specific to older people, though frail elderly people may be more vulnerable to negative effects of some conditions—for example, smog and air impurities. Younger people are more likely exposed to environmental hazards in the workplace and other areas and are more subject to negative health effects because of prolonged exposure. A full examination of environmental health issues related to age is beyond the scope or expertise of this chapter. Instead, this section touches on a few points that seem particularly important to older people, and which may push the envelope of environmental health. They are ethical issues because they raise questions about what should be promoted as environments for older people and which values should take precedence in social policy.

Built Environments

The built environment could be more conducive to meeting the needs of people as they age and acquire disabilities. This includes housing stock, furniture, public buildings, transportation systems, and the like. Signs could be easier to read, bus terminals and airports easier to navigate, and phones easier to use. New sensitivities to Americans with disabilities may result in environments that minimize excess disability in the very high proportion of older disabled people.

Noxious Living Environments for Old People

In long-term care programs in the United States, nursing homes predominate. More by happenstance than deliberate design, nursing homes are constructed with double occupancy and hospital-like designs. They are also organized with rigid routines, the latter reinforced by regulations. People with Alzheimer disease are mingled with cognitively intact people—sharing programs, common living space, meals, and often rooms. Privacy is rare. Few opportunities exist for nursing home residents to exercise their capabilities for independent functioning in simple matters like bathing and housekeeping activities. Fewer opportunities are present for meaningful intellectual and social activities.

Protective environments such as the traditional nursing home could be considered truly unhealthy when they constrain individual initiative and energy and dampen the human spirit. As Brody and colleagues pointed out three decades ago (Brody et al., 1974), "excess disability" results when older people are overprotected and when no goals are set to actively encourage functional abilities.

M. Powell Lawton's seminal theories about competence in older people speak to the importance of environments that combine sufficient support with sufficient challenge (Lawton, 1982). Writing about intervention strategies for health promotion and disease prevention in the elderly, George Maddox (1985) zeroed in on strategies to change residential environments. He wrote: "Whether the behavior of older individuals can be changed through purposive interventions is largely irrelevant if the staff, policies, and programs in the relevant milieu do not promote or promise the continuation of the interventions. Interventions designed to modify organizations and institutional structures are as vital as interventions designed to change individuals" (p. 1028). Maddox's essay also emphasizes the importance of applying research from social science about family behavior to fashion interventions that take into account the family as part of the milieu of the older person.

The views of ethicists who have considered long-term care are consistent with Maddox's analysis. In his insightful monograph about autonomy in long-term care, philosopher George Agich (1993) suggested that appropriate respect for personal autonomy would call for creating environments where real and meaningful choices are possible. This would seem to be a public health mission though it expands the traditional boundaries of environmental health. Traditional nursing homes are an obvious target. However, board-and-care homes, often seen as alternatives to nursing homes, may be equally unlikely to promote the full health and functioning of elderly residents.

The importance of family, which Maddox brings up as a social scientist, has also been emphasized by ethicists. Here, however, ethicists raise questions about how right it is to maximize the full health and well-being of an elderly person at the possible expense of family caregivers whose own sacrifices may be needed to achieve this standard (Collopy, Dubler, and Zuckerman, 1990). Regarding "high tech" care at home, Arras and Dubler argued for an "aggregate best interest standard," which takes into account interests of involved family members as well as those of the patient. In an extremely thoughtful essay on conflicts of interest within long-term care, Arras (1995) wrote of the inevitability that the interests of various family members will collide and calls for a midway position between accommodation of family interests and the claims of the primary patient or client. He argues that the danger is still present that the wishes of competent elderly clients are given insufficient weight. This seems to be an arena that would profit from collaborative work of gerontologists (particularly those who study family dynamics and family care), ethicists (who are working out the duties and rights of the persons involved from a philosophical standpoint), and public health researchers and practitioners, who are concerned with promoting health and functioning and preventing excess disability or handicap.

Noxious Decision-Making Environments

Related to noxious living environments is the broader topic of noxious decision-making environments. Arguably, when older people are forced to make important life decisions quickly and when incentives are present to force them to choose a nursing home placement, the conditions should be a public health concern. (*Choice* of nursing home *placement* is somewhat of an oxymoron.)

Older people often make (or have made for them) important decisions at time of crisis. They often choose a place to live in a debilitated condition from a hospital bed. Hospital staff, who have every incentive to get the older person out of the hospital, may advise the easiest placement solution.

Ethicists assert that an autonomous decision must be made without coercion and with information about the available alternatives and their likely effects. The decision maker must then apply his or her own preferences and values to these alternatives. In fact, older people often make health decisions without such information. To exacerbate matters, trusted decision-counselors often feel constrained in their ability to give real information about community resources, including nursing homes, lest they be accused of interfering with trade or dispensing opinions that cannot be substantiated.

Thus, older people often make important life decisions without considering a range of choices. Either no choices exist, or subtle coercion and persuasion narrows the considerations. Hospital discharge planning is an arena notorious for short-circuiting individual decision making on the part of seniors (Coulton et al., 1982). But it is also true that community-based case managers and home health authorities constrain decision-making of older people, partly out of concern that they take undue risks (Kane and Caplan, 1993; Wetle, 1995). Clemens and colleagues (1994) detailed the many ways that the espoused values of respect for autonomy were contradicted in the daily practices of a long-term care case-management agency. Unfortunately, a hasty decision to enter a nursing home may be irreversible if family members act to remove the "escape routes" back to the community—for example, by selling houses and furniture and closing apartments.

So far, the discussion has concentrated on major decisions that are usually discernible to the parties involved—decisions where a choice must be made among possible courses of action. Choices among specific medical treatments, or advance directives about whether or not to forgo life-extending treatments under specified circumstances, are decisions where choices are put upon the older individual or made for them. Similarly, the decision to relocate physically in a long-term care setting is a major life choice. However, the numerous small decisions made in the course of daily life, which Kane and Caplan (1993) called "everyday" decisions and which Agich (1995) called "interstitial" as opposed to "nodal" decisions, may be no less important. Elderly people with impaired physical or cognitive abilities may lose the opportunity to make such decisions, with resulting negative effects on their perceived control and their health.

Public Health Regulation and Quality Assurance

In most states, the state and local health departments are responsible for regulation of and quality assurance in health programs that affect the elderly. This means that state health departments, often with designated responsibilities to local health departments, may license nursing homes, board-and-care homes, adult foster homes, day care settings, and home care. Typically, they are also designated by the federal government to certify nursing homes for payment in the Medicare and Medicaid programs. Health departments also perform quality assurance tasks such as reviewing the appropriateness and quality of care given by various providers. In conjunction with state professional groups and boards, health departments also develop policy for licensure of health occupations.

These roles carry enormous power and importance. In helping set and guard standards for good care, public health authorities play a time-honored role related to protecting and promoting public safety. In long-term care in particular, these responsibilities are onerous because of the presumed vulnerability of the clientele. The pendulum here tends to swing between underregulated programs where no protections exist to overregulated programs where the very regulations designed to protect the elderly end up curbing their freedoms and limiting their options. Some critics believe that long-term care is now regulated too closely. A recent consensus conference on enhancing autonomy for nursing home residents (Gamroth, Semradek, and Tornquist, 1995) concluded that regulation aimed at safety at all costs was part of the problem. Sometimes the difficulties are less in the regulations as written than in the way they are applied by both providers and inspectors, but the end result may be undue restriction.

Regulation and New Care Paradigms

At present, a wide variety of regulations affecting services to the elderly, particularly long-term care, are under scrutiny. The much-heralded 1987 reforms on federal nursing home regulations, which stemmed, in part, from a study by the Institute of Medicine (1986), moved quality assurance and regulation in nursing homes toward patient-centered policies. It did so by creating new Conditions of Participation (i.e., conditions required before a nursing home could receive federal payments) concerning Residents' Rights, Quality of Life, and Functional Assessment. It also ushered in a revised survey (i.e., inspection) process, in which information is gathered directly from observing and interviewing a sample of residents, as well as new enforcement regulations that differentiate on the severity and duration of problems. In the long implementation period for this legislation, an enormous change has come about in the use of physical restraints in nursing homes. Once perceived as a proper tool of management with a need to justify failure to restrain a patient who subsequently is injured, physical restraints are now understood to cause as many injuries and deaths as they prevent (Miles and Irvine, 1992). Moreover, they can be deeply injurious to the human spirit of the person restrained, and they negatively alter the perceptions of caregivers who encounter the person in restraints (Kane et al., 1993).

Despite the accomplishments of the 1987 changes in the regulations of nursing homes, some authorities question whether we use an appropriate regulatory paradigm for long-term care. Noting that the services are so attuned to everyday life, ethicists and gerontologists alike are beginning to question the premises on which regulations are based. Collopy, a philosopher, has urged rethinking the predominant view of safety as the consummate value for long-term care consumers (Collopy, 1995a, 1995b). Kane (1995c) attempted to parse out distinctions between regulations that promote autonomy and those that impede it. At a consensus conference on "Quality, Autonomy, and Safety in Home and Community-Based Long-Term Care," conferees were overwhelmingly in favor of a new model of quality assurance and regulation that placed consumer preferences at the center and countenanced informed risk-taking on the part of vulnerable people using long-term care services (Kane, 1995d). From a legal perspective, Kapp and Detzel (1992) also argue for informed risk-taking on the part of consumers, noting that providers' fears of legal liability are overblown; even for clients who cannot fully make informed decisions because of cognitive incapacities, they advocate less intrusive alternatives to guardianship. Furthermore, commentaries on regulations for emerging forms of long-term care, such as assisted living, highlight the tensions between protective regulation and development of innovative consumer-friendly programs (Kane and Wilson, 1993; Mollica, 1995). On another front, the regulation of nursing practice must come under scrutiny; various states have proposed modifications to nursing practice acts so that unlicensed personnel can provide nursing services after instruction from a nurse (Kane, O'Connor, and Baker, 1995; Kane, 1995d). Finally, requirements for occupational health and safety are unexpectedly colliding with the ability to offer consumer-centered care at home and in assisted living settings; the issue here is whether the private home or the apartment in an assisted living complex is viewed as a workplace where the inhabitant must meet all Occupational Safety and Health Administration (OSHA) standards for products that in-home workers might use. A related issue is whether new models of personal assistant services (which largely bypass home care agencies and in which the consumer is construed as an employer of the worker) must require those consumer-employers to meet OSHA requirements when their private homes become workplaces for health workers.

The question here is how open-mindedly and thoroughly public health officials will explore the calls for a new paradigm of regulation. Public health officials need to consider where they stand on balancing consumer freedom and consumer risk. Risk is very much a public health term, but it is usually thought of in terms of risk factors to be mitigated rather than risks to be deliberately accepted in order to lead as normal a life as possible. This will be especially pertinent as new forms of long-term care are considered by state regulators.

One argument holds that if the program serves people with impairments similar to those of nursing home residents, it follows that all nursing home regulations should apply to the alternative programs or settings. An opposite view holds that new service models must be permitted to emerge, and that one should not use regulation to force all care into old molds. New paradigms to consider safety and protection will also be pertinent as standards for nursing practice and other professional practices are reviewed. At times the breaking point in the high costs of home and community-based care (and therefore the recommendations to enter a nursing home) is propelled by the need for routine nursing services and the lack of any relative to provide it. Clearly, altered personnel policies that allow non-nurses to perform the same kind of nursing functions family members would perform will drive down the costs, but will it be sufficiently safe? These questions pose a clear agenda for public health authorities—and one that involves an ethical issue at its very core.

Although the issue does not directly concern physical health and safety, arguably public health officials have a moral obligation to speak out against standard services of care that perhaps meet care and safety standards, but fall way below levels of privacy and dignity and individualization that older people arguably have a right to expect. For example, public health has not been in the forefront of the arguments in favor of single occupancy as a minimum standard for any residential long-term care program. Standard settings for minimal environments for care financed with public money are based on underlying assumptions about resource constraints. Moreover, efforts to change those standards usually meet with heavy lobbying from affected interest groups—for example, owners of board-and-care homes or nursing homes. The responsibilities of public health officials to take stands on these issues have not been well delineated.

Paradoxically, although the thrust toward environmental standards for living tends to be minimalist (i.e., there is resistance to mandating privacy and autonomy-enhancing features in services to the elderly), the thrust on educational and other standards for staffing is the opposite. It is typically assumed (often without data) that certain training and credentials lead to better results for clientele and are worthwhile, even if they drive up prices for public and private payors in situations in which the guild interests of various professional groups (nurses and social workers and others) often carry the day. Again, these topics are the rightful province of public health, they have no easy answers, and they are ethical problems as well as practice problems. They strike to the heart of the kind of society and lives envisaged for older people with infirmities.

Conclusions

Population aging is, in a way, a triumph of public health. Now public health officials and aging professionals need to join together to give emphasis to some value-laden, ethical issues related to public health in an aging society. The questions raised in the various sections of this chapter have no easy answers. They require ongoing attention to the way older people are valued in society and the values (individual and collective) of older people. They require balancing principles of respect for personal autonomy of old people and beneficent efforts to protect old people. They require considering, in the name of justice, the claims of people of various ages (in families and society as a whole). Public health, with its historical concern for the well-being of populations, could play a leading role in this analysis and can bring ethically tinged issues to the attention of policy makers and the general public. And in designing, conducting, and reporting epidemiological and health services research, public health scholars need to take care to examine any hidden assumptions about older people that might detract from their well-being.

In conclusion, several points related to ethics and public health of older people are stressed:

1. Attention should be given to everyday issues associated with living with care. These are as important as issues surrounding the good death, which ethics have consistently been emphasized. Aging and public health professionals should guide bioethics into these arenas.

2. Respect for autonomy should not be a passive, reactive approach only. Noninterference is cold comfort. An ethic is needed that takes into account intimate relationships involved in care of the elderly.

3. Public health personnel should take care about how issues are framed and whether these are research issues or policy issues. This care needs to occur even at the level of specifying variables and designing studies, because value judgments lurk in these seemingly technical decisions.

4. Public health officials need to reconsider the best ways to assure the quality of services and life to older people needing care, including the extent and nature of

protective regulation. Regulation must be recognized as a two-edged sword that limits the freedoms of the very people being protected.

This chapter has applied a biomedical ethics lens to the general functions of public health as they affect or might affect elderly persons. None of the issues raised has been analyzed in depth, and, indeed, relatively little of such analysis has been done. Those who hold simultaneous interests in public health, bioethics, and aging have interesting work ahead.

References

Agich, G. 1993. *Autonomy and Long-Term Care*. New York: Oxford University Press.

American Association of Homes and Services for the Aging. 1994. *Making Ethical Decisions in Long-Term Care*. Washington, DC.

Agich, G. 1995. Actual autonomy and long-term care decision making. In McCullough, L. B. and Wilson, N. L., eds., *Long-Term Care Decisions: Ethical and Conceptual Dimensions* (pp. 113–36). Baltimore: Johns Hopkins University Press.

Arras, J. 1995. Conflicting interests in long-term care decision-making: Acknowledging, dissolving, and resolving conflicts. In McCullough, L. B., and Wilson, N. L., eds., *Long-Term Care Decisions: Ethical and Conceptual Dimensions* (pp. 197–220). Baltimore: Johns Hopkins University Press.

Avorn, J. 1984. Benefit and cost analysis in geriatric care: Turning age discrimination into health policy. *New England Journal of Medicine* 310:1294–1301.

Avorn, J. L., and Soumerai, S. M. 1983. Improving drug therapy decisions through educational outreach: A randomized controlled trial of academically based "detailing." *New England Journal of Medicine* 308:1457–63.

Beauchamp, D. E. 1995. Philosophy of public health. In Reich, W. T., ed., *Encyclopedia of Bioethics, Revised Edition Vol. 4* (pp. 2161–65). New York: Simon & Schuster Macmillan.

Beauchamp, T. L., and Childress, J. F. 1994. *Principles of Biomedical Ethics* (4th ed.). New York: Oxford University Press.

Brody, E. M., Kleban, M. H., Lawton, M. P., and Moss, M. 1971. A longitudinal look at excess disabilities in the mentally impaired aged. *Journal of Gerontology* 11:124–32.

Callahan, J. J. Jr. 1982. Elder abuse programming: Will it help the elderly? *Urban and Social Change Review* 15:15–16.

Clemens, E., Wetle, T., Feltes, M., Crabtree, B., and Dubitzky, D. 1994. Contradictions in case management: Client-centered theory and directive practice. *Journal of Aging and Health*, 6:70–88.

Collopy, B. J. 1988. Autonomy in long term care: Some crucial distinctions. *Gerontologist* 28(Suppl.):10–17.

Collopy, B. J. 1993. The burden of beneficence. In Kane, R. A., and Caplan, A. L., eds., *Ethical Conflicts in the Management of Home Care: The Case Manager's Dilemma*. New York: Springer Publishing Company.

Collopy, B. J. 1995a. Safety and independence: Rethinking some basic concepts in long-term care. In McCullough, L. B., and Wilson, N. L., eds., *Long-Term Care Decisions: Ethical and Conceptual Dimensions* (pp. 137–52). Baltimore: Johns Hopkins University Press.

Collopy, B. J. 1995b. Power, paternalism, and the ambiguities of autonomy. In Gamroth, L. M., Semradek, J., and Tornquist, E. M., eds., *Enhancing Autonomy in Long-Term Care: Concepts and Strategies* (pp. 3–14). New York: Springer Publishing Company.

Collopy, B. J., Dubler, N., and Zuckerman, C. 1990. The ethics of home care: Autonomy and accommodation. *Hastings Center Report* 20(2):S1–16.

Coulton, C. J., Dunkle, R. E., Goode, R. A., and MacIntosh, J. 1982. Discharge planning and decision-making. *Health and Social Work* 253–61.

Denton, F. T., Li, S. N., and Spencer, B. G. 1987. How will population aging affect the future costs of maintaining health-care standards? In Marshall, V., ed., *Aging in Canada* (2nd ed.). Markham, Ontario: Fitzhenry and Whiteside.

Gamroth, L. M., Semradek, J., and Tornquist, E. M., eds. 1995. *Enhancing Autonomy in Long-Term Care: Concepts and Strategies.* New York: Springer Publishing Company.

Geron, S. M., and Chassler, D. 1994. *Guidelines for Case Management Practice Across the Long-Term Care Continuum.* Washington, DC.

Institute of Medicine. 1986. *Improving the Quality of Care in Nursing Homes.* Washington, DC: National Academy Press.

Jameton, A. 1988. In the borderlands of autonomy: Responsibility in long term care facilities. *Gerontologist* 28(Suppl.):18–23.

Kane, R. A. 1993. Dangers lurking in the "continuum of care": Repertoire of services is a better goal. *Journal of Aging and Social Policy* 5(4):1–7.

Kane, R. A. 1995a. Assessment of social functioning: Recommendations for comprehensive geriatric assessment. In Rubenstein, L. Z., Wieland, D., and Bernabei, R., eds., *Geriatric Assessment Technology: The State of the Art* (pp. 91–110). Milan: Editrice Kurtis.

Kane, R. A. 1995b. Decision making, care plans, and life plans in long-term care: Can case managers take account of clients' values and preferences. In McCullough, L. B., and Wilson, N. L., eds., *Long-Term Care Decisions: Ethical and Conceptual Dimensions.* Baltimore: Johns Hopkins University Press.

Kane, R. A. 1995c. Autonomy and regulation in long-term care: An odd couple, an ambiguous relationship. In Gamroth, L. M., Semradek, J., and Tornquist, E. M., eds., *Enhancing Autonomy in Long-Term Care: Concepts and Strategies* (pp. 68–86). New York: Springer Publishing Company.

Kane, R. A. 1995d. *Quality, Autonomy, and Safety in Home and Community-Based Long-Term Care: Toward Regulatory and Quality Assurance Policy.* Report of a National Mini-Conference held February 11–12. Minneapolis: University of Minnesota National LTC Resource Center.

Kane, R. A., and Caplan, A. L., eds. 1993. *Ethical Conflicts in the Management of Home Care: The Case Manager's Dilemma.* New York: Springer Publishing Company.

Kane, R. A., and Wilson, K. B. 1993. *Assisted Living in the United States: A New Paradigm for Residential Care for Frail Older Persons?* Washington, DC: American Association of Retired Persons.

Kane, R. L., Kane, R. A., and Arnold, S. 1985. Prevention and the elderly: Risk factors. *Health Services Research* 19:945–1006.

Kane, R. L., Williams, C. C., Williams, T. F., and Kane, R. A. 1993. Restraining restraints: Changes in a standard of care. *Annual Review of Public Health.* 14:545–84.

Kane, R. A., O'Connor, C., and Baker, M. O. 1995. *Delegation of Nursing Activities: Implications for Patterns of Long-Term Care.* Washington, DC: American Association of Retired Persons. Minneapolis: University of Minnesota National LTC Resource Center.

Kapp, M. B., and Detzel, J. A. 1992. *Alternatives to Guardianship for the Elderly: Legal Liability*

Disincentives and Impediments. Dayton, OH: Wright State University School of Medicine.

Lawton, M. P. 1982. Competence, environmental press, and adaptation of older people. In Lawton, M. P., Windley, P. G., and Byerts, T. O., eds., *Aging and the Environment: Theoretical Approaches.* New York: Springer Publishing Company.

Macklin, R. 1990. Good citizen, bad citizen. In Kane, R. A., and Caplan, A., eds., *Everyday Ethics: Resolving Dilemmas in Nursing Home Life.* New York: Springer Publishing Company.

Maddox, G. L. 1985. Intervention strategies to enhance well-being in later life: The status and prospect of guided change. *Health Services Research* 19:1007–32.

McCullough, L. B., and Wilson, N. L., eds. 1995. *Long-Term Care Decisions: Ethical and Conceptual Dimensions.* Baltimore: Johns Hopkins University Press.

McCullough, L. B., Wilson, N. L., Teasdale, T. A., Kolpakchi, A. L., and Skelly, J. R. 1993. Mapping personal, familial, and professional values long-term care decisions. *Gerontologist* 33:324–32.

Menzel, P. T. 1990. *Strong Medicine: The Ethical Rationing of Health Care.* New York: Oxford University Press.

Miles, S. H., and Irvine, P. 1992. Deaths caused by physical restraints. *The Gerontologist* 32(6):762–66.

Mollica, R. 1995. *A Guide to Assisted Living and State Policy.* Portland, ME: National Academy for State Health Policy.

Montgomery, R. J. V. 1995. Examining respite care: Promises and limitations. In Kane, R. A., and Penrod, J. D., eds., *Family Caregiving in an Aging Society: Policy Perspectives* (pp. 29–45). Thousand Oaks, CA: Sage Publications, Inc.

National Association of Private Geriatric Care Managers. 1990. *Standards and Practices for Private Geriatric Care Managers* [Brochure]. Tucson, AZ.

Szwabo, P. A., and Grossberg, G. T. 1993. *Problem Behaviors in Long-Term Care: Recognition, Diagnosis, and Treatment.* New York: Springer Publishing Company.

Wetle, T. 1995. Ethical issues and value conflicts facing case managers of frail elderly people living at home. In McCullough, L. B., and Wilson, N. L., eds., *Long-Term Care Decisions: Ethical and Conceptual Dimensions* (pp. 63–86). Baltimore: Johns Hopkins University Press.

Williams, E. I. 1989. *Caring for the Elderly in the Community* (2nd ed.). London: Chapman and Hall.

Chapter

15

Implications of an Aging Society
for the Preparation of Public
Health Professionals

Thomas R. Prohaska, Ph.D., and Steven P. Wallace, Ph.D.

Public health, as an academic discipline and as a practice, offers a unique contribution to the health and well-being of older adults. It is the only health profession that is grounded in a philosophy of dealing with populations rather than individuals, and it is unique in specializing in promoting and protecting health rather than treating disease. This perspective will become increasingly important for older people as modern medicine reaches its limits in treating chronic illness and we increasingly look toward primary prevention. As more older adults live to older ages, there will also be an increasing emphasis on maintaining functional independence and maximizing the quality of life rather than extending the average life expectancy. Public health is positioned to be especially useful in addressing these quality-of-life issues.

Applying the principles of public health to older persons requires some knowledge and skills in both public health and gerontology. In this chapter we refer to this combination of knowledge and skills as "public health and aging," to distinguish it from "geriatrics," which focuses more on disease and pathology, and from "gerontology," which encompasses all topics that are significant to the older population. We need to be deliberate in transmitting the increasing knowledge of public health and aging to future public health practitioners. In the following historical review of training in public health and aging, we argue that education on the topic has *not* de-

veloped according to employment demands for public health practitioners in gerontology. We then predict how past trends are likely to influence future training in
public health and aging. Finally, we offer suggestions about how training might better be structured to improve the applicability of the knowledge, skills, and attitudes
that future public health practitioners will need to work with programs and policies
that affect older Americans.

The Origins and Growth of Public Health Gerontology

The field of public health gerontology is quite recent. While professional research and practice in general public health fostered the founding of the American
Public Health Association in 1872, the Gerontological Society of America (the primary scientific organization for researchers and educators in gerontology) was not
founded until 1945. By 1964 there were still only two schools of public health with
courses in public health gerontology (Magee, 1985). Growth in the field led to the
formation of a Gerontological Health section in the American Public Health
Association in 1982, and section membership grew to 1000 in the following ten years.
By 1992, twenty-one of twenty-three accredited U.S. schools of public health surveyed had one or more courses in gerontological public health (Prohaska, 1993).

This rapid growth in public health gerontological research and training within
ten years was the result of a number of contributing forces: the demographic shift
of the population; the development and growth of federal- and foundation-
sponsored research in aging; the recognition of geriatrics as a medical specialty; and
the recognition of the need for health professionals who can address issues of long-
term care, community-based health education interventions, and epidemiological
health risk factors in older populations.

Demography and Disease

Most courses on aging start with an overview of the historic demographic changes
occurring in technologically advanced countries. At the turn of the twentieth century,
40 percent of the U.S. population was under age 18, while only 4 percent was age 65
or older (U.S. Senate, 1989). During that time, public health emphasized improved
sanitation, decent housing, and the control of communicable diseases for all ages, but
the young were the most vulnerable. Maternal and child health was an appropriate
priority for public health, given the size and risks of that group.

Since the early twentieth century there has been a shift in the leading causes of
death from infectious diseases (e.g., pneumonia/influenza, tuberculosis) to chronic
diseases (e.g., heart disease, cancer, stroke) (McKinlay, McKinlay, and Benglehold,

1989). It is now recognized that behavioral risk factors such as tobacco use, diet, and exercise significantly contribute to these chronic conditions. There has also been significant growth in the older population since the early twentieth century. Currently over 12 percent of the U.S. population is 65 years of age or older. The majority of these older adults (80%) have one or more chronic conditions or diseases (National Center for Health Statistics, 1993). Public health has taken a primary role in documenting the incidence and prevalence of chronic conditions in the population, identifying risk factors associated with these chronic diseases, and designing strategies to reduce the risk of these chronic diseases.

Politics and Public Health

Through the first half of the twentieth century, the primary political involvement of and for older persons centered on pensions (Wallace et al., 1991). Social movements of the aged during the Depression focused on federally guaranteed pensions. For a variety of political and economic reasons, Social Security and Old Age Assistance (state-administered welfare for aged persons) were established at that time (Quadagno, 1988). As pensions became a less critical issue, health care for elderly persons rose in prominence. Work-based health insurance became the norm in the United States during the 1940s and 1950s. Unfortunately, older adults were generally excluded because of their high medical expenses and separation from the labor force (Fein, 1989). Advocates of national health insurance, having been defeated for years by the medical profession and other special-interest groups, shifted their focus to health insurance problems of the older population as a vehicle for developing support for a national health program (Starr, 1982). The political legitimacy of the elderly, their need for health insurance, and the social activism of the early 1960s helped the passage of Medicare and Medicaid (Wallace and Williamson, 1992) and boosted awareness of health and aging issues in public health. But Medicare is acute care insurance, and although Medicaid has become a dominant payer of long-term care for those over age 65, the public health needs of elderly persons have been unaddressed to a large extent.

Medicare spending increased from $7.5 billion in 1970 to $114 billion in 1991 (Haber, 1994). The rapid growth in Medicare and Medicaid expenditures has created political pressure to reduce the use of hospitals and nursing homes (Estes et al., 1993), helping to stimulate interest in the public health community for chronic disease prevention and ways of maximizing the independence of the functionally disabled. In addition, the public concern that has been generated regarding Alzheimer disease has led to increased public health interest in this incurable condition (Fox, 1989). The high cost associated with chronic conditions such as Alzheimer disease and the competition for limited health care dollars has contributed to a search for cost-effective community-based public health alternatives to institutionalization.

Growth by Research Funding

The demographic patterns and politics of aging have also shaped the research agenda of our country. Federal involvement in health research began in a substantial way with the founding of the National Institutes of Health in 1943 via the Public Health Service Act of 1943 and 1944 (Snyder, 1994). In response to the growing recognition of aging research issues, the National Institute on Aging (NIA) was added to NIH in 1977 (Lockett, 1983).

While much of NIA's funding goes for biomedical and clinical research, the behavioral sciences section funds a large amount of research that is consistent with a public health perspective. The NIA has sponsored the Established Populations for Epidemiologic Studies of the Elderly to provide detailed prospective information about the health status of defined older populations. The NIA has also been instrumental in funding national surveys with older populations, including the Longitudinal Study of Aging (1984–1990) and the National Caregiver Study (1982–1988). In addition to funding large, national, longitudinal studies, the NIA also funds smaller investigator-initiated proposals that address specified priority areas, including those relevant to public health—such as falls in older adults and physical frailty in older minorities. Education is encouraged through research training grants to institutions, including four in epidemiology and several in other areas of public health (U.S. Senate, 1994).

The large national surveys funded in part by the NIA have often been conducted by the National Center for Health Statistics (NCHS). As the nation's central health statistics collector, NCHS began gathering information on nursing home residents in 1973. During the 1980s the center's interest in aging increased as it produced research and reports on issues of aging and health including determinants of health, use of community-based and long-term care health care services, and assessment of costs associated with the use of such services (NCHS, 1993). Researchers (and program planners) in public health and aging continue to examine these national data sources to better understand the nature of illness and disability in the older population (Harris and Kovar, 1992). Publications based on these data sources also help provide the knowledge base used in teaching about health and aging.

While the NIA is a major resource for funding public health research with older populations, it is not the only resource contributing to the proliferation of research in public health and aging. Other major research funding sources include the Health Care Financing Administration (HCFA), Agency for Health Care Policy and Research (AHCPR), the Centers for Disease Control (CDC), the Administration on Aging (AoA), and the Social Security Administration (U.S. Senate, 1994). Private foundations that have been funding aging research since the 1960s include the Retirement Research Foundation, the Robert Wood Johnson Foundation, and the American Association of Retired Persons (AARP). Together, these groups have provided extensive resources that have nurtured gerontological public health research and broadened our knowledge of the health and well-being of older adults.

Research has played an important role in the development of gerontological public health training, since almost all schools of public health, and most other Masters of Public Health (M.P.H.) programs, are located in large research-oriented universities. As a result, the growing number of researchers in gerontological public health have provided many faculty dispersed over most schools who have been interested in developing public health courses in their area of research expertise.

Geriatrics, Gerontology, and the Professionalization of Aging Services

Several conditions make it possible for a profession to dominate a service sector. Professional dominance generally involves a claim of unique and specialized knowledge, a level of monopoly control over the market for their expertise, required advanced training, and often some type of certification or licensure (Larson, 1977). Allopathic medicine, nursing, and social work have all followed the path of professional licensure and state regulation that provides them with protected access to a number of gerontological jobs. General gerontology and public health both have accreditation standards for specialized degrees (the Master of Science in Gerontology (M.S.G.) and Master of Public Health (M.P.H.), respectively), but neither discipline has the type of privileged access to jobs in the way the other disciplines do.

Allopathic medicine is often used as the exemplar of how a profession develops and lays claim to the exclusive exercise of a set of skills (Starr, 1982). Having solidified its position among the healing professions in the early part of the century, it has worked to expand the areas over which it can claim expertise. The medical field showed interest in aging issues early on, focusing on "senescence" and the diseases of elderly persons. Despite this early start, payment for geriatric services has been generally low and, until Medicare, uncertain. The limited development of medical training in geriatrics contributed to the establishment in 1979 of the Geriatric Education Center program, which funds the development and provision of geriatric education nationally. Geriatrics has only recently come to be an area of certification of added qualifications, with certification in geriatric medicine provided by the American Board of Internal Medicine and Family Practice beginning in 1988.

Similarly, nursing identified a specific body of clinical expertise that distinguishes it from lay nursing in the early 1900s (Larson, 1977). It has been interested in the care of elderly persons at least since the 1950s, when Montefiore Medical Center in New York began an innovative home health care program, but it took many years before nursing schools initiated formal gerontological health tracks.

Similar to public health and nursing, social work began primarily as a profession devoted to child and family welfare. Social workers have been widely employed in human service programs, and the growth of services for older adults through the Older Americans Act and Medicare has increased the ability of social workers to claim special expertise in aging. In the health care field, the needs for hospital discharge planning, nursing home social work, and case management have fit the social work model and provided areas of growth for the profession.

Programs in gerontology, especially at the master's level, are a relatively recent development. The Older Americans Act, first passed in 1965 and expanded since then, has created an "aging network" (or aging enterprise) that requires knowledge in aging policy and services that can be met with a degree in gerontology (Estes, 1979). But gerontology has not developed an exclusive franchise on this knowledge, and has not developed a guaranteed occupational niche like the earlier professions.

Public health is like gerontology in being an interdisciplinary field. However, it is different in having identified a unique methodological tool (epidemiology) and a characteristic population-based intervention approach. Public health claims that its specialized body of knowledge involves (1) a broad focus on health and well-being, not just the absence of disease and disability; (2) a focus on the aggregate population rather than a clinical one-on-one approach; (3) an emphasis on primary and secondary prevention; and (4) interventions at all levels, including the person, the family, the community, health care systems, government, and society. The special contribution of this public health approach to aging was codified in a 1990 training curriculum produced for the U.S. Bureau of Health Professions (1990). That curriculum, which was targeted at health department employees, covers:

1. aging, demography, biology, and epidemiology,

2. psychosocial issues in aging and health,

3. financing the health care of older adults,

4. continuum of care services for older adults, and

5. health promotion for older adults.

Similar to general gerontology, public health education in general has a limited penetration into the workforce, since many public health jobs do not require accredited M.P.H. degrees. The one job that requires a special, accredited degree is that of nursing home administrator. The specific nature of nursing home administrator accreditation requirements, however, results in those degrees being offered more commonly in non–public-health administration programs than in schools of public health (Infeld and Kress, 1989).

Overall, while the process of professionalization has occurred in many of the occupations that work with elderly persons, the discipline of gerontology and the field of public health have yet to sufficiently convince employers that they command a *unique* body of knowledge, to develop singular control over the market for their expertise, or to require licensure for the practice of their skills. Both do require advanced training to obtain the M.S.G. and M.P.H. degrees, but those degrees are not necessary requirements for many jobs.

Summary of Historical Influences

Demography, disease patterns, politics, research funding, and the professionalization of some aging-related disciplines have all contributed to the development of the field of aging and gerontology within public health. These factors also contribute to the potential for instability in the growth of training in public health and aging. While the demographic shifts and disease patterns are likely to occur as predicted, politics, research funding, and professional turf battles are unpredictable. For example, if research funding opportunities in aging significantly shift from being compatible with a public health perspective to being more clinical or basic biomedical, there may be a corresponding shift in interest in curriculum and training in public health and aging.

One important factor does *not* currently exist that would encourage training in public health gerontology: a strong demand for health professionals trained specifically in gerontological public health. "Generally speaking, job opportunities are excellent in geriatrics and somewhat unpredictable in gerontology. A strong demand continues for licensed health professionals. The demand is softer for personnel in administration, planning, policy analysis, and service delivery jobs for which hiring requirements are less stringent" (Kahl, 1992, p. 4). At least two changes could make the labor market play a more central role in defining training in health and aging. First, public health organizations and agencies could emphasize perspectives compatible primarily with public health gerontology (e.g., community-based health promotion and disability prevention for older populations). A beginning of this exists in the form of a prevention block grant provided to states by the federal government. The demand for those trained in gerontological public health is unlikely to catch the attention of educators and students, however, until funding reaches the magnitude of smoking control or HIV/AIDS prevention. The second change that could lead the labor market to encourage training in aging and public health would be for jobs in working with older adults to give a clear preference to those with gerontological training. Either of these two changes is likely to lead public health educators to shape curricula to more directly meet the needs of public health *practice* with older adults.

Curriculum Content and Training in Public Health and Aging

The 1980s saw a strong national growth in the availability of course work in public health and aging. A summary of course offerings in aging in U.S. schools of public health is provided in Table 15.1. These findings are based on an assessment of programs and course offerings and related materials describing the curriculum content within each school of public health in 1992. A total of 96 course offerings with content in gerontology were reported by schools of public health in 1992 (Prohaska, 1993), compared to 63 course offerings reported by Magee in 1985—an increase of 52 percent over the seven-year period. There is a considerable range between universities in the number of aging-related course offerings in schools of public health (0 to 11), with all but two schools offering at least one course in aging.

Table 15.1 also provides a distribution of public health gerontology courses offered in 1992 by content area. These courses were categorized into six general topic areas: introduction or overview of gerontology; processes of aging (including biology and nutrition in aging); epidemiology; psychosocial issues of aging; organizational finance and delivery of care; and health education and promotion. The content areas were similar to the curricula content areas used in the Geriatric Training Curriculum for Public Health Professionals (U.S. Bureau of Health Professions, 1990). Based on this classification, courses in organizational finance and delivery of care were the most common aging courses offered in Schools of Public Health (34 of 96 courses). Seventeen of the twenty-three Schools of Public Health surveyed had one or more courses in the finance and delivery of care to older populations. The least common public health gerontology course focused on health education and health promotion of older adults (six courses) (Prohaska, 1993).

While individual courses in health and aging are common, coordinated programs on the subject are less common. A review of program literature provided by twenty-three schools of public health revealed that two offered a special degree in gerontological public health (Table 15.2). Eight programs reported a gerontology concentration or track. Of the twenty-two schools that specifically mentioned continuing education, only two discussed gerontology as part of this continuing education, and only four of the twenty-one schools that reported offering any certificate programs mentioned a certificate in gerontology (Prohaska, 1993). This suggests that for most of the schools with limited courses in gerontological public health, only a few courses are offered by faculty with research or applied interests in aging. It appears that most of the gerontological teaching responsibilities in schools without a formal concentration fall on one or a small number of faculty. Thus, the courses may be limited in scope and vulnerable to retirements, changing research interests, and sabbaticals.

TABLE 15.1. Number and Distribution of Gerontology Courses, by School of Public Health and Course Content Area, 1992

School of Public Health	A	B	C	D	E	F	Total	Magee 1985
University of Alabama–Birmingham					1	1	2	0
Boston University	1		1		2		4	2
University of California–Berkeley		1		1	3	1	6	3
University of California–Los Angeles	1		1	3	3	1	9	2
Columbia University	1	3		2	5		11	8
Harvard University							0	1
University of Hawaii	2	1		1	1		5	6
University of Illinois–Chicago	1	1	1	2	3	1	9	4
Johns Hopkins University	1	1	1		1	1	5	4
Loma Linda University	2	1	1	1			5	3
University of Massachusetts					1		1	0
University of Michigan		2	1	2	1		6	8
University of Minnesota	2	2			2		6	4
University of North Carolina	1	1		1	4		7	4
University of Oklahoma			1	1	1	1	3	4
University of Pittsburgh			2	1	1		4	2
San Diego State University							0	0
University of South Carolina		2	1		1		4	0
University of South Florida		1					1	0
University of Texas					1		1	2
Tulane University	1				3		4	0
University of Wastington							1	1
Yale University	1		1				2	5
Total	14	16	11	15	34	6	96	63

A. Introduction/overview of aging
B. Processes of aging
C. Epidemiology of aging
D. Psychosocial issues of aging
E. Organizational finance/delivery of care
F. Health education/health promotion in aging

Since there are many different ways to teach each course topic, Wallace (1994) conducted a content analysis of seventy-six syllabi from eighteen of the twenty accredited public health programs reporting course work in public health and aging (seventy-one contained useable information). The most common topics receiving full class sessions in these courses were: a general overview of health policy and aging (39%); noninstitutional care of elderly persons (38%); and normal psychology and mental health (37%) (Table 15.3). Fewer courses devoted one or more class sessions to special populations such as minorities, women, the poor, or the oldest-old.

TABLE 15.2. Characteristics of Gerontology Programs for Schools of Public
Health, 1992

School of Public Health	Degree Programs	Track, Concentration, Specialization	Continuing Education	Certificate Programs
University of Alabama–Birmingham	No	No	No	No
Boston University	No	Yes	No	No
University of California–Berkeley	No	No	No	No
University of California–Los Angeles	No	Yes	No	No
Columbia University	Yes	Yes	Yes	No
Harvard University	No	No	No	No
University of Hawaii	No	No	No	No
University of Illinois–Chicago	No	Yes	Yes	Yes
Johns Hopkins University	Yes	*	*	Yes
Loma Linda University	No	Yes	*	*
University of Massachusetts	No**	No	*	*
University of Michigan	No	No	No	No
University of Minnesota	No	Yes	No	No
University of North Carolina	No	No	No	No
University of Oklahoma	No	No	No	No
University of Pittsburgh	No	Yes	No	No
San Diego State University	No	No	No	No
University of South Carolina	No	No	*	Yes
University of South Florida	No***	Yes	No	Yes
University of Texas	No	No	No	No
Tulane University	No	No	No	No
University of Washington	No	No	No	No
Yale University	No	No	No	No
Total	2	8	2	4

*Unable to determine from materials
**Ph.D. in Gerontology (graduate school, not school of public health)
***M.A. in Gerontology (College of Arts and Sciences, not school of public health)

Table 15.3 also shows the relative emphasis placed on a broad understanding of health status in older populations in the courses. General health status of older adults is presented in 28 percent of the courses, while issues associated with mental health (23%), chronic physical diseases (15%), and Alzheimer disease (13%) are also frequently addressed in public health and aging curricula. Extensive course work was also found in the long-term care of chronic conditions including nursing homes (31%), community-based care (38%), and informal care (35%). Overall, Wallace (1994) concluded that most of the existing course work is aimed at students with

TABLE 15.3. Content Areas Covered in One or More Public Health and Aging Class Sessions ($n = 71$)

Health Problems and Health Services	
Health status, general	20 (28%)
Mental health, psychology	25 (35%)
Mental illness	16 (23%)
Alzheimer's disease and dementias	9 (13%)
Chronic disease	11 (15%)
Dying	5 (7%)
Health care organization, general	8 (11%)
Acute care	4 (6%)
Nursing homes	22 (31%)
Alternative (community) services	27 (38%)
Informal care/family	25 (35%)
Disease Prevention and Health Promotion	
Health promotion/prevention	17 (24%)
Teaching methods	3 (4%)
Normal/successful aging	15 (21%)
Autonomy and independence	5 (7%)
Health behavior	17 (24%)
Social construction of aging or health	15 (21%)
Social issues (e.g., retirement)	12 (17%)
Policy Issues	
Health policy—overview	28 (39%)
Regulation	11 (15%)
Finance, general	16 (23%)
Cost-containment	6 (8%)
Medicaid/Medicare	6 (8%)
Private insurance	6 (8%)
Policy process	10 (14%)
Political power—elderly, organizations	8 (11%)
Practice Issues	
Program planning	8 (11%)
Program evaluation/assessment	7 (10%)
Administration/management	8 (11%)
Quality assurance/quality of care	16 (23%)
Ethics	14 (20%)
Special Populations	
Minority aged	14 (20%)
Older women	6 (8%)
Socioeconomic status	7 (10%)
Oldest old (85+)	2 (3%)
Other Issues	
Demography of aging	20 (28%)
Epidemiology	15 (21%)
Biology of aging	18 (25%)
Gerontological and related theory	14 (20%)
Research methods in aging	11 (15%)
International issues	1 (1%)

limited knowledge or experience in gerontology. This means that most students who receive training in aging and public health are receiving a low level of specialization rather than a rigorous preparation in applying public health concepts to the elderly population. We will argue later that this approach is appropriate for most public health programs, although there is a need to maintain several advanced centers where students can obtain more in-depth training.

In addition to course content, the way in which courses are taught is important. One major deficiency in public health training, according to the Institute of Medicine's (IOM) report on the Future of Public Health (1988), is a lack of sufficient interaction with agencies and programs addressing the health and social needs of individuals in the community. This failure is also common to courses on health and aging (Wallace, 1994). Only one-quarter of the courses reviewed required any first-hand experience (e.g., site visit, interview) with older adults or an organization that works with them. While this type of assignment can be relatively easy to structure, the low incidence of such assignments reflects a broader problem in academic public health of a distancing from the communities and populations served.

The findings from the Prohaska (1993) and Wallace (1994) surveys show that aging curricula in public health have grown over the years since Magee (1985). The content analysis by Wallace indicates that, while there is considerable variability in content, curricula are compatible with public health in that they are generally focused on populations rather than individuals and tend to broadly define health in the aggregate population.

These two surveys also demonstrate that the growth in aging and public health is not uniform across either schools of public health or accredited public health programs outside schools of public health. Prohaska (1993) found that eight of the twenty-three schools of public health surveyed had two or fewer aging courses in their school of public health. Similarly, Wallace (1994) found that six of the twenty-two accredited programs in public health outside of schools of public health did not report any formal course content in aging. It is clear that there is little movement to develop credentialing or specific degrees in aging and public health at this time.

Findings from both these surveys should be interpreted cautiously. The school of public health program catalogs and printed descriptions used by Prohaska (1993) may be dated and may not include new course offerings. It is also possible that as faculty leave, some course offerings that were listed are no longer offered. The survey by Wallace (1994) was based on a content analyses of public health and aging syllabi offered. While this method allowed for a detailed examination of aging course content, it did not adjust for the number of times a specific course was offered in a given academic year or the extent of coverage of a specific topic within a course. Unpublished data, for example, show that, despite the wide availability of course offerings in accredited M.P.H. programs nationally, only 5 percent of M.P.H. students enroll each year in a class on public health and aging.

The two analyses of gerontological public health curricula just reviewed reflect forces that have encouraged the development of the field. The demographic and disease patterns of older adults generated from national data are well reflected in public health curricula. The considerable research in long-term care services and political and public concern over funding health services for the older population are reflected in the large proportion of public health and aging courses in organization, finance, and delivery of care. The politics of aging has helped produce more course content on Alzheimer disease than on death and dying, but overall the focus of courses is even more likely to reflect central public health concerns such as successful or "healthy" aging and health promotion through modified health behavior. Finally, the limited professionalization in public health (not to mention gerontological public health) has resulted in a plethora of introductory aging courses in public health training programs but few advanced courses and little exposure to field experience and public health practice in aging.

Future Directions for Training in Public Health and Aging

The forces that we have identified as shaping existing training in public health and aging are likely to continue to shape curriculum development in the future. The demographic and disease patterns of the population will continue to create a need for professionals with knowledge and skills relevant to the aged. In addition, the growing numbers and high medical care use by older Americans will also continue to generate political pressure for both continued research in health problems faced by the aging population, as well as continued attempts at cost containment.

Past trends in the professionalization of occupations that serve older adults suggest that some fields, such as social work, will consolidate their position in some aging services (e.g., case management). However, it is unlikely that public health, let alone public health gerontology, will arrive at a position anytime soon where a large number of jobs will require *licensed* public health practitioners (although there is a movement in this direction in the subfield of health education with the Certified Health Education Specialist (CHES) accreditation program). Given that, there will be no compelling reason for public health programs to establish specific degrees in public health gerontology. The growth of the aging population and its complicated health and disease issues, however, will continue to generate a demand for health professionals with *some* knowledge of gerontology and geriatrics. Thus, the current pattern of most schools of public health having some introductory course work in health and aging, and a few with well-developed concentrations, is likely to be sufficient to meet the demand for public health practitioners in the aging-services and policy workforce in the near future.

The potential for future growth in health and aging is more likely to come from research than from practice. Research funding through the NIA and other federal agencies appears to be on a continuing growth curve. NIA funding grew to $420 million in FY1994 during a period of severe pressure to limit discretionary federal expenditures (U.S. Senate, 1994). As long as this growth continues, we can expect that the field of public health and aging will also continue to grow as more faculty members in public health schools and programs continue to have research experience in gerontological public health. Similarly, increased funding for research on health services organization and delivery is likely, especially in the expensive and expanding field of long-term care. On the other hand, the funding for practice-oriented training is unstable. In 1995 the U.S. Congress proposed eliminating the Geriatric Education Center program, one of the few education (versus research) programs that target health professionals who work with older adults. These trends will provide incentives for the continued growth in the production of public health and aging *researchers*, and in turn, continued growth in the information base for gerontological public health curricula.

Perhaps the largest challenge in the coming years is to ensure that all professional public health students have *some* exposure to the field of aging. Current accreditation standards require that public health professional students receive training in five core areas of public health: epidemiology, biostatistics, behavioral sciences, environmental health, and health services. While each of these areas is important to older persons, there is no guarantee that students will receive any training in how to apply those subject areas to policies and programs for elderly persons. It is important that older adults be referenced throughout the core curriculum so that students develop an awareness of elderly persons as a significant target of all public health measures, and not simply a group that is of concern only to hospital and nursing home administrators. The other chapters in this volume attest to the wide range of public health interventions that can promote and protect the health of adults at all ages.

Because a significant proportion of the public health workforce does not have a strong public health background, it is also important that continuing education be available and encouraged for those already in the workforce. Perhaps most surprising in the review of aging courses in schools of public health (Prohaska, 1993) was the limited availability of continuing education training in the area. The absence of licensure requirements guarantees that people from a variety of backgrounds will be in positions that involve public health and aging. This can be good when it brings a variety of perspectives and experiences that are useful in problem solving and program development. But, it creates a problem when the diversity of training brings uneven levels of knowledge about the issues facing the aged, limited knowledge about what has worked and not worked in the past, and/or a lack of appreciation of how generic programs and policies need to be modified to best address the aging population. In the aging network (primarily Area Agencies on Aging), employees report a high level of need in job-relevant continuing education, including information on aging policies and regulations, data on community resources and funding, and knowledge about alternative ways of meeting the needs of older adults (Peterson, Wendt, and Douglass, 1991). These are areas that would also be relevant to public health professionals who work in the aging field.

The primary problem with relying on researchers to define public health and aging according to their research interests is that they typically focus on a defined topic, while there are a variety of approaches that can contribute to the improvement of the lives of older Americans. The review of courses and course topics reflects the large amount of research on long-term care and other medical care for elderly people. However, it also reflects the limited attention to health promotion and quality of life issues in aging research.

To expose students to the strengths of a public health approach to aging, a group of public health educators gathered in 1992 and developed a model course outline for an introductory Public Health and Aging course (Wallace and Prohaska, 1993). The consensus of the group was that the objectives for an introductory course on health and aging should include:

1. A basic understanding of biological, psychological, social, and environmental aspects of health and illness in the aging process

2. An understanding of the changing aging population and its interaction with society and the health care system

3. An appreciation of the heterogeneity of the older adult population and the aging process

4. The ability to integrate research into practice

5. Skills and knowledge in the organization and delivery of services to older adults

6. A sensitivity to moral, ethical, and legal issues in aging

Experience to date suggests that many students in M.P.H. programs will take only a single class, at most, in health and aging. These six objectives are important for public health practitioners regardless of their specific employment responsibilities. To meet those ends, the workshop recommended that a one-semester course on public health and aging cover the following topics:

1. Theories of aging and normal aging (including basic biology of aging)

2. Epidemiology

3. Aging and a healthy environment

4. Health promotion in aging populations

5. The older adult and the acute care system

6. Chronic illness

7. Organization, financing, and delivery of long-term care

8. Mental health and mental illness

9. Informal support and family systems

10. Death and dying

11. Organizational cultures and health care

12. Diversity issues (race, ethnicity, gender)

13. Politics of aging

14. Issues in research, program design, and education of elderly persons

15. Ethics of health and aging

Conclusion

Schools of public health advance the health of the public by conducting research and by training public health practitioners with skills and knowledge necessary for conducting assessment, policy development, and assurance activities (Institute of Medicine, 1988). These objectives should be followed for public health and aging students. A number of schools of public health have programs to educate students to work in agencies that deliver services to older adults. This is particularly true of Master of Public Health (M.P.H.) and Doctor of Public Health (Dr.P.H.) degrees, which are primarily directed toward students interested in service and administrative positions.

A fundamental shortcoming of academic education and training of gerontology public health professionals is that it often fails to adequately communicate with the community agencies providing health and social services for older adults. A reciprocal exchange of information and expertise would benefit students, professionals in community agencies serving older populations, and ultimately, older community residents.

If public health expects to be effective in responding to the needs of older adults in the community, graduate public health programs need to work more with programs and community groups that historically have not been the focus of academic public health. In particular, public health and aging need to reach out to organizations that are outside of the traditional public health system of health departments, including government-funded agencies such as Area Agencies on Aging and Medicaid-funded long-term care programs, and the large number of voluntary, community-based, and religious organizations that have historically been important sources of aid to older persons and their families. "To achieve public health objectives, public health will need to serve as leaders and catalysts of private efforts as well as performing those health functions that only government can perform" (Institute of Medicine, 1988, p. 31).

The increase in research and information on aging and public health has resulted in the development of curriculum resource materials tailored to specific health care disciplines within public health (e.g., U.S. Bureau of Health Professions, 1990; Haber, 1994). However, we do not recommend that every school of public health or program in public health should have a degree or a track, concentration, or specialization in aging in public health. Given the demographic and historical influences discussed earlier, all programs should offer at least one elective and include material on elderly people as examples of how to implement programs and policies relating to each of the core areas in required core courses. We may not be able to guarantee that everyone working in public health and aging has specialized in the field, but we should make sure that all public health professionals are at least sensitive to the issues of this growing population.

References

Estes, C. 1979. *The Aging Enterprise.* San Francisco: Jossey-Bass.

Estes, C., Swan, J., et al., 1993. *The Long-Term Care Crisis: Elders Trapped in the No-Care Zone.* Newbury Park, CA: Sage.

Fein, R. 1989. *Medical Care, Medical Costs.* Cambridge, MA: Harvard University Press.

Fox, P. 1989. From senility to Alzheimer's disease: The rise of the Alzheimer's disease movement. *Milbank Quarterly* 67(1):58–102.

Haber, D. 1994. *Health Promotion and Aging.* New York: Springer.

Harris, T., and Kovar, M. 1992. Data sets for research in aging: The National Center for Health Statistics. In Wallace, R., and Woolson, R., eds., *The Epidemiologic Study of the Elderly* (pp. 248–61). New York: Oxford University Press.

Infeld, L., and Kress, J. 1989. *Crisis or Quality: Management for Long-Term Care.* McLean, VA: Association of University Programs in Health Administration.

Institute of Medicine. 1988. *The Future of Public Health.* Washington, DC: National Academy Press.

Kahl, A. 1992. Career preparation in public health and aging. In Wallace, S. P., and Prohaska, T., eds., *Proceedings from the Aging and Public Health Curriculum Development Workshop.* Los Angeles: California Geriatric Education Center and UCLA School of Public Health.

Larson, M. 1977. *The Rise of Professionalism.* Berkeley: University of California Press.

Lockett, B. 1983. *Aging, Politics, and Research: Setting the Federal Agendas for Research on Aging.* New York: Springer.

Magee, J. 1985. *Gerontology Programs and Curricula in U.S. Schools of Public Health. Bureau of Health Professions.* DHHS Publication No. 84-213. Washington, DC: Association of Schools of Public Health.

McKinlay, J., McKinlay, S., and Benglehold, R. 1989. Trends in death and disease and the contribution of medical measures. In Freeman, H., and Levine, S., eds., *Handbook of Medical Sociology,* (4th ed., pp. 14–45). Englewood Cliffs, NJ: Prentice Hall.

National Center for Health Statistics. 1993. Van Nostrand, J., Furner, S., and Suzman, R. eds. Health Data on Older Americans: United States 1992. *Vital and Health Statistics* 3(27).

Peterson, D., Wendt, P., and Douglass, E. 1991. *Determining the Impact of Gerontology Preparation on Personnel in the Aging Network: A National Survey.* Washington, DC: Association for Gerontology in Higher Education.

Prohaska, T. 1993. The current status of training in aging and public health. In Wallace, S. P., and Prohaska, T., eds., *Proceedings from the Aging and Public Health Curriculum Development Workshop.* Los Angeles: California Geriatric Education Center, UCLA.

Quadagno, J. 1988. *The Transformation of Old Age Security.* Berkeley: University of California Press.

Snyder, L. 1994. Public health service act, 1944. *Public Health Reports* 109(4):468–71.

Starr, P. 1982. *The Social Transformation of American Medicine.* New York: Basic Books.

U.S. Bureau of Health Professions. 1990. *Geriatric Training Curriculum for Public Health Professionals.* Washington, DC: Department of Health and Human Services, Health Resources and Services Administration.

U.S. Senate, Special Committee on Aging. 1989. *Aging America, Trends and Projections.* Washington, DC: U.S. DHHS.

U.S. Senate, Special Committee on Aging. 1994. *Developments in Aging: 1993.* Washington, DC: U.S. Government Printing Office.

Wallace, S. 1994. The contribution of public health to gerontology: An evaluation of public health curricula on aging. *Gerontology and Geriatrics Education* 14(4):21–37.

Wallace, S., and Lubben, J. 1995. *Preliminary findings from the 1994 Social Work—Public Health Gerontology Curriculum Survey.* Los Angeles: California Geriatric Education Center.

Wallace, S., and Prohaska, T. 1993. *Proceedings from the Aging and Public Health Curriculum Development Workshop.* Los Angeles: California Geriatric Education Center, UCLA.

Wallace, S., and Williamson, J. 1992. The senior movement in historical perspective. In Wallace, S. P., and Williamson, J. B., eds., *The Senior Movement.* New York: G.K. Hall.

Wallace, S., Williamson, J., Lung, R., and Powell, L. 1991. A lamb in wolf's clothing? The reality of senior power and social policy. In Minkler, M., and Estes, C. L., eds., *Critical Perspectives on Aging* (pp. 95–114). Amityville, NY: Baywood.

Chapter

16

■ Implications of an Aging Society
for the Organization
and Evaluation
of Public Health Services

Elizabeth A. Kutza, Ph.D.

While the demographic changes reflective of our aging society are routinely cited and readily observable, their impact on our social and service systems is largely unknown. Most observers do expect, however, that increased survivability among the old-old will certainly affect the need for and use of health care services. This expectation is based on the relationship between age and the use of health care.

As we live longer, we require more health care services. People over 65 now constitute 12.4 percent of our population, yet they account for nearly one-third of national expenditures for health care (Havlik, Liu, and Kovar, 1987). Increases in life expectancy at age 85 would indicate that the oldest-old are living longer (Cohen, Van Nostrand, and Fumer, 1993). In addition, problems with activities of daily living (ADLs) increase with advanced age. While 15 percent of males and 16 percent of females in the 65 to 69 age group have difficulty performing at least one ADL, by age 85 and over the figures are 35 percent and 48 percent, respectively (Cohen, Van Nostrand, and Fumer, 1993). Between the years 1980 and 2040, although the total population will increase by two-fifths, the number of noninstitutionalized elderly needing assistance with one or more ADLs is estimated to double (Rogers, Rogers, and Belanger, 1990). Thus, the sheer weight of tomorrow's older population is likely to place critical demands on existing health care delivery systems, both acute and long-term care. How these changes will impact on one part of our service system, our public health system, is harder to predict, however, without analyzing how vulnerable the public health system is to influences in its environment.

Every organization sits within and is affected by an environmental context. Hall (1987) identified seven dimensions that may change over time. These include technological conditions, legal conditions, demographic conditions, political, economic and cultural conditions, as well as ecological conditions. The more dependent the organization is on one or another of these environmental dimensions, the more vulnerable it is to its changing conditions. This chapter will examine how vulnerable our public health system is to changing demographics and will explore what other environmental conditions may lead to or impede the development of a public health agenda for an aging society.

An Aging Society and Public Health Goals

The first relevant question to ask as we explore these issues is: "What are the appropriate goals of a public health system in an aging society?" An Institute of Medicine study on "The Future of Public Health" defines the mission of public health to be "the fulfillment of society's interest in assuring the conditions in which people can be healthy" (Institute of Medicine, 1988). Thus, a public health system is built upon a systematic identification of health problems and development of means to solve these problems.

Broadly speaking, public health systems have two major goals. The first, the systematic identification of health problems within society, is accomplished through surveillance, the collection and interpretation of data, and case-finding activities. In addition to assessing the health status of the population through epidemiological means, a second goal is to maintain or improve the health status of the population through the implementation of programs directed at disease prevention and health promotion.

Over time, success in public health's disease-prevention strategies has resulted in a shift in mortality from acute disease to a rise in chronic illnesses and a resultant increase in morbidity. The most striking effect of morbidity in old, as compared with younger, adults, is the resulting chronic disability. Population aging thus challenges public health goals in some fundamental ways. The shifts that are required for a public health system to be responsive to an aging society are summarized in Table 16.1.

For a public health agenda in an aging society to emerge, public health systems must engage in a paradigm shift. To date, the dominant paradigm used for understanding the majority of health problems in the United States is that held in the

TABLE 16.1. Population Aging Shifts Public Health Goals

From	To
Acute disease focus	Chronic disease focus
How to prevent disease	How to prevent/delay chronic illness
Keeping people disease free	Increasing active life expectancy
Understanding patterns of illness	Understanding patterns of behavior that determine active life expectancy

acute-care community—that is, the disease model. Yet this approach is increasingly seen as inadequate in meeting the needs of people with disabilities and those at risk of disability (Caplan, 1988; Mold, 1995; Zola, 1988).

Berg and Cassells (1990) noted that for a number of reasons an acute-care framework provides a poor view of disability. First, it is restricted to somatic conditions. But disability includes phenomena that go well beyond this sphere. Second, it is associated with a curative bias that assumes that health and the absence of disease are essentially synonymous. And finally, acute disease classification systems are static and abstract while "the social manifestations of disability must be understood relative to the particular abilities an individual hopes to maintain or achieve" (p. 24). To be useful for older people, Mold (1995) noted, "a paradigm for health must incorporate a definition of health that is both optimistic and achievable and values individual variation" (p. 88). He argues that rather than a "problem-oriented model," what is needed in an aging society is a "goal-oriented model." In this paradigm, the primary purpose of health care is to help each individual set and achieve personal health-related goals—that is, ones that will enhance active life expectancy.

This concept of "active life expectancy" also is one that requires a paradigm shift in the epidemiology of public health. Active life expectancy—the expected time in years of functional well-being—measures not only how long a subpopulation can expect to live at each age, but also what fractions of this expected remaining lifetime will be spent in independent and dependent status. Rogers and colleagues (1990), using multistate analysis, have found that many individuals are living long and active lives, and that many individuals who become dependent are dependent only temporarily and then return to an independent status. For example, an independent 72-year-old in 1984 could have expected to live another 12.2 years, 8.9 (73 percent) of them in continued independent status. The comparable figures for an independent 92-year-old would be 4.9 years and 2.6 years (53 percent), respectively.

To summarize, then, public health goals in an aging society will require a shift from a narrow disease-control paradigm to how to prevent or delay chronic illness and from a traditional disease-oriented model (i.e., keeping people disease free) to a health promotion model (i.e., how to increase the span of a healthy life by maximizing functioning). In addition, the patterns of disease that characterize public health will be less relevant than understanding the pattern of behaviors that determine active life expectancy. Predictors of high levels of physical functioning and the risk factors that compromise that functioning need to be better identified. The age-specific incidence of physical conditions and social events that impact on late-life health status will require better understanding, and health behaviors that promote normal or successful aging will have to be encouraged.

The Organization of Public Health Services in the United States

The public health system, if it alters its goals in response to an aging society, will change another part of its environment, its inter-organizational relationships. All organizations have relationships with other organizations. Some are relatively trivial while others are of central importance to the parties involved (Hall, 1987). The two primary organizations that serve the aged's health and health-related needs and that may have overlapping goals with a new public health focus are the Health Care Financing Administration (HCFA) and the Administration on Aging (AoA). A brief overview of the current organization for health and health-related services will make clear what changes will be needed to meet a public health agenda for an aging society. A more extensive description of both the public health service system and the aging network of services can be found in this book in Chapter 2, by Balsam and Bottum. The first distinction that can be made in the health services arena is between publicly provided health services and privately financed health services.

Publicly Provided Health Services

The public health system is organized through federal, state, and local structures. Public health responsibility at the federal level is lodged within the Public Health Service of the U.S. Department of Health and Human Services. It sets goals for national health, funds research, and develops policy and program directions. Through its activity, the federal government provides consumer health protection, broadly defined. It contracts with the states and local areas for actual health service provision.

States are central authorities in the nation's public health system. States involve themselves in assessment, policy development, and assurance of access to health services.

Finally, the local health agencies are the critical components of the public health system. They directly deliver public health services to citizens. They conduct communicable disease programs, provide screening and immunizations, provide health education services, run school health programs, conduct sanitation inspections, and deliver maternal and child health services, home care, and other ambulatory care services (Institute of Medicine, 1988).

Two other publicly provided health care systems serving special populations also should be involved in the setting of a public health agenda for an aging society—the Veterans Affairs system and the Indian Health Service system. The Department of Veterans Affairs (VA) extends eligible veterans free or highly subsidized health care services, including hospitalization, ambulatory, and nursing home care. The VA provides most of its care in its 172 hospital centers, where it also operates outpatient clinics, and 101 nursing home units. Most long-term care services, however, are either provided under contract in community nursing homes or subsidized in state veterans homes (U.S. Congress, Congressional Budget Office, 1994).

The aging of America's population is accelerated in the veterans population because of its unique composition. By 1990, one out of four veterans were 65 years of age or older; by 2000, the figure will be one out of three; and by 2020, the figure will reach nearly one out of two. The number of elderly "at risk" for frailty, those 75 years of age and older, in the veterans population will increase more than fourfold between 1980 and 2000. By the year 2020, veterans over the age of 75 will account for 47.8 percent of all aged veterans and 21 percent of the total veterans population (U.S. Veterans Administration, 1984).

A major difference between the general population and the VA population is in composition by sex. In the general population, services for the aged will deal with a predominantly female base of patients, while in the veterans population, males will dominate. In addition, proportionally more nonwhites turn to the VA as their source of care than whites. Although nonwhites constitute only about 9 percent of the veteran population, some figures estimate that 31 percent of all veterans who rely on the VA as their sole source of care are nonwhite (U.S. Veterans Administration, 1984).

Another publicly provided health care system is found in the Indian Health Service (IHS). The issue of long-term health care in reservation settings is in its early development. Furthering the discussion has been the IHS Workgroup on Aging, an interagency task force that was organized in 1991 to assess and recommend means by which the IHS could begin to address the needs of American Indian aged. Reporting in 1992, the Workgroup found the Indian aged population rapidly increasing and at significant health risk. The 1990 Census reported more than 165,000 Indians over the age of 60 years, a 52 percent increase from 1980. A survey of 369 aged living within the IHS service delivery areas and representing eight tribes was conducted in 1991 and 1992 under the Tribal Elders Entitlement Project, a project funded by the Administration on Aging. About one-quarter of these aged were found to be in poor health, and one-quarter had a moderate to high level of mobility limitation. Nearly one-half (45 percent) had high blood pressure and one-third (34 percent) had diabetes. Overall, 13 percent of respondents reported one or more personal care needs due to health problems. Most of these aged (78 percent) used IHS for their primary health care (Funk, 1993).

While Indian aged comprise only about 6 percent of the Indian Health Service user population, they represent 20 percent of hospital stays, 10 percent of outpatient visits, and 38 percent of Community Health Representative services (National Council on Indian Aging, 1993). It is clear from these data that Indian aged are another subgroup among the aged whose health care needs require consideration in any public health agenda for an aging society. While small in number, Indian aged, especially those on reservations, demonstrate a high incidence of chronic illness and will be at increasing risk for health and long-term care services in the future.

Publicly Financed Health Services

Most aged persons receive their health services not under a publicly provided system of care, but rather through a publicly financed system of care. The two primary publicly financed but privately provided systems of health care are Medicare and Medicaid, both of which are administered by the federal Health Care Financing Administration (HCFA).

Medicare is a federally funded health insurance plan for persons 65 years of age and older. It mirrors private insurance plans and has two parts—Part A pays for hospital care costs, and Part B pays for supplemental medical costs incurred outside the hospital setting. In 1993, Medicare covered 32.1 million older persons and paid for $147.5 billion of their medical expenses (U.S. Social Security Administration, 1994).

Given its size, Medicare is the primary driver in the health care delivery of aged persons. Reimbursement policies under Medicare are developed with no health goals in mind for the population as a whole. This is in sharp contrast to the behavior of public health systems. Rather, what care is paid for is that which is ordered by a physician for each individual Medicare enrollee. Services to the aged are provided by individual practitioners working primarily in a fee-for-service system. The focus in this system is on tertiary, not primary care (i.e., disease prevention) and it does not routinely address health promotion activities.

Title XIX of the Social Security Act, Grants to States for Medical Assistance, more commonly known as Medicaid, is a federal-state program that pays for medical services for persons of low income or those who are "medically needy." Since Medicare covers most aged persons for their acute care needs, Medicaid's role in the health care delivery system of the aged is primarily in long-term care. Medicaid is the health financing mechanism that drives long-term health care for the frail aged. It serves only those who meet its income eligibility criteria, and services under this financing plan are primarily delivered in institutional, not community or home-based, settings. Seventy-five percent of Medicaid expenditures for long-term care in 1993 supported nursing home care for the aged, 25% supported community-based care. Like Medicare, this health-financing mechanism has no explicit health or rehabilitative goal embedded in its reimbursement policies.

Publicly Funded Aging Services

Social services to the aged, an important adjunct to a public health system for the aged, are provided through an alternate local delivery system, the Area Agencies on Aging (AAAs). These are funded through a distinct federal agency, the Administration on Aging, under authority found in the Older Americans Act.

Much like public health services, Older Americans Act services are organized into a federal, state, and local service delivery structure. Also like the public health system, it is the local organizational entity that delivers services, or contracts for the delivery of them. These local organizations are legislatively identified as Area Agencies on Aging, or AAAs, although locally they may have other names.

AAAs are local planning and coordinating bodies with responsibility for information and referral (I & R) services, linkage activities (e.g., transportation), congregate and home-delivered meal programs, and some "gap filling" services that may be health related. In only a few states, where the AAA has responsibility for community long-term care services, does the AAA address the health care needs of the aged in any extensive way. Even in those cases, however, the organizational culture of the AAA is based more upon a social work model of service delivery than a medical model.

Goals versus Current Organizational Structure

The organizations described above, all directed at providing health or health-related social services to older persons, are not organizationally connected in any significant way. Their authority rests in discrete legislative mandates. They do not *directly* compete against each other for budgetary allocations. And, their successful functioning requires no interdependence, although occasionally they may cooperate on some local endeavor. An analysis of this current organizational map points to several issues that hinder our reaching the public health goals of an aging society described above. Four issues stand out: budgetary allocations, a retreat from neighborhood-based services, lack of program integration, and the sovereignty of individual providers and provider organizations.

Current financing mechanisms for health services are not directed toward specific health goals. In fact, expenditure data reveal a dominance of investment in institutionally based tertiary care at the expense of community-based primary care.

Budgetary allocations for services under community-based models (i.e., public health services, AAAs) are shrinking; budgetary allocations under individual, health care financing models (i.e., Medicare, Medicaid) are growing. When adjusted for medical care inflation over time, for example, outlays for maternal and child health services under public health authority declined by 20 percent between 1975 and 1990, while outlays for Medicaid during the same period increased by 235 percent.

At the federal level, there is some movement to reverse this trend, but it is nascent and minimal. Examples include encouragement of HMO participation, health care reforms that are structured around a managed care concept with a primary care physician as gatekeeper and case manager, and physician payment reforms in Medicare that are altering the reward structure from specialty to primary care and patient education. But until and unless budgetary allocations support broad public health goals, the meeting of these goals will be hampered.

A second issue, America's retreat from neighborhood-based community services, also will hinder reaching our public health goals in an aging society. At an earlier time in American history, health care and social service providers were neighborhood based. Home visits were commonplace and continuity of care the norm. Today, however, the office or the hospital has become the primary site of health care delivery for Americans. This pattern of health care delivery presents disadvantages for older persons in several ways.

First, large numbers of the aged live alone and often don't stray far from their communities. The percentage of older people living alone increases with age. Of older people aged 65 to 74, one out of four lives alone. Among those 85 and older, almost half do (Kasper, 1988). Three percent of those 65 to 74 have chronic conditions that restrict them to traveling within their own neighborhoods. Over 24 percent of those 85 and older are limited in this way (National Research Council, 1988). Such isolation suggests that outreach services into the home are vitally important in order to do case findings of health problems.

Second, the aged are a population who can benefit greatly from health monitoring and early intervention, two tasks better accomplished through home visiting and community nursing. Yet only 4 percent of older people living alone in 1984 received home health services, a smaller than expected number given that the majority of both black and white older people who are poor and who are not in good health live alone (Kasper, 1988). Early identification of treatable chronic diseases and home safety reviews to reduce the incidence of falls are two examples of how a modest community investment can reap large health care cost savings in the future. A major advantage to such an environmental or community-based approach is that the effectiveness of the intervention is not limited to the currently "at risk" portion of the population at the time of intervention but will, ideally, extend forward as new persons enter the "at risk" group (Ory and Bond, 1989).

Finally, mobility problems can isolate the aged and restrict their access to health care in clinic and hospital settings. With limited access to transportation, seeking care outside the home becomes difficult. Today, for example, it is the suburbs and small towns that are experiencing the fastest growth of their older adult populations. Between 1960 and 1980, the number of persons 65 and older living in central cities increased by 42 percent, while gaining by 90 percent in the suburbs. In 1980, for the first time, a greater number of the aged lived in the suburban ring (10.1 million) than in the central cities (8.1 million) (Fitzpatrick and Logan, 1985). And it is in these areas that public transportation is lacking and the aged's access to a doctor's office is compromised. While transportation planners now realize that the majority of trips by older persons are not into or out of the city, but rather between two suburban locations, the population density in the suburbs is generally too low for transit systems to serve these areas (National Research Council, 1988).

A lack of program integration is the third issue of importance. Meeting the public health goals of an aging society requires the integration of health and social services, an integration that does not currently exist. At the present time, health and health-related programs for the aged in the United States provide a patchwork of inefficient, unevenly distributed and poorly coordinated services (Phillips, 1985). As noted above, few of the organizations providing health and health-related social services to the aged are integrally linked. Each of these organizations claims its own domain or market, and there is consensus among them as to the right that each has to operate in a particular way and in a particular area. Organizational theorists call this "domain consensus," while it is more commonly known as organizational "turf" (Hall, 1987). With no environmental imperative to integrate or coordinate, these organizations are likely to continue on their individual paths.

Finally, effective goal attainment regarding public health for the aged requires a perspective that "emphasizes the role of community as problem solver rather than the sovereignty of individual providers and provider organizations" (Kaluzny and Fried, 1985, p. 283). Yet, within our health financing programs, the programs that dominate the provision of health care for the aged, it is individual practitioners that dictate the health goals of the older person within a narrow disease prevention paradigm. The larger public health goals of the population as it ages are not the focus of attention.

These, then, are the four issues that challenge the attainment of a public health goal in an aging society. One might regard these as environmental issues; that is, issues in the larger society that affect whether broad public health goals can be reached by our existing organizational net. Of equal importance are intraorganizational barriers that prohibit or at least restrict change within organizations. In order to pursue new goals, organizations must change. They will be asked to redirect their mission and alter their internal organizational objectives. They also will be asked to reallocate their scarce resources away from established programs—many of them legislatively mandated—and do something new. Significant barriers challenge any organization that attempts such changes.

Organizational Change

For illustrative purposes, we will focus specifically on what barriers would be faced by the public health system if it wanted to alter the organizational mission so as to be responsive to the needs of an aging society. Five barriers stand out.

Organizational Culture

While the community-based organizational structure of public health services is appropriate to meet the needs of an aging society, its organizational culture is not. Organizational culture is rooted in historical patterns of organizational belief structures and behaviors and is difficult to change. The organizational culture of the public health system is rooted both in the belief that scientific knowledge can provide a means of controlling disease as well as in the value of public responsibility for disease control. These "taken-for-granted" beliefs are rarely if ever questioned, and yet they would need to be if the goals of the organization were to shift in the ways displayed in Table 16.1.

For the culture of an organization to change, something must occur that puts into question these basic assumptions and beliefs. Dyer and Dyer (1989) identify six stages of culture change. First, a crisis calls into question these organizational assumptions, followed by a breakdown of symbols, beliefs, and structures. Next, new leadership emerges with a new set of assumptions. Fourth, conflict occurs between the old and new culture, and a modified culture emerges. Finally, new symbols, beliefs, and structures develop to sustain the new culture. In the case of public health systems, it is not obvious what kind of crisis would provoke such a culture shift. The demographic changes now occurring in society would seem insufficient to provoke such a crisis of organizational culture.

Professional Orientation

Related to organizational culture is the orientation of the professional staff within an organization and its impact on change. Public health systems are staffed by health care professionals who focus on population and social/environmental aspects of health and less on individuals in a clinical context. And as one critic has noted, "the division between public health and medicine has implicitly absolved medicine of responsibility for clinical prevention" (Coye, 1994). Public health professionals also are not attentive to social or rehabilitative models of care, although these two models are more appropriate when dealing with an aging and frail population who suffers from chronic illnesses. Compromises in a person's ADLs do not lend themselves to a quick medical "fix" but can be responsive to rehabilitative, restorative, and environmental interventions, interventions more consistent with a social model of care.

Thus, the continued recruitment into the public health system of individuals whose professional orientation is toward a disease-care paradigm rather than a disability paradigm presents a significant barrier to organizational change. And, differing professional orientations in each of the health and social service systems stand in the way of joint goal-seeking behavior. Team approaches to meeting public health goals of an aging society are needed but are not in place.

Separate Funding Streams

Separate funding streams through local health agencies, area agencies on aging, and most especially through Medicare and Medicaid make concerted action around health goals for an aging society difficult. Each stream of money is authorized through individual pieces of legislation and carries with it restrictions for how the money can be used.

Related to the issue of multiple funding sources is the issue of categorical eligibility. Categorical eligibility within public programs presents a barrier to meeting broad national goals. A focus on those over 65, for example, leaves the group 50 to 65 years of age vulnerable. A focus on a disease category, for example, AIDS or Alzheimer's, distracts from health promotion activities for the larger population. As long as multiple funding sources and categorical eligibility remain, organizations will have little incentive to change what they are doing.

Organizational Jurisdiction

Rigid jurisdictional lines of authority stand in the way of coordinated planning for and service delivery to the older population. The public health system has its jurisdiction defined by federal legislation that mandates it to do surveillance of communicable diseases and to provide maternal and child health services, for example. The Area Agencies on Aging are mandated to provide meal programs for seniors and to provide "linkage services" like transportation. Incentives to bridge these jurisdictional boundaries through joint planning and service coordination do not exist. In fact, it is probably rare for these two systems to interact at all. When AAAs plan health screening or health promotion activities, they are more likely to reach out to a local hospital than they are to reach out to the local health department. Their narrow jurisdictional focus often leads these organizations to see each other as irrelevant to their own missions.

America's Political Culture

Unlike in other developed Western countries, the notion in the United States of "public" as regards health services does not include an acceptance of universal and comprehensive, society-wide interventions. Thus, developing a national "public" health strategy will be difficult, and finding political support for funding such a strategy is uncertain. For example, the Public Health Service produced a report entitled *Healthy People 2000: National Health Promotion and Disease Prevention Objectives* (1991). This report sets out health goals for the nation, goals that are consistent with the needs of an aging society. Yet the biggest health funders, Medicare and Medicaid, do not operate in ways that will make these goals realizable. And more importantly, the Public Health Service has no way to prevail upon these health funding systems to alter their behavior so as to meet the goals set forth in the *Healthy People 2000* report. Thus, while the ideal model of assuring that all persons receive health services that will foster "active life expectancy" is a neighborhood, community-based one, the size, complexity, and individual orientation of American society (as exhibited in its major health financing program) inhibits implementation of this model.

Implications for Research and Practice

It has been argued here that there are significant environmental and organizational barriers to implementing public health goals that are appropriate to an aging society. But progress can be made to bring down these barriers if the public health system assumes leadership and makes a commitment to try to influence its policy environment, its organizational environment, and its professional environment.

The policy environment can be influenced in several ways. Indirectly, it can be influenced through public education. As Americans are made more aware of how their individual actions can lead to a healthier old age, two outcomes may occur. One, individuals may actually alter their behavior, and two, they may start to influence the behavior of their individual physicians in a new direction. They may demand that their physicians order interventions that can improve the quality of their lives, even in the face of chronic illness.

Take a common problem in late life like incontinence. An educated population may well no longer tolerate a physician who adopts an ageist attitude (e.g., "Just use Attends,™ there is not much that can be done") or who perhaps just prescribes a medication. Instead, the educated consumer may demand the full range of options to deal with incontinence, from exercise, to behavior modification, to surgery if appropriate. Thus, patient education can alter the behavior of individual practitioners and, over the long term, modify Medicare and Medicaid reimbursement policies.

More directly, the public health service can use its "bully pulpit" to highlight the need to change government policy in ways that support a public health agenda in an aging society. The *Healthy People 2000* report is a start. By setting national goals, this report encourages a conscious and systematic assessment of needs and provides a way to monitor progress. These goals need to be kept in the national focus and used as a benchmark when policies are developed or modified, whether these policies relate to health financing issues, health service issues, or environmental issues.

The organizational environment can change only when the issues of organizational domain are addressed. Organizational domain is characterized by one or more of the following attributes—exclusiveness, autonomy, and dominance (Benson, 1973). Issues of domain have been particularly troublesome in service delivery to the aged. Because these services span health and social service agencies, organizational coordination is important. Yet coordination is possible only if there is "high mutual awareness." As Kaluzny and Fried (1985) noted: "It is impossible to effectively coordinate a group of agencies that are individually unaware of services provided by other organizations in the group" (p. 285). These authors go on to observe that it is generally easier to achieve coordination if the organizations share a common philosophical and service orientation and have similar structural characteristics. As the earlier analysis of the public health agencies and area agencies on aging show, while their structural characteristics may be similar, their organizational cultures are not. Therefore, leadership on the part of the public health service in setting a public health agenda for an aging society would involve greater awareness of the services provided by AAAs, as well as a recognition that different organizational cultures will make coordination more challenging but not necessarily impossible.

Of course, injunctions to coordinate are only marginally effective. It would be more effective if the federal legislation that provides authorization to these two agencies would actually require collaboration. For example, under the Older Americans Act, area agencies on aging are required to develop health promotion activities for seniors. If the legislation required that such activities must be done in concert with local public health agencies, stronger incentives would be in place to assure coordination.

In addition, the professional environment needs to be changed. More attention needs to be paid to aging and health issues in public health curricula. Chapter 15 in this volume, by Prohaska and Wallace, provides a detailed road map for how these educational changes can take place.

How will we know if we have met our goals? Evaluation of success in meeting public health goals in an aging society is challenging. Moving from a disease to a disability focus, public health professionals will need to develop clear goal specifications and definitions of "active life expectancy." They will need to encourage more research on the age-specific incidence of disabling conditions, not just diseases, and they will need to develop more objective measures of individual functioning. Current self-report data do not allow reliable population-based estimates of incidence.

But, ultimately, we will know we are successful if there is a new commitment to overcoming the organizational barriers now found among the health financing, health delivery, and social service delivery systems now serving the aged. When public health agencies reorient themselves to a community-based intervention model and join hands with the aging services network, a health agenda for an aging society will naturally emerge.

References

Benson, J. K. 1973. The inter organizational network as a political economy. *Administrative Science Quarterly* 20:229–49.

Berg, R. L., and Cassells, J. S. 1990. *The Second Fifty Years: Promoting Health and Preventing Disability.* Washington, DC: National Academy Press.

Caplan, A. L. 1988. Is medical care the right prescription for chronic illness? In Sullivan, S., and Lewin, M. E., eds., *The Economics and Ethics of Long Term Care and Disability* (pp. 73–89). Lanham, MD: University Press of America.

Cohen, R. A., Van Nostrand, J. F., and Fumer, S. E. 1993. *Chartbook on Health Data on Older Americans, United States, 1992.* National Center for Health Statistics. Vital Health Statistics 3 (29).

Coye, M. J. 1994. Our own worst enemy: Obstacles to improving the health of the public. In Coye, M. J., Foege, W. H., and Roper, W. L., eds., *Leadership in Public Health* (pp. 1–11). New York: Milbank Memorial Fund.

Dyer, W. G., and Dyer, W. G., Jr. 1989. Organizational development: System change or culture change? In French, W. L., Bell, C. H., and Zawocki, R. A., eds., *Organizational Development: Theory, Practice, and Research* (pp. 643–49). Homewood, IL: Richard D. Irwin, Inc.

Fitzpatrick, K. M., and Logan, J. R. 1985. The aging of the suburbs, 1960–1980. *American Sociological Review* 50:106–17.

Funk, P. E. 1993. Long term care needs of tribal elders (Preliminary report). Washington State Indian Council on Aging, Tribal Elders Entitlement Survey.

Hall, R. H. 1987. *Organizations: Structures, Processes, and Outcomes* (4th ed.). Englewood Cliffs, NJ: Prentice-Hall.

Havlik, R. J., Liu, M. G., and Kovar, M. G. 1987. *Health Statistics on Older Persons, United States 1986.* (Vital and Health Statistics, 3 [25]). Washington, DC: Government Printing Office.

Institute of Medicine. 1988. The Future of Public Health. Washington, DC: National Academy Press.

Kaluzny, A. D., and Fried, B. J. 1985. Interorganizational coordination of services to the elderly. In Phillips, H. T., and Gaylord, S. A., eds., *Aging and Public Health* (pp. 267–92). New York: Springer.

Kasper, J. 1988. *Aging Alone: Profiles and Projections.* (A report of the Commonwealth Fund Commission on Elderly People Living Alone). New York: The Commonwealth Fund.

Mold, J. W. 1995. An alternative conceptualization of health and health care: Its implications for geriatrics and gerontology. *Educational Gerontology* 21:85–101.

National Council on Indian Aging. 1993. *National Indian Aging Agenda Issues for the Indian Health Service.* (Available from the National Indian Council on Aging, Albuquerque, NM.)

National Research Council. 1988. *Transportation in an Aging Society: Improving Mobility and Safety for Older Persons.* (Special report 218). Washington, DC: Transportation Research Board.

Ory, M. G., and Bond, K., eds. 1989. *Aging and Health Care: Social Science and Policy Perspectives.* London: Routledge.

Phillips, H. T. 1985. Organizing community health services for the elderly. In Phillips, H. T., and Gaylord, S. A., eds., *Aging and Public Health* (pp. 251–66). New York: Springer.

Rogers, R. G., Rogers, A., and Belanger, A. 1990. Active life among the elderly in the U.S.: Multistate life-table estimates and population projections. *Milbank Quarterly* 67 (3-4):370–411.

U.S. Congress, Congressional Budget Office. 1994. Veterans Administration Health Care: Planning for Future Needs. Washington, DC: U.S. Congress.

U.S. Department of Health and Human Services, Public Health Service. 1991. *Healthy People 2000: National Health Promotion and Disease Prevention Objectives.* Washington, DC: Government Printing Office.

U.S. Department of Health and Human Services, Social Security Administration. 1994. *Annual Statistical Supplement to the Social Security Bulletin, 1994.* Washington, DC: Government Printing Office.

U.S. Veterans Administration. 1984. *Caring for the Older Veteran.* Washington, DC: Government Printing Office.

Zola, I. K. 1988. Policies and programs concerning aging and disabilities: Towards a unifying agenda. In Sullivan, S., and Lewin, M. E., eds., *The Economics and Ethics of Long Term Care and Disability* (pp. 90–98). Lanham, MD: University Press of America.

Part

V

Conclusion

Chapter

17

Toward a Synthesis of a Public Health Agenda for an Aging Society

Ronald Andersen, Ph.D., and Nadereh Pourat, Ph.D.

What might be helpful in planning a public health agenda for an aging society? Let us start with the underlying assumptions that provided impetus for this collaborative effort. These assumptions produce a rationale for merging perspectives and activities of public health and aging as well as increasing the interaction of researchers and academics with policy makers and practitioners.

The first assumption is that these merges and interactions are in the best interests of older people as well as society as a whole and should have taken place long ago. Second, there is a demographic imperative based on increasing numbers and proportions of older people in the population that requires new ways of thinking about and meeting the needs of the older population. Finally, the very needs of older people and their demands on our society are changing as well as their actual and potential contributions to that society. At the same time, society's perspectives of what it is able or willing to provide to older people may be changing as well. New ways of understanding and facilitating this exchange between older people and the rest of society are required.

This book is part of a process, itself a call to what the philosopher of science Thomas Kuhn (1970) referred to as a "scientific revolution." A scientific revolution comes about when new paradigms are created (Figure 17.1). In seeking a synthesis of a public health agenda for an aging society this book is exploring how the para-

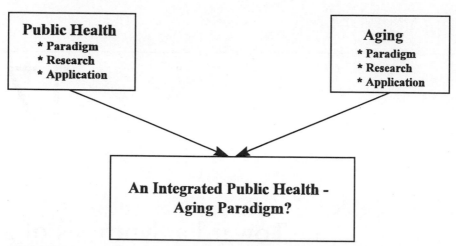

FIGURE 17.1 Toward a synthesis of a public health agenda for an aging society.

digms of public health and aging along with their related research and knowledge base and applications in practice might merge to create what we have referred to as an integrated public health–aging paradigm.

Kuhn noted that a paradigm has two essential characteristics. One is that scientific achievements and core principles are accepted and shared by a scientific community and its practitioners. A paradigm includes laws, theories, applications, and instrumentation. A second characteristic is that a paradigm is sufficiently open ended to leave all sorts of problems for its adherents or practitioners to resolve. It helps to define the problems and suggest the methods that its practitioners will use to solve those problems.

New paradigms emerge, according to Kuhn, through a process when anomalies are observed—occurrences that cannot be explained by the old paradigm. Problems present themselves for which the old paradigm seemingly suggests no methods or means to resolve. A crisis develops as anomalies increase and new research discoveries are at odds with the dominant ways of thinking. The result may be a new paradigm with new adherents. Its success and growth depends on its ability to better explain anomalies and offer solutions to previously insolvable problems in a field of inquiry.

Kuhn's original work was based on observations in the physical sciences. Although his ideas have also proved helpful in understanding new developments in the biological and social sciences, some might question whether or not there are really current paradigms in the applied and multidisciplinary fields of public health and aging—let alone the possibility of a new paradigm based on the merging of the two. The chapters presented in this collection suggest that the idea of old paradigms being replaced by new might be helpful in seeking a synthesis of a public health agenda. We seek an integrated paradigm because our society is aging and the traditional approaches of public health and aging are not adequately dealing with the resulting problems we face.

The upper left box in Figure 17.2 provides suggestions based on our deliberations of what some key elements of the more traditional public health paradigms might be and how elements of those paradigms might be synthesized to move toward a new integrated paradigm of public health and aging. The components of a traditional public health paradigm emphasize younger people, a traditional focus on infectious disease, concentration on primary prevention, a community orientation, and population-based needs assessments and interventions. In contrast, an aging paradigm might be characterized as focusing on older people, secondary and tertiary prevention, chronic disease, an individual patient or client orientation, and direct personal services as shown in the upper right box in Figure 17.2.

An integrated paradigm will be composed of selected elements of each of the two older paradigms (lower box in Figure 17.2). From the aging paradigm comes a focus on older people, chronic disease, and secondary and tertiary prevention. From the public health paradigm comes a community orientation and a focus on population-based assessments and interventions. A successful new integrated paradigm would not simply select and utilize those components in the same fashion they were used in the old paradigms but would foster new ideas, research, and applications as these elements are integrated into the new paradigm.

This concept of a new integrated paradigm can be related to the purpose of bringing together researchers, teachers, policy makers, and practitioners to better understand each other's needs and the opportunities to collaborate fruitfully. Figure

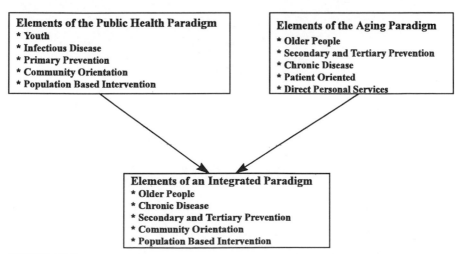

FIGURE 17.2 Elements of the public health, aging, and integrated paradigms.

17.3 provides some perspectives on such linkages. An integrated paradigm draws on the current research findings and available knowledge base, as well as related policy and practice. It is also the source of new ideas and research directions.

One way of viewing and classifying the chapters in this book is to consider whether they contribute primarily to development of an integrated paradigm, provide the knowledge base and insight about current research that might have implications for new policy and practice, or inform us about current policies and practices. The latter classification criterion suggests what practitioners need in the way of new knowledge or research efforts to aid them in planning or implementing, what evaluation research is necessary to assess how well programs or policies are working, what changes might improve those programs or policies, or to what extent they can be successfully applied in other settings.

Of course, the book chapters are multifaceted and could be classified in many different ways, but here are some suggestions as to ways they contribute toward a synthesis and needed research for policy and practice in an aging society.

Contributions Toward an Integrated Paradigm

Box 1 in Figure 17.4 suggests the way in which each of four chapters makes a significant contribution toward an integrated paradigm. Fernando Torres-Gil in the Foreword outlined rather elegantly the logic and necessity for the public health and

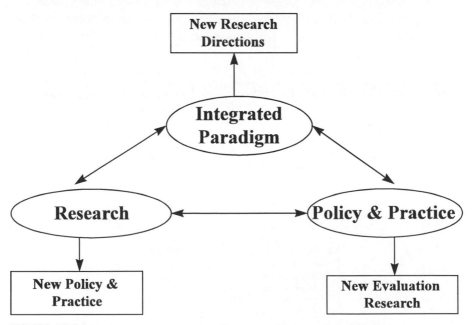

FIGURE 17.3 Identifying needed research, policy, and practice for an aging society.

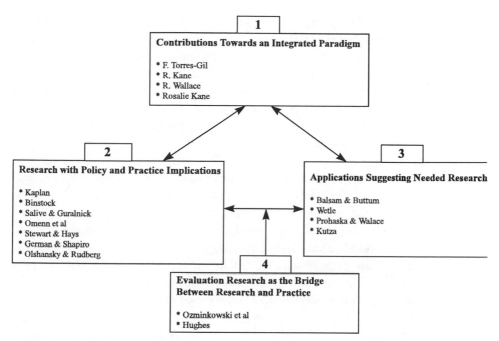

FIGURE 17.4 Contributions toward an integrated paradigm, research, and policy and practice.

aging networks to work together and pointed out the necessity for change at the institutional level. He reviewed the challenges facing public health in an aging society as how to: improve the access of the diverse elderly population; share information across organization borders; recognize the mutuality of public health and aging infrastructure and efforts; build a coalition to generate resources; demonstrate the necessity of quantifiable outcome measures; and realize the advantages of working together as opposed to competing for limited resources.

Robert Kane provides the major elements of the public health paradigm and its links to an aging perspective. Kane discusses how aging elements can be identified or developed in public health policy and planning activities. For example, in surveillance activities, he highlights the importance of identifying disease and disability rates particular to the aged. Similarly, while planning programs, special service configurations are necessary. Quality assurance activities such as monitoring programs should be done with appropriate quality of care measures for the elderly. Kane goes on to discuss the implications of a chronic disease model for public health to include an emphasis on chronic causes; a shift in prevention efforts to earlier phases of life and the potential for intervention in later life; the challenge in demonstrating the effectiveness of prevention; the effectiveness of new approaches to care, such as the success of managed care in promoting health of the elderly; the inclusion of elderly in community trials; the need for targeting subgroups of elderly prone to disease versus just reducing the risk factors; screening the elderly; and confronting elderly stereotypes and misinformation. Kane also points out that a chronic disease model for academic public health requires a strong research base, similar to what was done in maternal and child health in early public health efforts. This chronic disease model includes an emphasis on theories of aging not simply applied research; an emphasis on public health skills and knowledge in aging research; and the need for special curriculum including aging majors, core public health and aging courses, and introducing aging content into regular courses.

Robert Wallace contributes effectively to the new paradigm by summarizing the clinical aging perspective as he discusses variability of disease manifestations and some of its public health implications. After providing a biological definition of aging he examines the mechanisms that affect clinical disease in aging. He also considers some of the behavioral dimensions of aging and their relationship to interpopulation variation in disease and disability. Wallace contends that interpopulation or international comparative work on disability is needed to overcome some of the measurement difficulties of practicing public health in an aging society. However, not only the way information on older and disabled populations is acquired has to change, but also the taxonomy and nomenclature of public health surveillance systems will need to incorporate multiple interactive conditions in longitudinal studies. Such surveillance systems would allow us, for example, to monitor long-term disability in aging populations. Furthermore, a new set of tertiary prevention programs should be developed to increase emphasis on preventing the progression of chronic conditions. Finally, a good understanding of the importance of providing primary and secondary prevention in elderly, from the efficacy and cost-benefit perspectives, is necessary.

Rosalie Kane's discussion of bioethical issues is integral to this new paradigm because it emphasizes the point that, while paradigms are based on scientific findings, other issues including ethics play an important role in their definition. She identifies five substantive areas in public health—prevention, health services research, health education, environmental health, and regulation/licensure—and illustrates the ethical dilemmas in applying this new paradigm to the aged population. The ethical dilemmas in prevention concern the effectiveness of prevention in older adults. Little is known about the effectiveness of prevention, and many moral decisions have to be made on how much prevention and screening affect the quality of life.

Kane notes that health services research is also riddled with value judgments in studies of the elderly populations. Some topics such as prevalence of marital discord and effectiveness of psychotherapy are virtually ignored, and studies of social well-being neglect other potentially rewarding aspects of life. Health services researchers should reevaluate their assessment of other areas of research such as outcome measures and personal preferences.

Another substantive area of public health where additional sensitivity is needed is health education. The aging of the population and the negative way this information is conveyed to the public is yet another example of ethical and moral issues to be dealt with in an aging society. Environmental health, the fourth substantive area of public health, might be expanded to include the living environments of the elderly. For example, nursing homes are generally designed like hospitals with no attention to privacy and the need for independent living. Similarly, decision-making environments are often subtly coercive, with little chance for freedom in major life-change decisions such as being institutionalized or living with others. Finally, Kane stressed that the fifth area of public health, regulation and licensure requirements in nursing homes, impedes autonomy and consumer preferences, and informed risk taking should be considered in regulatory activities.

Research with Policy and Practice Implications

Box 2 in Figure 17.4 lists those chapters that emphasize research findings with policy and practice implications and applications. George Kaplan provides a revealing perspective on what is known on how social, behavioral, and environmental factors are related to health, life expectancy, and quality of life for older persons. Such knowledge has implications for both applications and new research directions. He highlights the importance of prevention in older adults and provides the needed evidence that prevention can work for older people as support for his argument. He argues that prevention can help postpone the onset of disease, slow its progression, minimize impairment, and delay disability. He groups the support for the link between risk factors and health of older adults into benefits of eliminating or improving behavioral factors such as smoking; social factors such as lack of social networks; socioeconomic factors such as lack of education and low incomes; and socioenvironmental factors such as living conditions in crime-ridden neighborhoods.

However, Kaplan's review of evidence also serves to point out the many gaps in the current knowledge about public health efforts in an aging society. For example, relatively little is known of the natural history of risk factors, risk-factor changes, functional problems, and health transitions in elderly persons. Furthermore, the ways in which behavioral, social, and socioenvironmental factors interact with diagnosed and preclinical disease should be studied, as well as comorbidities and their synergistic effect on longevity and quality of life. Overall, prevention programs are needed for the elderly based on systematic morbidity and disability data collected at the state and local level.

Robert Binstock discusses resource allocation in the health sector according to age. His work certainly suggests the need for additional research on the relationship between growing numbers and proportion of older people in the population and health care spending. He argues that policy makers and the public should be informed about the realistic choices for limiting medical care to the adults. An agenda for research on such choices is needed. Simultaneously, political leadership is required to unite disparate constituencies in support of a long-term care policy. In addition, the federal government should explore the value of nonmedical technologies to help the frail elderly in the community. Finally, priorities in biomedical research should be set for treatment, prosthetics, and rehabilitation techniques for nonfatal conditions.

Marcel Salive and Jack Guralnik present fascinating findings concerning disability outcomes, particularly deficiencies in sensory functions, for older people with chronic disease. These findings have a number of implications for public health practice and important directions for new research. The research to date suggests that priority should be given to additional studies of exercise intervention and their impact on sensory functions and disability. Preliminary work suggests that these interventions can reduce disability. The longer-term impact may be to reduce nursing home admissions. By limiting disability, older individuals may enjoy extended independence through additional home care and social support. The authors point out that this research agenda might be of considerable help to practitioners. For example, it may indicate how practitioners can provide medical and technical help with sensory functioning, informal support, and exercise programs. It might also assist in the formulation of guidelines for medical doctors and nurses to improve quality-of-life outcomes for older persons.

Gilbert Omenn and colleagues provide some very encouraging research findings about how community-based interventions can modify risk factors related to health promotion and disease prevention. Their findings show the potential for joining fields of public health and aging. The authors demonstrate how epidemiological studies of prevalence of risk factors can be combined with studies of risk-factor modification in order to reduce frailty and disability. They also suggest how interventions might incorporate outcomes and effectiveness measures. Intermediate endpoints and various biomarkers of behavior change and early disease states can add substantially to the value of epidemiological studies and prevention trials. A simple but important message is to include older adults in prevention studies and conduct well-monitored and well-controlled studies in community settings to contact hard-to-reach individuals and elderly population subgroups.

Anita Stewart and Ron Hays give a well-organized and enlightening assessment of the state of the art in measuring health status of older populations, which is highly relevant to aging studies and evaluation of programs targeting older adults. They discuss how a variety of measurement issues are age related. For example, reliability may diminish among the older age groups; measures of health status must be sensitive to both improvement and deterioration in well-being of the elderly; and common summary indicators of health status may be inappropriate for older persons because they do not include components of geriatric health.

Next, the authors discuss the practical issues in measuring health status of older age groups, such as methods of survey administration. While self-administered surveys are less expensive, they may be more difficult to complete for those with vision problems. In those cases, the more costly and effort-intensive phone surveys may be preferred. Issues in use of proxy respondents and difficulties in selecting appropriate measures of health in older adults are other examples of practical issues to be considered. Stewart and Hays conclude that health status of older adults is best defined from the perspective of the individual as opposed to that of clinicians, particularly because of the diversity in health status of elderly.

Pearl German and Sam Shapiro emphasize the heterogeneity of risk factors in aging populations and point out some of the implications for research and intervention trials. First, research hypotheses should reflect that outcomes are broad and varied in the elderly population, and methods of data collection should define and measure characteristics of this target population. Next, interventions must identify the appropriate population with the problem as well as the strategy that will help alleviate the problem. In addition, the strategy should be operationalized while keeping the different characteristics and cumulative risks of the target population in mind. The goals of the intervention should vary based on the heterogeneity of elderly. Finally, evaluations should include control or comparison groups so that between-group differences can be studied with respect to heterogeneity and cumulative risks. Attention to analytic details will help facilitate generalizations from the study for future interventions in other populations.

Jay Olshansky and Mark Rudberg deal effectively with the critical issue of postponing disability in older persons and what the research findings might mean for potential interventions. The authors argue that today's elderly are a genetically robust subgroup of the population that are more likely to survive into advanced ages. They predict that the mortality and disability risks facing future cohorts of elderly are different, and even new, compared to those observed in the past. Consequently, public health efforts in an aging society face new challenges. For example, methods of measuring disability influence the trends observed nationally and internationally and should be reevaluated. Similarly, age at onset of disease and disability may have changed with the new medical methods and interventions as compared to the past. Hence, the appropriate time for intervention has also changed. The traditional intervention methods deal with fatal disease such as cancer. Yet the aging of the population has exposed it to an increased risk of nonfatal diseases such as osteoporosis. However, morbidity may be compressed or forestalled through targeting of appropriate public health intervention strategies.

Applications Suggesting Needed Research

While much of this collection dwells on research implications for practice, there was also concern for understanding the current state of practice and how research can or might help the practitioners to perform more effectively and efficiently (Figure 17.4, Box 3). Balsam and Bottum describe both aging and public health networks and possible common grounds between them. In their view, the Area Agencies on Aging (AAA) and public health networks can collaborate in many ways. Collaboration can take place in need assessment, planning, implementation, and evaluation phases of various programs. At the program-planning stage, data systems can be linked, report forms can be standardized, and access to data networks can be provided for maximum exchange of information. At the implementation phase, public health programs can be conducted in elder service sites and senior housing, access to existing public health facilities for elders can be enhanced, and AAA and public health dollars can be supplemented or joined together to initiate new programs. Individual care plans for elders can be coordinated, for example, in the shape of single intake and assessment forms. During the evaluation phase, research results can be shared through providing program models for AAA and public health networks, holding joint conferences and professional meetings, and publishing in journals read by professionals in both networks to disseminate information. The gaps between the two networks can be narrowed, and duplication can be eliminated by redefining the roles and responsibilities in both networks, coordinating efforts by creating offices for coordination, cross-training professionals, and providing informal technical consultation to each other.

Terrie Wetle provides an informative commentary on program planning and development for aging populations that has important implications for related evaluation research efforts. Through the use of two case studies, Wetle points out the importance of the need for multifaceted, multidimensional approaches to program planning and policy development for aging. This research should target specific heterogenous elderly populations to develop a knowledge base of resources in both aging and public health networks. Researchers should not only be sensitive to the constraints and values of each component of the network, they should also take into consideration the efficiency and effectiveness of the interventions while targeting programs. Development of nontraditional partnerships and tracking outcomes to provide feedback is essential to these program-planning efforts. Wetle reemphasizes the need to overcome the barriers to mutual understanding and cooperation between the academic researchers and policy makers and practitioners.

Thomas Prohaska and Steven Wallace provide us with some research on how public health professionals are trained in issues of aging. Their work has implications for new directions in training in response to an aging society. The authors predict that schools of public health will face a growing demand for health professionals with some knowledge in gerontology and geriatrics. The growth of trained individuals is influenced more by availability of research funding than by practice jobs. Still, it is important to ensure that all public health professionals have some training in this field, and there is continuing education for those already in the workforce. Prohaska and Wallace contend that curriculum should be planned with more attention to health promotion and quality-of-life issues. Overall, the introductory courses in public health should be well rounded in all aspects of aging, population changes, heterogeneity of the older adults, integration of research and practice, skills in delivery of care, and sensitivity to moral, ethical, and legal issues. At least one elective course should be offered in all programs so that public health professionals are sensitive to the issues of this growing population. In addition, students should be educated to work in agencies delivering services to older adults. Such education depends on adequate communication between research and community agencies providing care to the elderly.

Elizabeth Kutza gives us a broader perspective on the organization of public health services and new classification forms that might be appropriate for our aging society. Kutza suggests that in order to answer the needs of an aging society the current system of care has to change. This can be done by an overhaul of the organizational culture. Organizational belief structure and behavior of the public health service have to change to emphasize coordinated services, goal-directed financing mechanisms, and neighborhood-based community services. HMO participation and Medicare physician payment reforms are examples of how major changes in the system of care can be accomplished. Social services should be integrated with medical services and the role of community as problem solver should be emphasized. The success of meeting the public health needs of an aging society should be evaluated through clear goal specification, more research on age-specific disabling conditions, and more objective measures of individual functioning. To accomplish these goals, a number of organizational barriers to reform should be overcome: domain conflict and rigid jurisdictional lines of authority, separate funding mechanisms and lack of goals and incentives to cooperate by the largest funders of services, different professional orientations among providers, and categorical eligibility among programs.

Evaluation Research as the Bridge between Research and Practice

The final category of contributions (Box 4 in Figure 17.4) supports a particular bias of ours. We would like to propose that evaluation research is the meaningful bridge between research and practice. Ozminkowski and Branch provide a good basic primer on the principles of evaluation research and its usefulness to policy and practice. They illustrate some important applications of evaluation research to the elderly populations. For example, since the elderly have special health problems, careful problem identification and definition as well as clear differentiation of target populations are essential in evaluation research of older populations. Studies of the aged should have randomized designs or the appropriate statistical adjustments in absence of randomization to account for the heterogeneity of this population. Threats to internal validity are high because subject loss due to death is common in aging research. Similarly, threats to statistical conclusion validity and construct validity are particularly relevant. For example, use of proxy respondents for aged people or use of different methods for collecting the same kinds of information for intervention and control groups (e.g., institutional and noninstitutional populations) can significantly influence the findings. The external validity of the results can be threatened by changes in the setting for intervention. For example, interventions in a nursing home setting may produce different results from those in a hospital rehabilitation facility. Similarly, the results of interventions for the young-old may be different from those for the old-old. In studies of cost benefit and cost effectiveness, the discount rates chosen should match the nature of the program; for example, long-term programs require a different discount rate than short-term programs because the benefits of the intervention may be observed only in the long term.

Susan Hughes adds life to this message that evaluation research is the bridge between evaluation and practice by not only emphasizing principles of evaluation research but giving us examples of good evaluation research in aging populations. She summarizes current efforts by state departments of health, CDC, and NCHS to monitor incidence and prevalence rates of morbidity and mortality in older populations and emphasizes that surveillance/needs assessment in public health should stress issues relevant to the elderly (e.g., chronic disease and disability). Also, the type of disability or vulnerability being studied should be amenable to intervention. Finally, evaluation should be selected where there is potential to use the results to implement or alter programs to directly benefit older populations.

Conclusion

We have suggested only the beginnings of an integrated public health–aging paradigm. We have a long way to go to improve the collaboration between researcher and practitioner. We further realize that there are many political and economic issues that make the integration of public health and aging networks difficult. These issues impede the direct use of research and its findings to influence program planning, implementation, and evaluation. However, we are encouraged that this book points the way toward the integration of the work of a number of interest groups who do have the common goal of maintaining and improving the health and welfare of the older populations. Further, the exigencies of demographic change and growing economic constraints require that we take heed of Benjamin Franklin's sage advice from over 200 years ago: "We must hang together or we shall all hang separately."

Reference

Kuhn, T. 1970. *The Structure of Scientific Revolutions.* Chicago: University of Chicago Press.

Index

abuse and neglect, 21, 81, 261, 262
academic public health, 11, 286, 316
active life expectancy, 7, 46, 107–109, 262, 295, 296, 304, 305
activities of daily living (ADLs),
  and aging network needs assessments, 152–154
  and disability, 7, 88–89, 95, 96, 101, 243–244
  and frailty, 108, 110, 120
  and measurement variability, 181
  and Minimum Data Set, 152
  and need for interventions, 22, 293, 303
  and National Health and Nutrition Examination Survey (NHANES) I, 149
  and National Health Interview Survey (NHIS), 150
  and Women's Health and Aging Study, 193
  impact of smoking on, 41
Administration on Aging (AoA),
  and National Aging Program Information System, 30
  and network needs assessments, 153
  collaborative funding, 33, 134, 136, 278
  programs and services, 13, 17–22, 23, 255, 279, 287, 296–299, 306
Adult Day Health Care Program (ADHC), 207–208, 214
age-based rationing, 5
age-related changes, 76–79, 82, 169, 255
  in metabolism, 79
  in sensory function, 79

Agency for Health Care Policy and Research (AHCPR), 278
aging network,
  and health promotion, 159
  and health services, 296
  client data collection, 29–30
  collaboration with public health network, 32
  compared to public health network, 9
  preparing professionals for, 280, 289
  research collaboration, 141
  role in providing services, 13, 17, 18, 19, 22, 23, 34
  surveillance systems, 144, 148, 153, 155
alcohol, 81, 82, 98, 99, 113, 114, 199
alcohol and drug abuse, 146–147
Alzheimer's disease, 22, 68, 97, 134, 136
  and surveillance, 155, 259
  and supportive living environments, 265
  and training needs, 284, 287
  intervention programs, 134, 136
  patient service needs, 22
  research priorities, 68
  resources for care, 277
American Association of Retired Persons (AARP), 278
American Board of Internal Medicine and Family Practice, 279
American Public Health Association, 3, 276
angina (see cardiovascular disease)
Area Agency on Aging, 18, 20, 21, 137, 141, 154, 291, 299, 320
arthritis (see also osteoarthritis),

arthritis (*Cont.*)
  and aging changes, 77, 79
  and assessment, 247
  and death rates, 242
  and disability, 92, 93, 95, 98, 111–113,
    196
  and intervention, 157
  and prevention, 85, 155
assisted living, 28, 62, 63, 269
atherosclerosis, 76, 111, 112

behavior change, 7, 8, 12, 28, 119, 121–123,
    136, 158, 258
behavioral science, 12, 119
bioethics, 252, 254–257, 260, 271, 272, 316 (*see
    also* ethics)
biomarkers, 123, 318
biomedical research, 12, 119, 155, 318
biostatistics, 12, 288
blindness, 82, 95, 243
blood pressure, 30, 98, 111–113, 298
  and disability, 245
  assessment, 149
  intervention, 218
  medication effects on, 80
bone density, 80, 84

cancer,
  and biomedical research, 67
  and disability, 92–94, 237, 238, 246
  and mortality, 190–192, 276, 246
  and prevention, 147, 152, 155, 242, 245–247,
    249
  and smoking, 242
  breast and cervical, 147, 152
  cancer management, 82
  colorectal cancer, 147
  research priorities, 123
  risk factors, 195, 198, 319
  role of public health, 26–28
  screening, 259
cardiovascular accident (CVA), 93 (*see also*
    stroke)
cardiovascular disease, 85, 93, 155, 242 (*see also*
    heart disease)
  angina pectoris, 79, 94
  congestive heart failure, 98
  ischemic heart disease, 112
  myocardial infarction, 94

case-mix, 263
cataracts, 67, 93, 96, 98, 102, 123, 243, 246
Centers for Disease Control and Prevention
    (CDC), 25–28, 30, 137, 139, 145–150, 278,
    322
  Behavioral Risk Factor Surveillance System,
    146
cerebrovascular disease, 111, 112, 147 (*see also*
    stroke)
Channeling Project, (*see* National Long Term
    Care (Channeling) Demonstration
    Project)
cholesterol, 149, 202
chronic disease, 7, 14, 27, 87, 316
  and disability, 87
  etiology, 7
  model, 7, 315–316
  prevalence of, 199, 277
  prevention, 155, 159, 313
  risk factors, 192, 195, 198, 199
  surveillance, 147, 151–153, 322
chronic obstructive pulmonary disease
    (COPD), 98, 155, 211
cognitive functioning, 83, 84, 92, 164, 167, 169,
    176
cohort analysis, 194
community-based care, 270, 284, 299
community-based programs/services, 17, 64,
    75, 84, 134, 137, 154
comorbidity,
  and assessment, 247
  and cumulative risk, 195, 203–204
  and disability, 92, 97, 98, 100, 103, 243
  and disease manifestation, 79, 82, 84
  and prevention, 38, 48
comparison groups (*see also* control groups),
    157, 158, 213, 215, 217
congestive heart failure, 94, 98
construct validity, 322
continuing care retirement communities, 62
control groups (*see also* comparison groups),
    204, 212–218, 221, 222
cost-benefit analysis, 12, 227, 228, 316
cost-effectiveness, 10, 12, 85, 103, 117, 158,
    209, 228, 258
cost-utility analysis, 227–228

death rates (*see also* mortality),
  age-adjusted, 242
  and prevention, 38, 45
  and cancer, 191–192

and compression of morbidity, 237–238,
240–241, 245–247
and heart disease, 191–192
delirium, 83
dementia, 6, 37, 61, 63, 66, 97, 108, 110
interventions, 241–243
screening for, 248
demography, 12, 55, 240, 276, 280, 281
and disease, 276
demographic imperative, 311
Department of Veterans Affairs (*see* Veterans
Administration)
depression,
and disability, 97–98
and health promotion interventions, 114
and loss of functional capacity, 110
and needs assessments, 122
and prevention, 246
and screening, 259
and socioeconomic factors, 47
Geriatric Depression Scale, 177
measurement issues, 165, 169, 221
diabetes,
and aging changes, 78
and assessment, 175
and disability, 92, 93, 98, 241, 246
and prevention, 85, 155
and risk factors, 111, 112
and surveillance, 146
dietary fat and intake, 146, 149, 247
disability,
and environmental factors, 46, 47, 265–266
and falls, 116
and impairment, 39, 109, 110
and morbidity/comorbidity, 55, 95, 97–103,
123
and socioeconomic factors, 45
assessment of, 12, 82, 144, 145, 148–150,
153–155, 169, 182, 262
definition of, 241–242
epidemiology of, 5, 7, 92, 254, 257, 259, 278,
315, 316
heterogeneity, 202, 203, 228
intervention outcomes, 67, 84, 318
prevalence of, 60, 69, 83, 84, 88, 89, 260
prevention, 8, 48, 87, 140, 237–238, 240–241,
245–247, 260, 280, 281
risk of, 98, 191–193, 195–199, 319
WHO definition, 87
disease prevention (*see also* health promotion),
and aging, 8
and the public health system, 294, 298, 301,
304

effectiveness of, 11, 117
types of programs, 20, 27, 28, 30, 32,
107–108, 277
diversity, (*see* heterogeneity)
dyspnea, 82, 93

Educational Demonstration of Urinary
Continence Assessment and Treatment for
the Elderly (EDUCATE), 132, 133, 135,
137, 141, 290
EPESE, (*see* Established Populations for
Epidemiologic Studies of the Elderly)
epidemiology,
and gerontology/geriatrics, 12, 13, 84
and health services research, 260
and national surveys, 278
curriculum issues, 280, 282, 288, 289
methods, 5–7
of illness, 78
paradigm, 295
studies, 4, 6, 132
surveillance, 81
Established Populations for Epidemiologic
Studies of the Elderly (EPESE), 46, 91,
95–97, 99, 100, 135, 138, 139, 178, 278
ethics (*see also* bioethics), 5, 12, 13, 252–254,
256–259
and long-term case management, 267
procedural ethics, 256
evaluation, 8, 24, 32
comparison groups, 319
evaluation strategies, 132, 139
definition of, 208
impact analyses, 212
of prevention programs, 85
public health skills/training, 12
research, 155, 209, 215, 231, 314, 320–322
exercise (*see also* physical activity)
and disability, 247
and functional limitation, 43, 102, 110, 130
and mortality and morbidity, 28, 42, 43, 99
and prevention, 155–159, 199, 203, 258, 260,
318
benefits of, 7, 8, 114, 117
external validity, 216, 223, 322

falls,
and disability, 116
and functional decline, 110–113

falls (*Cont.*)
  and serious illness and injury, 83, 93, 120,
    300
  environmental hazards and, 47
  physical activity and, 43
  prevention of, 243, 260
Frailty and Injuries: Cooperative Studies of
    Intervention Techniques (FICSIT), 158,
    180
functional impairment, 38–41, 43–45, 76–79,
    92, 116
  and disability, 82, 83, 87, 95–99, 110, 261,
    262, 265
  and environmental factors, 47–48
  problems, 317
  surveillance, 145, 150, 154
functional measurement, 12, 13, 116, 262

geriatrics, 5, 12, 13, 137, 140, 245–247, 275, 276
  Geriatric Assessment Unit (GAU), 214
  Geriatric Education Centers, 279
  Geriatric Depression Scale, 177
Gerontological Society of America, 140, 276
glaucoma, 243, 246
glucose tolerance, 78, 79

Hartford Puerto Rican Alzheimer's Education
    Project, 133–135
Health Belief Model, 138
Health Care Financing Administration (HCFA),
    59, 67, 116, 148, 152, 278, 296, 298
health promotion,
  and public health goals, 294, 296, 303–305
  as a core area of public health, 254, 280–282,
    287, 289, 290, 318–321
  targeting risks for, 203
health care,
  access, 296
  costs, 53, 55–57, 59, 293
  delivery systems, 294
  policy, 13
  rationing, 59
health maintenance organizations (HMOs), 11,
    58, 59, 137
health promotion (*see also* disease prevention),
  Administration on Aging programs, 25, 28,
    30, 32
  and environmental factors, 47
  and program planning, 111, 113

and public health network, 17
  effectiveness of, 11, 107, 110, 113, 115–120
  in academic curricula, 13, 122
  Public Health Service programs, 20, 21
health services research, 12, 158, 217, 252–254,
    260, 271, 316
health status/measurement, 318–319
Healthy People 2000, 120, 124, 146, 147, 304,
    305
hearing impairment, 155, 246
heart disease (*see also* cardiovascular disease),
    38, 92, 93, 98
  and disability, 92, 93, 98, 99
  and risk factors, 111, 112
  death rates, 191–192, 241–242
  prevention of, 38, 107, 123, 147, 159, 246
heterogeneity, 23, 85, 190–191
  in interventions and evaluation, 202
  in research, 202
  typology of, 197
high blood cholesterol, 149
high blood pressure (*see also* hypertension), 30,
    98, 111–113, 149, 245, 298
hip fracture, 44, 45, 92, 93, 98, 110, 112, 148,
    243, 246
Hispanic Health and Nutrition Examination
    Survey, 149
Hispanic Health Council, 134
HIV, 27, 149
HMOs (*see* health maintenance organizations),
    11, 58, 59, 137
home and community-based services, 58, 64,
    154, 300
hypertension (*see also* high blood pressure), 28,
    80, 92, 146, 155, 176, 196, 218, 242
hypothyroidism, 68, 78

immunization, 8, 30, 82, 110, 149, 152, 155
impact analysis, 209
incidence of disease, 78, 81, 99, 113, 191
Indian Health Service, 25, 297, 298
infectious diseases, 7, 23, 24, 87, 245, 276, 313
Institute of Medicine, 151, 268, 286, 291, 294,
    297
instrumental activities of daily living (IADL),
    40–41, 88, 89, 95, 99, 101, 150, 154, 243
intellectual functioning, (*see* cognitive function-
    ing)
internal validity, 213, 215–217, 223, 224, 322
instrumental activities of daily living (IADL),
    154, 243

life expectancy, 7, 38, 43, 46, 103, 107–109
  and chronic disease, 7
  and decline in mortality, 38, 237, 242,
    248–249, 275, 304–305
  and education, 46
  and frailty, 108–109
  and health promotion, 107–109
  and physical activity, 43
  and surveillance systems, 153, 159
  by race and sex, 192–193, 196
  increases in, 275, 293, 295, 296
life satisfaction, 168, 172, 222, 262
Likert scales, 176
Longitudinal Study of Aging (LSoA), 42, 44,
  150, 278
long-term care,
  and frail elderly, 261
  and Medicaid, 63–65, 291
  case-mix and level of service, 263
  costs, 60, 61
  curriculum issues, 284, 287–291
  demographics, 276–278
  health systems and programs, 17, 27, 53–55,
    66–67, 248, 294, 297–299
  institutions, 81
  insurance, 62–64
  living environments, 265–270
  Medicaid-funded programs, 291
  model programs, 66–67
  policy, 5–7, 13
  research, 261

MacArthur Foundation Research Network on
  Successful Aging, 181
macular degeneration, 243, 246
mammography, 28, 81, 85, 146
managed care, 9–11, 59, 65–67, 202, 300, 315
Massachusetts Influenza Vaccination Project,
  135, 138
Master of Public Health (M.P.H.), 279, 290
Master of Science in Gerontology (M.S.G.), 279
measurement issues, 171–174, 318
Medicaid,
  and health status, 201
  and private insurance, 65
  and quality assurance, 268
  and rationing, 70
  and standardized assessment, 151 (*see also*
    Minimum Data Set)
  coverages, 53–55, 63–64
  demonstration programs, 65–67

expenditures, 64, 69
regulation, 6, 60
Medical Outcomes Study (MOS), 116, 117, 164,
  169, 171, 172
Medicare,
  and HMOs, 11
  and managed care, 9–11
  and prospective payment, 6
  and rationing, 70
  and standardized assessment (*see also*
    Minimum Data Set), 151
  coverages, 25–26, 53–55
  expenditures, 57, 58, 69
  funding, 7, 303
  history of, 298–300
  Prospective Payment System (PPS), 151
  reform, 58–60, 321
Minimum Data Set (MDS) for Resident
  Assessment and Care,
  Resident Assessment Instrument (RAI), 151
  Resident Assessment Protocols (RAPs),
    152
mobility problems, 41, 43, 47, 99, 301
morbidity, 48
  and aging, 78–79
  and comorbidity, 84
  and disability rates, 55, 69, 83, 84
  and functional status, 262
  and use of services, 5
  and risk factors, 199, 319
  and weight loss, 122
  compression of morbidity, 107, 152–153,
    238–241
  expansion of morbidity, 238–239, 294
  secondary prevention of, 258
mortality,
  and diet and exercise, 28, 122
  and disability, 100, 101
  and immune function, 78
  and physical activity, 42–43
  and smoking, 40
  and social functioning, 43–45
  and socioeconomic factors, 45–46, 182
  and socioenvironmental factors, 46–47,
    182
  causes of, 94
  data registries, 30–31
  postponing mortality, 199, 205, 237, 239,
    242, 248, 294
  rates, 38
  risks factors, 145, 147, 319
  summary measures of, 174, 262
  surveillance, 148, 151–154, 159

Multicenter Trials of Frailty and Injuries—
Cooperative Studies of Intervention
Techniques (FICSIT), 158

National Aging Program Information System,
30, 154
National Caregiver Study (1982–1988), 278
National Center for Health Statistics (NCHS),
38, 89, 148, 154, 277, 278
National Health and Nutrition Examination
Survey (NHANES), 99
NHANES I Epidemiologic Follow-up Study,
148, 149
NHANES II, 149
National Health Interview Survey (NHIS), 89,
111, 148, 149, 150, 182
National Institute on Aging (NIA), 89, 138,
278, 288
National Long Term Care (Channeling)
Demonstration Project, 207, 214
National Nursing Home Survey (NNHS), 89,
148, 151
needs assessments, 30, 144, 153, 159, 313
neighborhood-based community services, 300,
321 (*see also* community-based
programs/services)
New York Quality Assurance System, 207, 255
nutrition, 18–23, 115, 120, 122, 148, 149, 260,
282

Older Americans Act (OAA), 18–22, 30, 63,
255, 280, 299, 305
Omnibus Budget Reconciliation Act (OBRA),
151
osteoarthritis (*see also* arthritis), 77, 95, 98, 148,
153, 157, 238, 247
osteoporosis, 80, 93, 111, 112, 148, 149, 242,
243, 246, 319

passive smoking, 149
perceived health, 168, 179, 181
peripheral neuritis, 82
physical activity (*see also* exercise),
and functioning, 42, 43
and health promotion, 20, 48, 113, 117
and mortality, 42

and quality of life, 39
and risk of falls, 47, 48
evaluation, 158, 202–203
measurement and assessment, 146, 147, 153,
175
physical functioning, 23, 40–45, 94, 164–166,
169–174, 178–179, 225, 249, 296
policy development, 25, 132, 296
poliomyelitis, 82
politics of aging, 13, 278, 287, 290
population-based intervention, 313
power analysis, 232
prevalence, 81–83, 123, 137, 191
and disability, 87–106
prevention,
and health promotion training, 13
and living environments, 266–267
and program planning, 111
and public health and aging paradigm,
313–315, 318
and public health network, 17, 18, 20, 21, 26,
28, 30
and public health training, 280–281
and risk reduction, 99, 101–103, 107–109,
117, 123
as a core area of public health, 252–254, 257,
277, 294
community-based models/services, 301–304
cost-effectiveness of, 258
primary, 37–39, 48, 87, 101, 245–246, 280,
313, 316
secondary, 37–39, 85, 87, 155, 245–246, 258,
280, 313, 316
services, 200, 201, 203
surveillance systems, 144–148, 152–155, 158,
159, 257–260
tertiary, 48, 85, 87, 102, 243, 246, 260, 313,
316
preventive interventions, 8, 11, 48, 82, 84,
144–150, 153–155
formative evaluation of, 156–157
substantive evaluation of, 158–159
primary care, 27, 32, 113, 121, 181, 200, 258,
298–300
primary data collection, 224–225
Program of All-inclusive Care for the Elderly
(PACE), 207, 211
proxy respondents, 178
psychological well-being, 167, 169, 170
public health,
accreditation, 287–290
agencies, 305

and aging curriculum, 280, 282–283,
285–287
and environmental health, 265, 316, 317
disease and disability rates, 315
education, 264, 316
environmental health issues, 316, 317
ethics, 253
goals and mission, 294–295
intervention strategies, 319
network, 17, 23–25, 30–34, 320
paradigm for public health-aging, 312
policy, 315
politics, 277–279
prevention, 316
quality assurance, 268, 271, 315
regulation and licensure, 268, 315–317
services, 296–299, 316, 321
surveillance, 145–146, 294, 315–316
Public Health Service (*see* United States Public
Health Service)
Public Health Service Act, 278
pulmonary disease, 82, 98, 155, 211

Quality Adjusted Life Years (QUALYs or
QALYs), 6, 175, 262
Quality of Well-Being Scale (QWB), 204
quasi-experimental designs,
comparison groups, 215
regression-discontinuity design, 215
random assignment/sampling, 213–214
statistical processes, 215

resource allocation, 53, 54, 60, 84
Retirement Research Foundation, 278
risk factors, 144–149, 152–154, 190–194,
242–243
cumulative risk, 194
heterogeneity, 319
modification of, 318
prevalence of, 318
risk-factor changes, 317
Robert Wood Johnson Foundation, 65, 278

screening, 20, 28, 30, 38, 81, 109, 257–259
secondary analyses, 12, 14, 133, 225–226, 232
secondary infections, 83

self-care/maintenance, 43, 44, 88, 92, 157,
164–166, 177–178, 181, 193
self-esteem, 167
senescent diseases, 239–241, 249
Senior Health Watch, 200, 201, 203
sensory functions and impairments, 238, 242,
243, 246, 318
sexual functioning, 167
smoking,
and disability, 98–100, 242
and functioning, 40–41
and health promotion, 28, 257–258, 317
and mortality, 40–41
cessation, 7, 8, 28, 40, 99, 113, 123, 257–258
social factors of health, 43–45, 102, 317
Social Security and Old Age Assistance, 277,
278
social functioning, 166
social work, 255
Social/Health Maintenance Organization
(SHMO), 66
Minnesota Long-Term Care Options Project
(LTCOP), 66
On Lok Model, 66
socioeconomic factors and health, 45, 48, 215,
317
socioenvironmental factors and health, 46–48,
317
state units on aging, 18–20, 22, 29–31, 33, 153
statistical conclusion validity, 213, 216, 218,
223, 224, 322
stroke (*see also* cerebrovascular disease), 41, 45,
78, 82, 92–95, 98, 159, 241–246, 276
substance abuse, 81
Supplement on Aging (SoA), 150 (*see* National
Health Interview Survey)
surveillance systems, 84, 144–146 (*see also*
National Health and Nutrition
Examination Survey and National Health
Interview Survey)
survey methods, 319

tertiary care, 29, 299

urinary incontinence, 27, 95, 137, 138, 149, 152
United States Department of Health and
Human Services (USDHHS), 25, 30, 87,
146, 150, 203, 296

United States Public Health Service (USPHS), 24–25, 33, 108, 203, 278, 296, 304–305, 321

variability in disease manifestations, 316

Veterans Administration (VA), 53, 63, 207, 208, 214, 297
visual impairment, 93, 95, 96, 111, 112

World Health Organization (WHO), 5, 8, 25, 88, 107, 163, 241–242